MOSBY'S
POCKET GUIDE TO Fetal
Monitoring
A MULTIDISCIPLINARY APPROACH

EIGHTH EDITION

LISA A. MILLER, CNM, JD

Founder, Perinatal Risk Management and Education Services
Chicago, Illinois

DAVID A. MILLER, MD

Professor of Obstetrics, Gynecology, and Pediatrics
Keck School of Medicine
University of Southern California
Chief, Division of Maternal Fetal Medicine
Children's Hospital Los Angeles
Director, USC-CHLA Institute for Maternal Fetal Health
Los Angeles, California

REBECCA L. CYPHER, MSN, PNNP

Perinatal Nurse Practitioner
Department of Obstetrics and Gynecology
Maternal-Fetal Medicine Division
Madigan Army Medical Center
Tacoma, Washington

ELSEVIER

ELSEVIER

3251 Riverport Lane
St. Louis, MO 63043

MOSBY'S POCKET GUIDE TO FETAL MONITORING:
A MULTIDISCIPLINARY APPROACH, EIGHTH EDITION

ISBN: 978-0-323-40157-9

Notices

Knowledge and best practice in this field are constantly changing. As new research and experience broaden our understanding, changes in research methods, professional practices, or medical treatment may become necessary.

Practitioners and researchers must always rely on their own experience and knowledge in evaluating and using any information, methods, compounds, or experiments described herein. In using such information or methods they should be mindful of their own safety and the safety of others, including parties for whom they have a professional responsibility.

With respect to any drug or pharmaceutical products identified, readers are advised to check the most current information provided (i) on procedures featured or (ii) by the manufacturer of each product to be administered, to verify the recommended dose or formula, the method and duration of administration, and contraindications. It is the responsibility of practitioners, relying on their own experience and knowledge of their patients, to make diagnoses, to determine dosages and the best treatment for each individual patient, and to take all appropriate safety precautions.

To the fullest extent of the law, neither the Publisher nor the authors, contributors, or editors, assume any liability for any injury and/or damage to persons or property as a matter of products liability, negligence or otherwise, or from any use or operation of any methods, products, instructions, or ideas contained in the material herein.

Library of Congress Cataloging-in-Publication Data

Names: Miller, Lisa A. (Lisa Anne), 1958- author. | Miller, David A. (David Arthur), 1961- author. | Cypher, Rebecca L., author.
Title: Mosby's pocket guide to fetal monitoring : a multidisciplinary approach / Lisa A. Miller, CNM, JD, Founder, Perinatal Risk Management and Education Services, Chicago, Illinois, David A. Miller, MD, Professor of Obstetrics, Gynecology, and Pediatrics, Keck School of Medicine, University of Southern California, Chief, Division of Maternal Fetal Medicine, Children's Hospital Los Angeles, Director, USC-CHLA Institute for Maternal Fetal Health, Los Angeles, California, Rebecca L. Cypher, MSN, PNNP, Perinatal Nurse Practitioner, Department of Obstetrics and Gynecology, Maternal-Fetal Medicine Division, Madigan Army Medical Center, Tacoma, Washington.
Other titles: Pocket guide to fetal monitoring and assessment
Description: Eighth edition. | St. Louis, MO : Elsevier, [2017] | Revision of: Mosby's pocket guide to fetal monitoring / Susan Martin Tucker, Lisa A. Miller, David A. Miller. c2004. 5th ed. | Includes bibliographical references and index.
Identifiers: LCCN 2016002621 | ISBN 9780323401579 (pbk.)
Subjects: LCSH: Fetal monitoring—Handbooks, manuals, etc. | Fetal heart rate monitoring—Handbooks, manuals, etc.
Classification: LCC RG628 .T83 2017 | DDC 618.3/2075–dc23 LC record available at
http://lccn.loc.gov/2016002621

Senior Content Strategist: Sandy Clark
Content Development Manager: Laurie Gower
Senior Content Development Specialist: Lisa P. Newton
Publishing Services Manager: Hemamalini Rajendrababu
Project Manager: Andrea Lynn Villamero/Divya Krishna Kumar
Design Direction: Ryan Cook

Printed in the United States of America

Last digit is the print number: 9 8 7 6 5 4 3 2 1

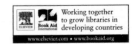

Working together to grow libraries in developing countries

www.elsevier.com • www.bookaid.org

HAYWOOD L. BROWN, MD
Professor & Chair, Obstetrics and Gynecology
Duke University School of Medicine
Durham, North Carolina

JANICE DENNY GIBBS, MSN, RNC-OB, C-EFM
Clinical Staff Educator, Women's Services
Norton Hospital
Louisville, Kentucky

JAMES M. KELLEY, JD
Elk & Elk
Mayfield Heights, Ohio

LU PERSHALL, RNC-OB
Scripps Memorial Hospital Encinitas
Encinitas, California

ACKNOWLEDGMENTS

The original author, Susan Martin Tucker, expresses her sincere and long overdue appreciation to Laurie Gower, Content Development Manager, for her outstanding guidance and expertise through multiple editions of this book. *Fetal Monitoring* was first published in 1978. The content was updated and revised in 1988 as part of the Pocket Guide Series. Publication of the eighth edition of this series provides an opportunity to acknowledge exceptional coauthors Lisa A. Miller and David A. Miller, whose unique expertise and collaboration have been exemplary. Rebecca L. Cypher has replaced Ms. Tucker as coauthor on this accomplished team, which will continue to produce an evidence-based, portable, and practical guide to safety-focused standards.

AirStrip Technologies, Inc.
San Antonio, Texas

Clinical Computer Systems, Inc.
Elgin, Illinois

GE Medical Systems Information Technologies
Milwaukee, Wisconsin

Hill-Rom Company, Inc.
Batesville, Indiana

Philips Medizin Systemes
Böblingen, Germany

Welcome to the eighth edition of *Mosby's Pocket Guide to Fetal Monitoring: A Multidisciplinary Approach*. Nursing, midwifery, and physician collaboration continues in this edition, as it should in a subject that is important to all disciplines. Conscientiously revised, this new edition includes standardized terminology and an evidence-based approach to interpretation and management. Providing real-world, clinically useful information on all aspects of fetal monitoring, including intermittent auscultation, the text continues to serve as a key resource for clinicians of all levels of experience. From birth center to tertiary care, this text provides a quick and current resource for your practice.

DESCRIPTION

Primarily an oxygen monitor, the electronic fetal monitor is a tool used to prevent fetal injury resulting from interruption of fetal oxygenation, whether used during labor or in the antepartum period. Key to this goal is standardization and simplification of clinical practices related to interpretation and management of fetal monitoring. This book provides clinicians with the tools needed to understand both the strengths and weaknesses of electronic fetal monitoring (EFM) and apply a collaborative approach to clinical practice that is evidence- and consensus-based. After a brief overview of the history of fetal monitoring, the text provides core clinical information on the physiologic basis for monitoring, reviews the newest instrumentation for uterine and fetal heart rate (FHR) monitoring, and identifies key factors in the evaluation of uterine activity. The National Institute of Child Health and Human Development (NICHD) definitions are presented and reviewed, and a standardized approach to interpretation and management is clearly outlined. The influence of gestational age on FHR is examined, along with the evaluation of fetal status outside the obstetric unit and in the antenatal setting. Documentation and risk management issues are delineated, including issues of informed consent in choice of monitoring modality. An overview of fetal monitoring in Europe provides clinicians with a look at fetal monitoring outside the United States. Patient safety, communication, and clinical collaboration are the cornerstones of each chapter, and suggestions for practice improvement make this edition an invaluable resource for the busy clinician.

FEATURES

This book has a number of distinctive features:

- Content is organized in a manner that allows clinicians to build on key fundamental concepts and progress logically to advanced principles, making the text suitable for novices needing basic information as well as experienced practitioners seeking greater insight into clinical practice issues.
- Critical information is highlighted using illustrations, tables, and illustrative fetal monitor tracings.
- FHR characteristics are explained and the supporting level of evidence is provided, revealing a number of common myths regarding fetal monitoring.
- Evidence levels are provided for information regarding various FHR patterns, and several common obstetric myths are laid to rest.
- Appendices now include self-assessment questions as well as fetal monitor tracings for practice in application of the NICHD definitions and principles of standardized interpretation.

ORGANIZATION

Chapter 1 traces the history of fetal monitoring from the use of auscultation in the 17th century to present-day practice and includes a discussion of the resurgence of intermittent auscultation for fetal monitoring in low-risk women.

Chapter 2 provides a review of the physiologic basis for monitoring. The oxygen pathway is discussed, as well as the fetal response to interrupted oxygenation. These core physiologic concepts provide clinicians with the fundamentals of fetal oxygenation that serve as the basis for current practice.

Chapter 3 offers a detailed look at instrumentation for both intermittent auscultation and EFM, including newer approaches such as abdominal electrocardiogram. Both external and internal monitoring devices and their application are covered in depth, including artifact detection, telemetry, and troubleshooting tips.

Chapter 4, on uterine activity, provides crucial information including a detailed discussion of normal versus excessive uterine activity and the limitations of the summary term *tachysystole*. New consensus guidelines for the diagnosis of active labor are presented, and the link between excessive uterine activity and fetal acidemia is elucidated. Evidence-based tips for managing uterine activity in clinical practice are offered, and oxytocin use is also addressed.

Chapter 5 breaks down clinical practice in fetal monitoring to its three core elements: definitions, interpretation, and management. This chapter includes the NICHD definitions with illustrations to aid in recognition and application. The role of NICHD categories is examined, and evidence- and consensus-based principles of interpretation are explained.

Chapter 6 presents the management of FHR tracings using a systematic approach based on principles of fetal oxygenation. This comprehensive model is based on EFM's value as a screening tool (rather than a diagnostic tool). The management algorithm uses NICHD categories and a structured approach based on the oxygen pathway. Evidence-based corrective measures for hypoxemia are provided in a checklist format. Chapter 6 elucidates the *primary objective* of intrapartum FHR monitoring: to prevent fetal injury that might result from the progression of hypoxemia during the intrapartum period.

Chapter 7 reviews FHR characteristics in the preterm, late-term, and postterm fetus, including implications for management in both antepartum and intrapartum settings. The chapter includes information on a variety of medications and clinical factors that can affect FHR at various gestational ages.

Chapter 8 explores nonobstetric settings and FHR evaluation, focusing on the importance of collaboration. Settings such as the emergency department, surgical suite, or intensive care unit are discussed with key points for clinical care and FHR assessment. Obstetric triage is reviewed, including the impact of the Emergency Medical Transport and Labor Act (EMTALA).

Chapter 9 focuses on antepartum testing, including the nonstress test, the contraction stress test, vibroacoustic stimulation, ultrasound, and the biophysical profile. Updated information regarding indication, frequency, and type of antepartum test based on the results of the most recent NICHD panel are provided in a clinically relevant manner.

Chapter 10 spotlights patient safety, risk management, and documentation. Common causes of error and principles of risk management are reviewed, and safety as an overriding concern in the clinical setting is introduced. Intermittent auscultation, EFM, and informed consent are discussed, with suggestions for inter- and intradisciplinary discussion points and patient education. Actual deposition testimony related to documentation reveals the importance of knowing both nomenclature and physiology in detail.

Chapter 11 provides a glimpse of FHR monitoring in select European countries, where paper speed is frequently 1 cm/minute versus the typical 3 cm/minute seen in the United States. Variations in obstetric care models and sample illustrations of a variety of fetal monitor tracings from our European colleagues are provided for review.

Appendix B has been updated and includes 20 new fetal monitoring tracings. Clinicians can use the tracings to practice application of the NICHD definitions, as well as the principles of standardized interpretation, and an answer key allows clinicians to evaluate their skills.

New to this edition, Appendix C offers a self-assessment consisting of multiple-choice questions related to the content of the textbook. Helpful for reinforcement of information presented herein, it can also be used to study for certification or credentialing examinations or to develop internal competency assessment tools for clinical practice.

Mosby's Pocket Guide to Fetal Monitoring: A Multidisciplinary Approach continues to be written by clinicians, for clinicians. Nurses, nurse-midwives, medical students, physicians, resident physicians, clinical specialists, educators, and risk management and medical-legal professionals will gain a clear perspective on modalities of fetal monitoring, the role of standardization, and the keys to successful collaboration. Designed for daily clinical practice, the text is a portable and practical resource for all obstetric clinicians.

LISA A. MILLER
DAVID A. MILLER
REBECCA L. CYPHER

CHAPTER 1

A Brief History of Fetal Monitoring

E lectronic fetal monitoring (EFM) today is but one aspect of a rapidly changing dynamic in obstetrics. What were once common practices, such as use of continuous EFM and the traditional labor progress curve, are now rightfully being examined with a keen scientific eye and a focus on patient safety. Women are being encouraged to participate in informed decision making during labor, which includes choice of monitoring modality. Intermittent auscultation (IA), for many years a neglected skill in many institutions, is making a return to daily practice, especially for low-risk women, and this shift is actively supported by professional organizations [1–3]. Much of this shift relates to these facts: research has been unable to definitively show that use of intrapartum fetal heart rate (FHR) monitoring leads to a significant reduction in neonatal neurologic morbidity [4], and both early randomized trials and meta-analyses have shown that women who have continuous EFM during labor have higher cesarean section rates than women who do not have continuous EFM [5]. Even with these shifts in practice, a majority of the approximately 4 million women giving birth each year in the United States will have EFM during some or all of their labor. Clinicians practicing today must be adept at both EFM and IA modalities, and for this reason, a brief overview of the history of FHR assessment is justified.

HISTORICAL OVERVIEW

In the seventeenth century, Jean Alexandre Le Jumeau, Vicomte de Kergaradec, used a stethoscope hoping to hear the noise of the water in the uterus, and identified the noise he heard as the FHR. Le Jumeau was the first person to speculate in print about potential clinical uses for FHR auscultation [6].

Early clinical use of determining the presence or absence of fetal heart sounds included confirmation of pregnancy, identification of twin gestation, and justification for a postmortem cesarean section. In 1833, William Kennedy, a British obstetrician, published

1

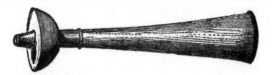

FIGURE 1.1 Early obstetric trumpet stethoscope. (Courtesy Wellcome Library, London.)

a description of "fetal distress" by describing what would later be identified as a late deceleration. Kennedy correctly associated late decelerations with poor prognoses, and he made the link between fetal head compression and decrease in FHR [7]. Other discoveries from early use of FHR assessment via IA included identification of fetal tachycardia in response to maternal fever, FHR decelerations following excessive uterine activity, and accelerations accompanying fetal movement (Figure 1.1) [6].

The head stethoscope, or DeLee-Hillis fetoscope, was first reported in the literature in 1917 [8]. During the 1950s physicians, including Edward Hon [9–11] in the United States, Caldeyro-Barcia [12,13] in Uruguay, and Hammacher [14] in Germany, developed electronic devices that were able to continuously measure and record the FHR and uterine activity. The simultaneous measurement of FHR and uterine activity came to be called EFM or cardiotocography. This new technologic capability permitted systematic study of the relationships between recorded FHR patterns and fetal physiology [10,11,15]. Different terms and definitions were developed worldwide as investigators made remarkably similar observations of FHR characteristics (Figure 1.2).

RANDOMIZED TRIALS OF ELECTRONIC FETAL MONITORING

Initially in the 1960s observational studies demonstrated a decrease in intrapartum stillbirth rates in settings that adopted continuous EFM [16–18]. Today, observational findings alone would not likely be sufficient to engender sweeping practice changes, but in the 1960s and 1970s these findings fueled widespread adoption of the technology into clinical practice. Although EFM was originally intended for use in high-risk laboring women, it was rapidly incorporated into the management of low-risk laboring women as well and quickly became ubiquitous.

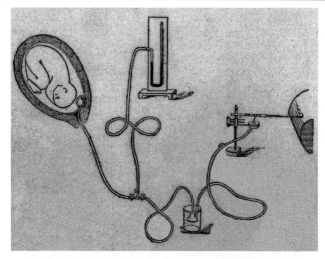

FIGURE 1.2 Apparatus for studying uterine contractions during childbirth. (Courtesy Wellcome Library, London.)

In the 1970s and 1980s, several randomized clinical trials* were conducted comparing continuous EFM with IA using a Pinard stethoscope or a handheld Doppler device. Continuous EFM was not associated with a decrease in low Apgar scores or perinatal mortality. However, there was an increase in the incidence of cesarean section in women who had continuous EFM. Despite these findings, use of continuous EFM did not decrease.

Meta-analyses have reviewed the results of trials comparing continuous intrapartum EFM to IA [5,28,29]. These studies included more than 37,000 women. Compared with IA, continuous EFM showed no significant difference in overall perinatal death but was associated with a significant reduction in neonatal seizures. No significant difference was detected in the incidence of cerebral palsy. However, there was a significant increase in cesarean sections associated with continuous EFM. Interestingly, none of the randomized trials published after 1980 demonstrated a statistically significant increase in the rate of cesarean section in electronically monitored patients. More important, the majority of newborns in the cohort who later developed cerebral palsy were not in the group of fetuses who had FHR tracings that were considered "ominous" [30].

---

*References 19-27.

RESEARCH AT THE END OF THE TWENTIETH CENTURY

What went wrong? Several things. Although the randomized controlled trials (RCTs) followed the usual guidelines for inclusion and exclusion of subjects and used recommended methods for the study protocols, the definitions of FHR patterns reflecting "fetal distress" varied among the different studies [23,25,31]. Many of the studies were conducted before the importance of FHR variability, a critical parameter, was recognized as significant related to fetal acid–base status. Outcome measures evaluated (Apgar scores, perinatal mortality, and cerebral palsy) were nonspecific indicators of the potential for hypoxic injury during the intrapartum period. Finally, the small sample size of published reports is an ongoing issue. It has been noted that more than 50,000 women would need to be randomized to show a difference in mortality [5]; the numbers that would be needed to show a reduction in neonatal encephalopathy related solely to intrapartum events are so high that RCTs for either EFM or IA become implausible [32]. As a result, the conclusions of these studies remain open to alternative interpretations [27,33], and a careful review of the oft-cited Cochrane Database meta-analysis by Alferic and colleagues reveals low-quality evidence for all conclusions, save the conclusion regarding neonatal seizures, which was found to be of moderate quality [5]. Clinicians may need to consider basing decisions regarding the use of continuous EFM on multiple factors, including forthright discussions of risks versus benefits with various patient populations. Informed consent regarding EFM versus IA is challenging with the state of current evidence and is discussed in more detail in Chapter 10.

In 1996, the National Institute of Child Health and Human Development (NICHD) Task Force met and made recommendations [34] for three important aspects of FHR monitoring for both research and clinical practice: (1) the task force developed standard definitions for FHR patterns; (2) they described the FHR pattern (normal baseline rate, moderate variability, presence of accelerations, and absence of decelerations) that consistently reflects an absence of asphyxia; and (3) they described FHR patterns (recurrent late or variable decelerations or substantial bradycardia with absent variability) that are "predictive of current or impending asphyxia" [34].

FETAL MONITORING IN THE TWENTY-FIRST CENTURY

In 2003, the Task Force on Neonatal Encephalopathy and Cerebral Palsy [35] was convened by the American Congress of Obstetricians and Gynecologists (ACOG) to review the world literature regarding the relationship between FHR patterns in labor and neonatal outcomes. The task force reviewed the literature on Apgar scores, neonatal encephalopathy and cerebral palsy, neonatal seizures, and umbilical cord gases. In 2010, a second task force was convened to update this important work, and in 2014 a second edition was published, which included the review of 1500 references by 17 task force members and 88 consultants [36]. This updated report focuses on neonatal encephalopathy in infants born at 35 weeks' gestation or greater and contains an in-depth review of intrapartum events and their relationship to newborn encephalopathy. Consensus from this work and others forms the basis of the principles of interpretation of EFM that will be elucidated later in this text.

Standardization in research in EFM has been aided by the NICHD definitions that were originally published in 1997 [34]. In 2008, a new NICHD panel on fetal monitoring was convened; the new panel confirmed and provided clarification of the definitions published in 1997 and provided a three-tiered categorization of FHR tracings to replace the traditionally used terms *reassuring* and *nonreassuring*. The panel also reviewed uterine activity and provided guidance for evaluation of uterine activity as well as definitions for summary terms. Finally, the 2008 NICHD workshop report provided important information regarding consensus on the validity of the negative predictive value of both moderate variability and/or FHR accelerations in relation to fetal metabolic acidemia [37]. Since the report, many healthcare systems have implemented multidisciplinary education and training related to the standardized NICHD definitions.

In an effort to find a more direct measure of fetal oxygenation to serve as an adjunct to EFM in the assessment of fetal acid–base balance, fetal pulse oximetry made a short-lived appearance on the clinical scene. The first randomized trial of fetal pulse oximetry demonstrated a reduction in the number of cesarean sections performed for "nonreassuring" FHR patterns but no overall reduction in cesarean sections [38]. At present, fetal pulse oximetry has been a useful tool for research but is no longer available for use in clinical practice. Computer analysis of the fetal electrocardiogram ST segment (STAN Neoventa Medical, Göteborg, Sweden), a technology based on evaluation of the ST segment and the T/QRS ratio of the fetal electrocardiogram complex, continues to be in use, primarily outside the United States, and is discussed in Chapter 11. The large, multicenter NICHD trial of ST analysis in the United States involving more than 11,000 patients failed to show any decrease in operative deliveries or any differences in perinatal outcomes [39].

SUMMARY

What began in 1822 with a stethoscope has evolved into a frequently used, and often misunderstood, technology. Today's clinicians need collaborative strategies for best practices in fetal assessment and monitoring. Clinicians must recognize the features of the EFM tracing that provide information regarding the absence of fetal metabolic acidemia, as demonstrated by the presence of accelerations and/or moderate variability, and must respond appropriately when those signs are absent. Although it is clear that more research is needed on EFM reliability (observer agreement), validity (association with neonatal outcomes), and efficacy (preventive interventions that work), the overall evidence suggests that extreme positions on EFM (either universal use or universal abandonment) are unwarranted. A middle path that encompasses appropriate patient selection, informed consent, and a clinical recognition of the limits of the technology is perhaps the most reasonable course for EFM in the near future. Women want and are entitled to complete information regarding fetal monitoring via auscultation as well as by electronic means [40,41]. As the history of EFM continues to unfold, one thing is certain: *research continues to be needed to identify best practices for EFM or IA in laboring women.* Technology alone will never be the answer. Standardization of terminology, multidisciplinary education regarding FHR interpretation and underlying physiology, and management based on collaboration and teamwork remain the best approach to safe passage for mother and child, regardless of the technology employed.

References

[1] American College of Nurse-Midwives, Intermittent auscultation for intrapartum fetal heart rate surveillance. ACNM Clinical Bulletin Number 13, J. Midwifery Womens Health 60 (2015) 626–632.

[2] American College of Obstetricians and Gynecologists, Intrapartum fetal heart rate monitoring: nomenclature, interpretation, and general

management principles, Obstet. Gynecol. 114 (2006) 192–202. Practice Bulletin no. 106, 2009.

[3] Association of Women's Health, Obstetric and Neonatal Nurses, Fetal heart monitoring, position statement, J. Obstet. Gynecol. Neonatal Nurs. 44 (5) (2015) 683–686, http://dx.doi.org/10.1111/1552-6909.12743.

[4] J.T. Parer, T.L. King, S. Flanders, et al., Fetal acidemia and electronic fetal heart rate patterns: is there evidence of an association? J. Matern. Fetal Neonatal Med. 19 (5) (2006) 289–294.

[5] Z. Alfirevic, D. Devane, G.M.L. Gyte, Continuous cardiotocography (CTG) as a form of electronic fetal monitoring (EFM) for fetal assessment during labour, Cochrane Database Syst. Rev. 5 (2013), http://dx.doi.org/10.1002/14651858.CD006066.pub2.

[6] C. Sureau, Historical perspectives: forgotten past, unpredictable future, Baillieres Clin. Obstet. Gynaecol. 10 (2) (1996) 167–184.

[7] E. Kennedy, Observations of Obstetrical Auscultation, Hodges & Smith, Dublin, 1833. p. 311.

[8] D.S. Hillis, Attachment for the stethoscope, JAMA 68 (1917) 910.

[9] E.H. Hon, Instrumentation of fetal heart rate and electrocardiography II: a vaginal electrode, Am. J. Obstet. Gynecol. 83 (1963) 772.

[10] E.H. Hon, The classification of fetal heart rate. I: a working classification, Obstet. Gynecol. 22 (1963) 137–146.

[11] E.H. Hon, The electronic evaluation of the fetal heart rate, Am. J. Obstet. Gynecol. 75 (1958) 1215.

[12] R. Caldeyro-Barcia, C. Mendez-Bauer, J. Poseiro, et al., Control of human fetal heart rate during labor, in: D. Cassels (Ed.), The Heart and Circulation in the Newborn and Infant, Grune & Stratton, New York, 1966.

[13] R. Caldeyro-Barcia, J.J. Poseiro, C. Negreierosdepaiva, et al., Effects of abnormal uterine contractions on a human fetus, Bibl. Paediatr. 81 (1963) 267–295. http://www.ncbi.nlm.nih.gov/pubmed/14065034 (accessed 05.08.15).

[14] K. Hammacher, New method for the selective registration of the fetal heart beat [German], Geburtshilfe Frauenheilkd. 22 (1962) 1542–1543.

[15] S.T. Lee, E.H. Hon, Fetal hemodynamic response to umbilical cord compression, Obstet. Gynecol. 22 (1963) 553–562.

[16] R. Errkola, M. Gronroos, R. Punnonen, et al., Analysis of intrapartum fetal deaths: their decline with increasing electronic fetal monitoring, Acta Obstet. Gynecol. Scand. 63 (5) (1984) 459–462.

[17] J.T. Parer, Fetal heart rate monitoring, Lancet 2 (8143) (1979) 632–633.

[18] S.Y. Yeh, F. Diaz, R.H. Paul, Ten year experience of intrapartum fetal monitoring in Los Angeles County/University of Southern California Medical Center, Am. J. Obstet. Gynecol. 143 (5) (1982) 496–500.

[19] A.D. Havercamp, M. Orleans, S. Langerdoerfer, et al., A controlled trial of differential effects of intrapartum fetal monitoring, Am. J. Obstet. Gynecol. 134 (4) (1979) 399–408.

[20] A.D. Havercamp, H.E. Thompson, J.G. McFee, et al., The evaluation of continuous fetal heart rate monitoring in high risk pregnancy, Am. J. Obstet. Gynecol. 125 (3) (1976) 310–320.

[21] I.M. Kelso, R.J. Parsons, G.F. Lawrence, et al., An assessment of continuous fetal heart rate monitoring in labor, Am. J. Obstet. Gynecol. 131 (5) (1978) 526–532.

[22] J. Leveno, F.G. Cunningham, S. Nelson, et al., A prospective comparison of selective and universal electronic fetal monitoring in 34,995 pregnancies, N. Engl. J. Med. 315 (10) (1986) 615–641.

[23] D.A. Luthy, K.K. Shy, G. van Belle, et al., A randomized trial of electronic monitoring in labor, Obstet. Gynecol. 69 (5) (1987) 687–695.

[24] D. MacDonald, A. Grant, M. Sheridan-Pereira, et al., The Dublin randomized controlled trial of intrapartum fetal heart rate monitoring, Am. J. Obstet. Gynecol. 152 (5) (1985) 524–539.

[25] S. Neldam, M. Osler, P.K. Hansen, et al., Intrapartum fetal heart rate monitoring in a combined low- and high-risk population: a controlled trial, Eur. J. Obstet. Gynecol. Reprod. Biol. 23 (1–2) (1986) 1–11.

[26] P. Renou, A. Chang, I. Anderson, et al., Controlled trial of fetal intensive care, Am. J. Obstet. Gynecol. 126 (4) (1976) 470–475.

[27] C.L. Winkler, J.C. Hauth, M.J. Tucker, et al., Neonatal complications at term as related to the degree of umbilical artery acidemia, Am. J. Obstet. Gynecol. 164 (2) (1991) 637–641. 1991.

[28] S.B. Thacker, D.F. Stroup, H.B. Peterson, Efficacy and safety of intrapartum electronic fetal monitoring: an update, Obstet. Gynecol. 86 (4 Pt 1) (1995) 613–620.

[29] A.M. Vintzileos, D.J. Nochimson, E.R. Guzman, et al., Intrapartum electronic fetal heart rate monitoring versus intermittent auscultation: a meta-analysis, Obstet. Gynecol. 85 (1) (1995) 149–155.

[30] S. Grant, N. O'Brien, M.T. Joy, et al., Cerebral palsy among children born during the Dublin randomized trial of intrapartum monitoring, Lancet 2 (8674) (1989) 1233–1235.

[31] C. Wood, P. Renou, J. Oats, et al., A controlled trial of fetal heart rate monitoring in a low risk obstetric population, Am. J. Obstet. Gynecol. 141 (5) (1981) 527–534.

[32] H.Y. Chen, S.P. Chauhan, C.V. Ananth, et al., Electronic fetal heart rate monitoring and its relationship to neonatal and infant mortality in the United States, Am. J. Obstet. Gynecol. 204 (6) (2011), http://dx.doi.org/10.1016/j.ajog.2011.04.024.

[33] J.T. Parer, T. King, Whither fetal heart rate monitoring? Obstet. Gynecol. Fertil. 22 (5) (1999) 149–192.

[34] National Institute of Child Health and Human Development Research Planning Workshop, Electronic fetal heart rate monitoring; research guidelines for interpretation, Am. J. Obstet. Gynecol. 177 (6) (1997) 1385–1390.

[35] American College of Obstetricians and Gynecologists Task Force on Neonatal Encephalopathy and Cerebral Palsy, Neonatal Encephalopathy

and Cerebral Palsy: Defining the Pathogenesis and Pathophysiology, ACOG, AAP, Washington, DC, 2003.

[36] American College of Obstetricians and Gynecologists, Task Force on Neonatal Encephalopathy and Cerebral Palsy, American College of Obstetricians and Gynecologists, American Academy of Pediatrics, Neonatal Encephalopathy and Neurologic Outcome, second ed., American College of Obstetricians and Gynecologists, Washington, DC, 2014. p. 7.

[37] G.A. Macones, G.D. Hankins, C.Y. Spong, et al., The 2008 National Institute of Child Health and Human Development workshop report on electronic fetal monitoring: update on definitions, interpretation, and research guidelines, J. Obstet. Gynecol. Neonatal Nurs. 37 (2008) 510–515.

[38] T.J. Garite, G.A. Dildy, H. McNamara, et al., A multicenter controlled trial of fetal pulse oximetry in the intrapartum management of nonreassuring fetal heart rate patterns, Am. J. Obstet. Gynecol. 183 (5) (2000) 1049–1058.

[39] G. Saade, Fetal ECG analysis of the ST segment as an adjunct to intrapartum fetal heart rate monitoring: a randomized clinical trial, Am. J. Obstet. Gynecol. 212 (1) (2015) S2.

[40] American College of Obstetricians and Gynecologists & Society for Maternal-Fetal Medicine, Safe prevention of the primary cesarean delivery: obstetric care consensus, Am. J. Obstet. Gynecol. 210 (3) (2014) 179–193.

[41] E.R. Declercq, C. Sakala, M.P. Corry, et al., Listening to mothers II: Report of the Second National U.S. Survey of Women's Childbearing Experiences. New York, October 2006. Childbirth Connection. Available from   www.childbirthconnection.org/listeningtomothers/   (accessed 02.05.11).

CHAPTER 2

Physiologic Basis for Electronic Fetal Heart Rate Monitoring

The objective of intrapartum fetal heart rate (FHR) monitoring is to prevent fetal injury that might result from interruption of normal fetal oxygenation during labor. The underlying assumption is that interruption of fetal oxygenation leads to characteristic physiologic changes that can be detected by changes in the FHR. Understanding the physiologic basis for electronic FHR monitoring requires a realistic appraisal of this basic assumption. The role of intrapartum FHR monitoring in assessing the fetal physiologic changes caused by interrupted oxygenation can be summarized as follows:

1. Fetal oxygenation consists of two basic elements:
   Transfer of oxygen from the environment to the fetus
   The fetal response to interruption of oxygen transfer
2. Certain FHR patterns provide reliable information regarding both of the basic elements of fetal oxygenation

This chapter reviews the physiology underlying fetal oxygenation, including transfer of oxygen from the environment to the fetus and the fetal response to interruption of oxygen transfer (Figure 2.1). Chapters 5 and 6 will review the relationship between fetal oxygenation and FHR patterns.

TRANSFER OF OXYGEN FROM THE ENVIRONMENT TO THE FETUS

Oxygen is carried from the environment to the fetus by maternal and fetal blood along a pathway that includes the maternal lungs, heart, vasculature, uterus, placenta, and umbilical cord, illustrated in Figure 2.1; this is a central concept in FHR monitoring. Interruption of oxygen transfer can occur at any or all of the points along the oxygen pathway. Therefore it is essential to understand the physiology and pathophysiology involved in each step.

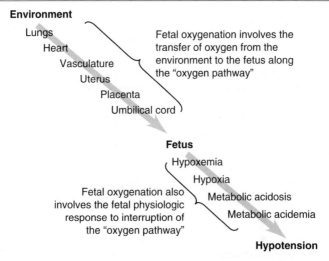

FIGURE 2.1 Physiology of fetal oxygenation. (Courtesy David A. Miller, MD.)

External Environment

Oxygen comprises approximately 21% of inspired air. Therefore, in inspired air, the partial pressure exerted by oxygen gas (Po_2) is approximately 21% of total atmospheric pressure (760 mm Hg) minus the pressure exerted by water vapor (47 mm Hg). At sea level, this translates to approximately 150 mm Hg. As oxygen is transferred from the environment to the fetus, the partial pressure declines. By the time oxygen reaches fetal umbilical venous blood, the partial pressure is as low as 30 mm Hg. After oxygen is delivered to fetal tissues, the Po_2 of deoxygenated blood in the umbilical arteries returning to the placenta is approximately 15 to 25 mm Hg [1–4]. The sequential transfer of oxygen from the environment to the fetus and potential causes of interruption at each step are described next.

Maternal Lungs

Inspiration carries oxygenated air from the external environment to the distal air sacs of the lung, the alveoli. On the way to the alveoli, inspired air mixes with less-oxygenated air leaving the lungs. As a result, the Po_2 of air within the alveoli (PAo_2) is lower than that in inspired air. At sea level, alveolar Po_2 (PAo_2) is approximately 105 mm Hg. From the alveoli, oxygen diffuses across a thin "blood-gas" barrier into the pulmonary capillary blood. The pulmonary blood-gas barrier consists of three layers: a single-cell layer of alveolar epithelium, a layer of extracellular collagen matrix (interstitium), and a single-cell layer of pulmonary capillary endothelium. Interruption of oxygen transfer from the environment to the alveoli can result from airway obstruction or depression of central respiratory control. Examples include maternal apnea during a convulsion and medications such as narcotics or magnesium. Interruption of oxygen transfer from the alveoli to the pulmonary capillary blood can be caused by a number of factors, including ventilation-perfusion mismatch and diffusion defects due to conditions such as pulmonary embolus, pneumonia, asthma, atelectasis, or adult respiratory distress syndrome.

Maternal Blood

After diffusing from the pulmonary alveoli into maternal blood, more than 98% of oxygen combines with hemoglobin in maternal red blood cells. Approximately 1% to 2% remains dissolved in the blood and is measured by the partial pressure of oxygen in arterial blood (Pao_2). The amount of oxygen bound to hemoglobin depends directly upon the Pao_2. Hemoglobin saturations at various Pao_2 levels are illustrated by the oxyhemoglobin dissociation curve (Figure 2.2). A normal adult Pao_2 value of 95 to 100 mm Hg results in hemoglobin saturation of approximately 95% to 98%, indicating that hemoglobin is carrying 95% to 98% of the total amount of oxygen it is capable of carrying. A number of factors affect the affinity of hemoglobin for oxygen and can shift the oxyhemoglobin dissociation curve to the left or right. In general, the tendency for hemoglobin to release oxygen is increased by factors that signal an increased requirement for oxygen. Specifically, oxygen release is enhanced by factors that indicate active cellular metabolism. These factors shift the oxyhemoglobin saturation curve to the right and include byproducts of aerobic metabolism (reflected by increased CO_2 concentration), byproducts of anaerobic metabolism (reflected by increased 2,3-DPG concentration), production of lactic acid (reflected by increased hydrogen ion concentration and decreased pH), and heat. Interruption of oxygen transfer from the environment to the fetus due to abnormal maternal oxygen carrying capacity can result from severe anemia or from hereditary or acquired abnormalities affecting oxygen binding,

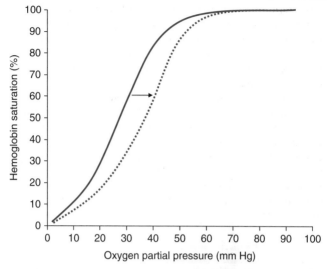

FIGURE 2.2 Fetal oxygen dissociation curve. The tendency for hemoglobin to release oxygen is increased by factors that signal an increased requirement for oxygen. Specifically, oxygen release is enhanced by factors that indicate active cellular metabolism. These factors shift the oxyhemoglobin saturation curve to the right and include anaerobic glycolysis (reflected by increased 2,3-diphosphoglycerate concentration), production of hydrogen ions (reflected by decreased pH), and heat. (Courtesy David A. Miller, MD.)

such as hemoglobinopathies or methemoglobinemia. In an obstetric population, reduced maternal oxygen carrying capacity rarely interferes with fetal oxygenation. Maternal hemoglobin saturation can be estimated noninvasively by transmission pulse oximetry (Spo_2). In recent years, investigators studying the efficacy of fetal oxygen saturation ($FSpo_2$) monitoring have provided valuable insights into fetal physiology (see Chapters 5 and 6).

Maternal Heart

From the lungs, pulmonary veins carry oxygenated maternal blood to the heart. Blood enters the left atrium with a Pao_2 of approximately 95 mm Hg. Oxygenated blood passes from the left atrium, through the mitral valve into the left ventricle and out the aorta for systemic distribution. Normal transfer of oxygen from the environment to the fetus is dependent on normal cardiac function, reflected by cardiac output. Cardiac output is the product of heart rate and stroke volume. Heart rate is determined by intrinsic cardiac pacemakers (SA node, AV node), the cardiac conduction system, autonomic regulation (sympathetic, parasympathetic), humoral factors (catecholamines), extrinsic factors (medications), and local factors (calcium, potassium). Stroke volume is determined by preload, contractility, and afterload. Preload is the amount of stretch on myocardial fibers at the end of diastole when the ventricles are full of blood. It is determined by the volume of venous blood returning to the heart. Contractility is the force and speed with which myocardial fibers shorten during systole to expel blood from the heart. Afterload is the pressure that opposes the shortening of myocardial fibers during systole and is estimated by the systemic vascular resistance or systemic blood pressure. Interruption of oxygen transfer from the environment to the fetus at the level of the maternal heart can be caused by any condition that reduces cardiac output, including altered heart rate (arrhythmia), reduced preload (hypovolemia, compression of the inferior vena cava), impaired contractility (ischemic heart disease, diabetes, cardiomyopathy, congestive heart failure), and/or increased afterload (hypertension). In addition, structural abnormalities of the heart and/or great vessels may impede the ability to pump blood (valvular stenosis, valvular insufficiency, pulmonary hypertension, coarctation of the aorta). In a healthy obstetric patient, the most common cause of reduced cardiac output is reduced preload resulting from hypovolemia or compression of the inferior vena cava by the gravid uterus.

Maternal Vasculature

Oxygenated blood leaving the heart is carried by the systemic vasculature to the uterus. The path includes the aorta, common iliac artery, internal iliac (hypogastric) artery, anterior division of the internal iliac artery, and the uterine artery. From the uterine artery, oxygenated blood travels through the arcuate arteries, the radial arteries, and finally the spiral arteries before exiting the maternal vasculature and entering the intervillous space of the placenta. Interruption of oxygen transfer from the environment to the fetus at the level of the maternal vasculature commonly results from hypotension caused by regional anesthesia, hypovolemia, impaired venous return, impaired cardiac output, or medications. Alternatively, it may result from vasoconstriction of distal arterioles in response to endogenous vasoconstrictors or medications. Conditions associated with chronic vasculopathy, such as chronic hypertension, long-standing diabetes, collagen vascular disease, thyroid disease, and renal disease may result in chronic suboptimal transfer of oxygen and nutrients to the fetus at the level of the maternal vasculature. Preeclampsia is associated with abnormal vascular remodeling at the level of the spiral arteries and can impede perfusion of the intervillous space. Acute vascular injury (trauma, aortic dissection) is rare. In a healthy obstetric patient, transient hypotension is the most common cause of interrupted oxygen transfer at the level of the maternal vasculature. Chronic vascular conditions can exacerbate this interruption and should be considered in the course of a thorough evaluation.

Uterus

Between the maternal uterine arteries and the intervillous space of the placenta, the arcuate, radial, and spiral arteries traverse the muscular wall of the uterus. Interruption of oxygen transfer from the environment to the fetus at the level of the uterus commonly results from uterine contractions that compress intramural blood vessels and impede the flow of blood. Uterine contractions and uterine injury (rupture, trauma) are the most common causes of interruption of fetal oxygenation at this level. Uterine activity is discussed in Chapter 4.

Placenta

The placenta facilitates the exchange of gases, nutrients, wastes, and other molecules (for example, antibodies, hormones, medications) between maternal blood in the intervillous space and fetal blood in the villous capillaries. On the maternal side of the placenta, oxygenated blood exits the spiral arteries and enters the intervillous space to surround and bathe the chorionic villi. On the fetal side of the placenta, paired umbilical arteries carry blood from the fetus through the umbilical cord to the placenta (Figure 2.3). At term, the umbilical arteries receive 40% of fetal cardiac output. Upon reaching the placental cord insertion site, the umbilical arteries divide into multiple branches and fan out across surface of the placenta. At each cotyledon, placental arteries dive beneath the surface en route to the chorionic villi (Figure 2.4). The chorionic villi are microscopic branches of trophoblast that protrude into the intervillous space. Each villus is perfused by a fetal capillary bed that represents the terminal distribution of an umbilical artery.

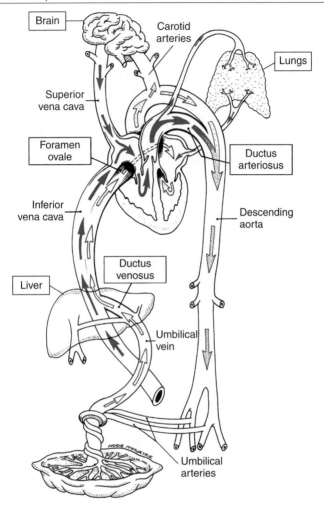

FIGURE 2.3 Fetal circulation. Oxygenated and nutrient-rich blood is carried to the fetus by the umbilical vein to the fetal heart. Oxygen-poor and waste product-rich blood circulates back to the placenta via the umbilical arteries. Three anatomic shunts (the ductus venosus, the foramen ovale, and the ductus arteriosus) permit fetal blood to bypass the liver and the lungs. (From R.S. Bloom, Delivery room resuscitation of the newborn, in: R.J. Martin, A.A Fanaroff, M.C. Walsh (Eds.), Fanaroff and Martin's Neonatal-Perinatal Medicine: Diseases of the Fetus and Infant, eighth ed., Mosby, Philadelphia, 2006.)

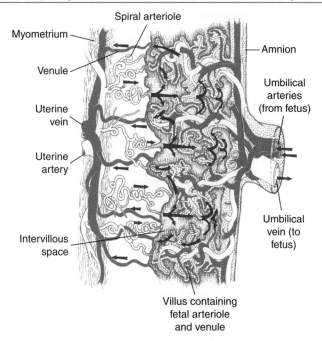

FIGURE 2.4 Schema of placenta. As maternal blood enters the intervillous space, it spurts from the uterine spiral arterioles and spreads laterally through the space. *White vessels* carry oxygenated blood. *Gray vessels* carry oxygen-poor blood.

At term, fetal villous capillary blood is separated from maternal blood in the intervillous space by a thin "blood-blood" barrier similar to the blood-gas barrier in the maternal lung. The placental blood-blood barrier is comprised of a layer of placental trophoblast and a layer of fetal capillary endothelium with intervening basement membranes and villous stroma. Substances are exchanged between maternal and fetal blood by a number of mechanisms, including simple diffusion, facilitated diffusion, active transport, bulk flow, pinocytosis, and leakage. These mechanisms are summarized in Table 2.1. Oxygen is transferred from the intervillous space to the fetal blood by a complex process that depends on the Pao_2 of maternal blood perfusing the intervillous space, maternal blood flow within the intervillous space, chorionic villous surface area, and diffusion across the placental blood-blood barrier.

TABLE 2.1 Mechanisms of Exchange Between Fetal and Maternal Blood

Mechanism	Description	Substances
Simple diffusion	Passage of substances from a region of higher concentration to one of lower concentration along a concentration gradient that is passive and does not require energy	Oxygen Carbon dioxide Small ions (sodium chloride) Lipids Fat-soluble vitamins Many drugs
Facilitated diffusion	Passage of substances along a concentration gradient with the assistance of a carrier molecule involved	Glucose Carbohydrates
Active transport	Passage of substances against a concentration gradient; carrier molecules and energy are required	Amino acids Water-soluble vitamins Large ions
Bulk flow	Transfer of substances by a hydrostatic or osmotic gradient	Water Dissolved electrolytes
Pinocytosis	Transfer of minute, engulfed particles across a cell membrane	Immune globulins Serum proteins
Breaks and leakage	Small breaks in the placental membrane allowing passage of plasma and substances	Maternal or fetal blood cells (potentially resulting in isoimmunization)

Intervillous Space Pao$_2$

As described previously, oxygenated maternal blood leaves the maternal heart with a Pao$_2$ of approximately 95 mm Hg. There are no capillary beds between the maternal heart and the spiral arteries, therefore the oxygenated maternal blood exiting the spiral arteries and entering the intervillous space has a Pao$_2$ of approximately 95 mm Hg. Oxygen is released from maternal hemoglobin and

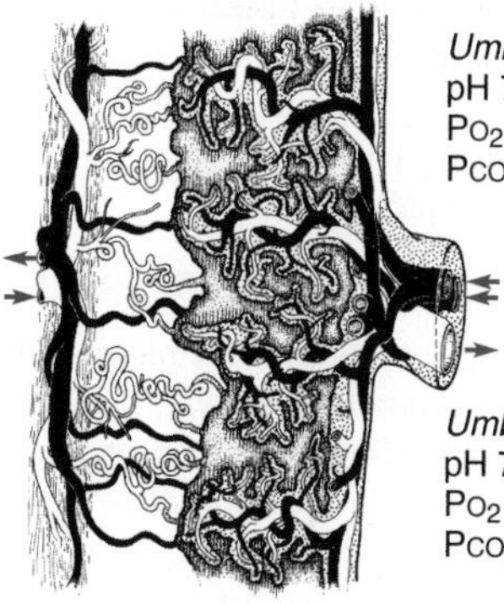

Uterine vein
pH 7.3
Po_2 40 mm Hg
Pco_2 40-50 mm Hg

Umbilical arteries
pH 7.2-7.3
Po_2 15-25 mm Hg
Pco_2 45-55 mm Hg

Uterine artery
pH 7.4-7.45
Po_2 95-100 mm Hg
Pco_2 30-35 mm Hg

Umbilical vein
pH 7.3-7.4
Po_2 25-35 mm Hg
Pco_2 35-45 mm Hg

FIGURE 2.5 Approximate maternal and fetal blood gas values.

diffuses across the placental blood-blood barrier into fetal blood where it combines with fetal hemoglobin. As a result, maternal blood in the intervillous space becomes relatively oxygen depleted and exits the intervillous space via uterine veins with a Pao_2 of approximately 40 mm Hg (Figure 2.5). Therefore the average Pao_2 of maternal blood in the intervillous space is between the Pao_2 of blood entering the intervillous space (95 mm Hg) and the Pao_2 of blood exiting the intervillous space (40 mm Hg). The average intervillous space Pao_2 is approximately 45 mm Hg. Interruption of fetal oxygenation can result from conditions that reduce the Pao_2 of maternal blood entering the intervillous space. These conditions have been discussed previously.

Intervillous Space Blood Flow

At term, uterine perfusion accounts for 10% to 15% of maternal cardiac output, or approximately 700 to 800 cc per minute. Most of this blood is located in the intervillous space of the placenta surrounding the chorionic villi. Conditions that can reduce the volume of the intervillous space include collapse or destruction of the intervillous space due to placental abruption, infarction, thrombosis, or infection.

Chorionic Villous Surface Area

Optimal oxygen exchange requires normal chorionic villous surface area. Normal transfer of oxygen from the environment to the fetus at the level of the placenta can be interrupted by conditions that limit or reduce the chorionic villous surface area available for gas exchange. These conditions can be acute or chronic and include primary abnormalities in the development of the villous vascular tree or secondary destruction of normal chorionic villi by infarction, thrombosis, hemorrhage, inflammation, or infection.

Diffusion Across the "Blood-Blood" Barrier

Diffusion of a substance across the placental blood-blood barrier is dependent on concentration gradient, molecular weight, lipid solubility, protein binding, and ionization. In addition, diffusion rate is inversely proportional to diffusion distance. At term, the placental blood-blood barrier is very thin, and the diffusion distance is short. Under normal circumstances, oxygen and carbon dioxide diffuse readily across this thin barrier. However, normal diffusion can be impeded by conditions that increase the distance between maternal and fetal blood. These conditions can be acute, subacute, or chronic and include villous hemorrhage, inflammation, thrombosis, infarction, edema, fibrosis, and excessive cellular proliferation (syncytial knots).

Interruption of Placental Blood Vessels

Rarely, fetal blood loss can be caused by injury to blood vessels at the level of the placenta. Damaged chorionic vessels can allow fetal blood to leak into the intervillous space, leading to fetal-maternal hemorrhage. This may be a consequence of abdominal trauma but can occur in association with abnormal placental development, placental abruption, or invasive procedures. A specific cause is not always identified. Ruptured vasa previa is a rare cause of fetal hemorrhage. Vasa previa is a placental vessel that traverses the chorioamniotic membrane in close proximity to the cervical os. Such a vessel may be damaged by normal cervical change during labor or injured inadvertently during membrane rupture or digital examination.

Summary of Placental Causes of Disrupted Oxygenation

Many conditions can interfere with the transfer of oxygen across the placenta. Those involving the microvasculature frequently are diagnosed by histopathologic examination after delivery. Clinically detectable causes, such as placental abruption, bleeding placenta previa, or vasa previa, should be considered but may not be amenable to conservative corrective measures.

Fetal Blood

After oxygen has diffused from the intervillous space across the placental blood-blood barrier and into fetal blood, the Pao_2 is in the range of 30 mm Hg and fetal hemoglobin saturation is between 50% and 70%. Although fetal Pao_2 and hemoglobin saturation are low in comparison to adult values, adequate delivery of oxygen to the fetal tissues is maintained by a number of compensatory mechanisms. For example, fetal cardiac output per unit weight is greater than that of the adult. Hemoglobin concentration and affinity for oxygen are greater in the fetus as well, resulting in increased oxygen carrying capacity. Finally, oxygenated blood is directed preferentially toward vital organs by way of anatomic shunts at the level of the ductus venosus, foramen ovale, and ductus arteriosus. Conditions that can interrupt the transfer of oxygen from the environment to the fetus at the level of the fetal blood are uncommon but may include fetal anemia (alloimmunization, infections, fetomaternal hemorrhage, vasa previa) and conditions that reduce oxygen carrying capacity (Bart's hemoglobinopathy, methemoglobinemia).

Umbilical Cord

After oxygen combines with fetal hemoglobin in the villous capillaries, oxygenated blood returns to the fetus by way of villous veins that coalesce to form placental veins on the surface of the placenta. Placental surface veins unite to form a single umbilical vein within the umbilical cord. Interruption of the transfer of oxygen from the environment to the fetus at the level of the umbilical cord can result from simple mechanical compression. Other uncommon causes may include vasospasm, thrombosis, atherosis, hypertrophy, hemorrhage, inflammation, or a "true knot."

From the environment to the fetus, maternal and fetal blood carry oxygen along the "oxygen pathway" illustrated in Figure 2.1. Common causes of interrupted oxygen transfer at each step along the pathway are summarized in Table 2.2. In the interest of simplicity, the foregoing discussion was limited to one gas, oxygen. It is critical to note that gas exchange also involves the transfer of carbon dioxide in the opposite direction—from the fetus to the environment. Any condition that interrupts the transfer of oxygen from the environment to the fetus has the potential to interrupt the transfer of carbon dioxide from the fetus to the environment. However, carbon dioxide diffuses across the placental blood-blood barrier more rapidly than

TABLE 2.2   Some Causes of Interrupted Transfer of Oxygen from the Environment to the Fetus

Oxygen Pathway	Causes of Interrupted Oxygen Transfer
Lungs	Respiratory depression (narcotics, magnesium)
	Seizure (eclampsia)
	Pulmonary embolus
	Pulmonary edema
	Pneumonia/ARDS
	Asthma
	Atelectasis
	Rarely pulmonary hypertension
	Rarely chronic lung disease
Heart	Reduced cardiac output
	Hypovolemia
	Compression of the inferior vena cava
	Regional anesthesia (sympathetic blockade)
	Cardiac arrhythmia
	Rarely congestive heart failure
	Rarely structural cardiac disease
Vasculature	Hypotension
	Hypovolemia
	Compression of the inferior vena cava
	Regional anesthesia (sympathetic blockade)
	Medications (hydralazine, labetalol, nifedipine)
	Vasculopathy (chronic hypertension, SLE, preeclampsia)
	Vasoconstriction (cocaine, methylergonovine)
Uterus	Excessive uterine activity
	Uterine stimulants (prostaglandins, oxytocin)
	Uterine rupture
Placenta	Placental abruption
	Rarely vasa previa
	Rarely fetal-maternal hemorrhage
	Placental infarction, infection (usually confirmed retrospectively)
Umbilical cord	Cord compression
	Cord prolapse
	"True knot"

ARDS, adult respiratory distress syndrome; *SLE,* systemic lupus erythematosus.

does oxygen. Therefore any interruption of the pathway is likely to affect oxygen transfer to a greater extent than carbon dioxide transfer. As summarized previously, oxygen transfer from the environment to the fetus represents the first basic component of fetal oxygenation. The second basic component of fetal oxygenation involves the fetal physiologic response to interrupted oxygen transfer.

FETAL RESPONSE TO INTERRUPTED OXYGEN TRANSFER

Depending on frequency and duration, interruption of oxygen transfer at any point along the oxygen pathway can result in progressive deterioration of fetal oxygenation. The cascade begins with hypoxemia, defined as decreased oxygen content in the blood. At term, hypoxemia is characterized by an umbilical artery Pao_2 below the expected range of 15 to 25 mm Hg. Recurrent or sustained hypoxemia can lead to decreased delivery of oxygen to the tissues and reduced tissue oxygen content, termed *hypoxia*. Normal homeostasis requires an adequate supply of oxygen and fuel to generate the energy required by basic cellular activities. When oxygen is readily available, aerobic metabolism efficiently generates energy in the form of adenosine triphosphate (ATP). Byproducts of aerobic metabolism include carbon dioxide and water. When oxygen is in short supply, tissues may be forced to convert from aerobic to anaerobic metabolism, generating energy less efficiently and resulting in the production of lactic acid. Accumulation of lactic acid in the tissues results in metabolic acidosis. Lactic acid accumulation can lead to utilization of buffer bases (primarily bicarbonate) to help stabilize tissue pH. If the buffering capacity is exceeded, the blood pH may begin to fall, leading to metabolic acidemia. Eventually, recurrent or sustained tissue hypoxia and acidosis can lead to loss of peripheral vascular smooth muscle contraction, reduced peripheral vascular resistance, and hypotension, in turn leading to potential hypoxic-ischemic injury to many tissues, including the brain and heart.

Acidemia is defined as increased hydrogen ion content (decreased pH) in the blood. With respect to fetal physiology, it is critical to distinguish between respiratory acidemia, caused by accumulation of CO_2, and metabolic acidemia, caused by accumulation of fixed (lactic) acid. These distinct categories of acidemia have entirely different clinical implications and are discussed later in this chapter.

Mechanisms of Injury

If interrupted oxygen transfer progresses to the stage of metabolic acidemia and hypotension, as described earlier, multiple organs and systems (including the brain and heart) can suffer hypoperfusion, reduced oxygenation, lowered pH, and reduced delivery of fuel for metabolism. These changes can trigger a cascade of cellular events, including altered enzyme function, protease activation, ion shifts, altered water regulation, disrupted neurotransmitter metabolism, free radical production, and phospholipid degradation. Disruption of normal cellular metabolism can to lead to cellular dysfunction, tissue dysfunction, and even death.

Injury Threshold

The relationship between fetal oxygen deprivation and neurologic injury is complex. Electronic FHR monitoring was introduced with the expectation that it would reduce the incidence of neurologic injury (specifically cerebral palsy) caused by intrapartum interruption of fetal oxygenation. In recent years, it has become apparent that most cases of cerebral palsy are unrelated to intrapartum events and therefore cannot be prevented by intrapartum FHR monitoring. Nevertheless, some cases of cerebral palsy may be related to intrapartum events and continue to generate controversy.

In 1999, the International Cerebral Palsy Task Force published a consensus statement identifying specific criteria that must be met to establish intrapartum interruption of fetal oxygenation as a possible cause of cerebral palsy [5]. In January 2003, the American College of Obstetricians and Gynecologists (ACOG) and the American Academy of Pediatrics Cerebral Palsy Task Force published a monograph titled *Neonatal Encephalopathy and Cerebral Palsy: Defining the Pathogenesis and Pathophysiology*, summarizing the world literature regarding the relationship between intrapartum events and neurologic injury [6].

In 2014, another publication from the ACOG Task Force on Neonatal Encephalopathy reevaluated and clarified the scientific evidence underlying the relationship among intrapartum events, neonatal encephalopathy, and neurologic outcome [7]. This publication, titled *Neonatal Encephalopathy and Neurologic Outcome* (second edition), was supported by the Royal College of Obstetricians and Gynecologists and endorsed by the American College of Nurse-Midwives, the American Gynecologic and Obstetrical Society, the American Society for Reproductive Medicine, the Association of Women's Health, Obstetric and Neonatal Nurses, the Australian Collaborative Cerebral Palsy Research Group, the Child Neurology Society, the Japan Society of Obstetrics and Gynecology, the March of Dimes Foundation, the Royal Australian and New Zealand College of Obstetricians and Gynaecologists, the Society for Maternal-Fetal Medicine, and the Society of Obstetricians and Gynaecologists of

Canada. Broad international consensus supports the conclusion that "in a fetus exhibiting either moderate variability or accelerations of the FHR, damaging degrees of hypoxia-induced metabolic acidemia can reliably be excluded."

SUMMARY

The physiology of fetal oxygenation involves the sequential transfer of oxygen from the environment to the fetus and the subsequent fetal response to interruption of this pathway (Figure 2.1). Interruption of oxygen transfer can occur at any point along the oxygen pathway. Examples of causes that might be encountered in a typical obstetric population are summarized in Table 2.2. Recurrent or sustained interruption of oxygen transfer can lead to progressive deterioration of fetal oxygenation and potential fetal injury. There is broad consensus in the literature that the presence of moderate variability or accelerations of the FHR reliably exclude hypoxic injury at the time they are observed. The physiologic basis of FHR monitoring can be summarized in a few key concepts (Table 2.3). Later chapters expand on these concepts and apply them to standardized interpretation and management of FHR patterns.

TABLE 2.3   Key Concepts of the Physiologic Basis of Intrapartum FHR Monitoring

1. The objective of intrapartum FHR monitoring is to assess fetal oxygenation during labor.
2. Fetal oxygenation involves the transfer of oxygen from the environment to the fetus along the oxygen pathway and the fetal physiologic response to interruption of the oxygen pathway.
3. Oxygen is transferred from the environment to the fetus by maternal and fetal blood along a pathway that includes the maternal lungs, heart, vasculature, uterus, placenta, and umbilical cord.
4. The fetal response to interrupted oxygen transfer involves the sequential progression from hypoxemia to hypoxia, metabolic acidosis, and metabolic acidemia.
5. Damaging degrees of hypoxia-induced metabolic acidemia can reliably be excluded in the fetus exhibiting either moderate variability or accelerations of the FHR.

References

[1] J.T. Helwig, J.T. Parer, S.J. Kilpatrick, R.K. Laros, Umbilical cord blood acid–base state: what is normal? Am. J. Obstet. Gynecol. 174 (1996) 1807–1812.

[2] A. Nodwell, L. Carmichael, M. Ross, B. Richardson, Placental compared with umbilical cord blood to assess fetal blood gas and acid–base status, Obstet. Gynecol. 105 (2005) 129–138.

[3] B. Richardson, A. Nodwell, K. Webster, M. Alshimmiri, R. Gagnon, R. Natale, Fetal oxygen saturation and fractional extraction at birth and the relationship to measures of acidosis, Am. J. Obstet. Gynecol. 178 (1998) 572–579.

[4] R. Victory, D. Penava, O. Da Silva, R. Natale, B. Richardson, Umbilical cord pH and base excess values in relation to adverse outcome events for infants delivering at term, Am. J. Obstet. Gynecol. 191 (6) (2004) 2021–2028.

[5] A. MacLennan, A template for defining a causal relation between acute intrapartum events and cerebral palsy: international consensus statement, BMJ 319 (7216) (1999) 1054–1059.

[6] American College of Obstetricians and Gynecologists' Task Force on Neonatal Encephalopathy and Cerebral Palsy, American College of Obstetricians and Gynecologists, American Academy of Pediatrics, Neonatal Encephalopathy and Cerebral Palsy: Defining the Pathogenesis and Pathophysiology, American College of Obstetricians and Gynecologists, Washington, DC, 2003.

[7] American College of Obstetricians and Gynecologists' Task Force on Neonatal Encephalopathy and Cerebral Palsy, American College of Obstetricians and Gynecologists, American Academy of Pediatrics, Neonatal Encephalopathy and Neurologic Outcome, second ed., American College of Obstetricians and Gynecologists, Washington, DC, 2014.

CHAPTER 3

Methods and Instrumentation

There are two primary methods for the evaluation of fetal heart rate (FHR) and uterine activity (UA): traditional auscultation of the FHR and palpation of UA or electronic fetal monitoring (EFM), which can involve external or internal monitoring methods or a combination of both. This chapter describes the methods of fetal monitoring and reviews the application and instrumentation of the various techniques.

INTERMITTENT AUSCULTATION OF FETAL HEART RATE

Description

Intermittent auscultation (IA) of the FHR may be performed non-electronically with a stethoscope, a DeLee-Hillis fetoscope, a Pinard stethoscope, or electronically using a Doppler ultrasound (US) device (Figure 3.1). If using a *stethoscope,* the end should be turned to the domed, or bell, side rather than the flat side. The domed side is then placed on the maternal abdomen over the fetal back, which is the location where the FHR is heard the loudest. Fetal ventricular heart valves are heard opening and closing with the stethoscope and fetoscope. The *fetoscope* should be worn on the listener's head because bone conduction amplifies the fetal heart sounds for counting. The *Doppler ultrasound* device transmits ultra high-frequency sound waves to the moving interface of the fetal heart valves and deflects these back to the device, converting them into an electronic signal that can be counted [1–3]. Although auscultation with Doppler technology is most frequently performed transabdominally in the first trimester, a transvaginal ultrasound (TVUS) probe may also be utilized to detect fetal cardiac activity by two-dimensional video or M-mode imaging [4] as well as cardiac sounds. TVUS provides closer proximity to the uterus, thus enabling the detection of fetal cardiac activity in clinically difficult examinations such as obese obstetric patients.

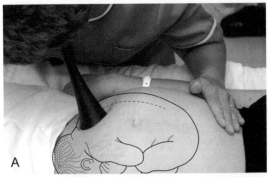

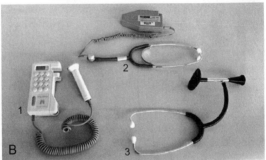

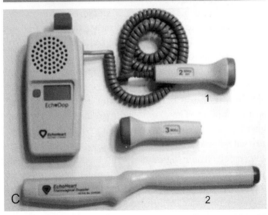

FIGURE 3.1 (A) Auscultation of the FHR with a Pinard stethoscope. Vertex left occipitoanterior. (B) 1, Ultrasound (US) fetoscope; 2, US stethoscope; 3, DeLee-Hillis fetoscope. (C) 1, Echoheart transabdominal US transducer; 2, Echoheart transvaginal probe (A, From D.M. Fraser, M.A. Cooper (Eds.), Myles Textbook for Midwives, fourteenth ed., Churchill Livingstone, London, 2003. B, Courtesy Michael S. Clement, MD, Mesa, AZ. C, Courtesy EchoHeart, Inc., Damariscotta, ME.)

Whereas EFM is based on visual assessment, auscultation is an *auditory* assessment in which an instrument or device is used to count the number of fetal heartbeats occurring in a prescribed amount of time at specified intervals and in relation to uterine contractions. IA is not simply EFM without a tracing because there are significant differences between IA and EFM [1,5]. These are summarized in Table 3.1. In addition to serving as the primary method of fetal assessment in labor, auscultation can assist clinicians with differentiation of maternal heart rate (MHR) from FHR and with correct placement of the external Doppler transducer used in EFM.

Procedure	Rationale
1. Perform Leopold's maneuvers (Figure 3.2) by palpating the maternal abdomen.	1. To identify fetal presentation and position.
2. Apply ultrasound gel to device if using a Doppler ultrasound. Place the listening device over the fetal back. If using a fetoscope or stethoscope, firm pressure may be needed.	2. To obtain the clearest and loudest sound (easier to count).
3. Count the maternal radial pulse.	3. To differentiate MHR from FHR.
4. Palpate the abdomen for the presence or absence of uterine activity.	4. To be able to count FHR between contractions.
5. Count the FHR for 30 to 60 seconds after a uterine contraction.	5. To identify the auscultated baseline rate as well as changes in the rate (increases or decreases).
6. Also auscultate the FHR before, during, and after a contraction.	6. To identify the FHR during the contraction as a response to the contraction and to assess for the absence or presence of increases or decreases in FHR.
7. When there are distinct discrepancies in FHR during listening periods, auscultate for a longer period during, after, and between contractions.	7. To identify significant changes that may indicate the need for electronic fetal monitoring (EFM).

TABLE 3.1   Fetal Heart Rate Characteristics Determined via Auscultation Versus Electronic FHR Monitor

FHR Characteristic[a]	Fetoscope	Doppler Without Paper Printout	Electronic FHR Monitor
Variability	No	No	Yes
Baseline rate	Yes	Yes	Yes
Accelerations	Detects increases[b]	Detects increases[b]	Yes
Decelerations	Detects decreases	Detects decreases	Differentiates types of decelerations
Rhythm[c]	Yes	Yes	Yes
Double counting or half-counting FHR	Can clarify	May double count or half count	May double count or half count
Differentiation of maternal heart rate and FHR	Yes	May detect maternal heart rate	May detect and record maternal heart rate

FHR, fetal heart rate.

[a] Definitions of each FHR characteristic per the National Institute of Child Health and Human Development 2008 criteria.

[b] Per method described by L.L. Paine, R.G. Payton, T. Johnson, Auscultated fetal heart rate accelerations, part I: accuracy and documentation, J. Nurse Midwifery 31 (1986) 68–72.

[c] Determined as regular or irregular. None of these devices can diagnose the type of fetal arrhythmia.

From American College of Nurse-Midwives, Intermittent auscultation for intrapartum fetal heart rate surveillance. ACNM Clinical Bulletin Number 13., J. Midwifery Womens Health 60 (2015) 626–632; M.M. Killion, Techniques for fetal heart and uterine activity assessment, in: A. Lyndon, L. Usher Ali (Eds.), Fetal Heart Monitoring Principles and Practices, fifth ed., Association of Women's Health, Obstetric and Neonatal Nurses, Washington, DC, 2015.

Leopold's Maneuvers

Leopold's maneuvers is a systematic abdominal assessment technique that includes four separate actions to determine the presentation, position, and lie of the fetus. This organized approach also facilitates optimal placement location of the auscultation or Doppler device [2,6].

Ensure the woman's bladder is empty.

Position woman supine with one pillow under her head and with her knees slightly flexed.

Place small rolled towel under her right hip to displace uterus (prevents supine hypotensive syndrome).

If right-handed, stand on woman's right, facing her:

1. Identify fetal part that occupies the fundus. The head feels round, firm, freely movable, and palpable by ballottement; the breech feels less regular and softer (identifies fetal lie [longitudinal or transverse] and presentation [cephalic or breech]; see Figure 3.2A).

2. Using the palmar surface of one hand, locate and palpate the smooth convex contour of the fetal back and the irregularities that identify the small parts (feet, hands, elbows). This assists in identifying fetal presentation (see Figure 3.2B).

3. With the right hand, determine which fetal part is presenting over the inlet to the true pelvis. Gently grasp the lower pole of the uterus between the thumb and fingers, pressing in slightly (see Figure 3.2C). If the head is presenting and not engaged, determine the attitude of the head (flexed or extended). This is referred to as Pallach's maneuver.

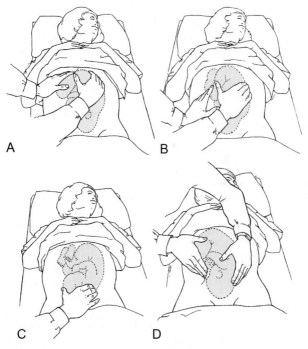

A   B

C   D

FIGURE 3.2 Leopold's maneuvers. (From D.L. Lowdermilk, S.E. Perry, K. Cashion, et al., Maternity & Women's Health Care, tenth ed., Mosby, St. Louis, 2012.)

4. Turn to face the woman's feet. Using both hands, outline the fetal head (see Figure 3.2D) with palmar surface of fingertips. When the presenting part has descended deeply, only a small portion of it may be outlined.

   Palpation of cephalic prominence assists in identifying attitude of head.

   If the cephalic prominence is found on the same side as the small parts, the head must be flexed, and the vertex is presenting. If the cephalic prominence is on the same side as the back, the presenting head is extended and the face is presenting.

Utilization, Procedure, and Frequency of Intermittent Auscultation

Some clinicians prefer IA to continuous EFM in women without risk factors because IA promotes mobility in labor, is less distracting, may be utilized with hydrotherapy, and provides a more natural birthing experience without the use of electronic devices. Reliance on the electronic monitor is more prevalent in the United States, most likely because of staffing patterns, staffing mix, and the increased use of defensive practices in a litigious environment [2,5]. The American College of Obstetricians and Gynecologists (ACOG) suggests continuous monitoring for patients with high-risk conditions, noting the uncertainty regarding the safety of IA in high-risk pregnancies [7].

Suggested IA counting techniques in the literature are typically based on protocols evaluated in randomized trials [1,8]. At this time, there is insufficient evidence on the best counting method for auscultating FHR characteristics. One suggested method to identify the rate is to auscultate the FHR for 15 to 60 seconds when the fetus is not moving and between uterine contractions. The rhythm (regular or irregular) is typically identified during this time. This is the first element of auscultation. Auscultation should also be done immediately after a contraction to identify the fetal response. A multiple-count strategy is the second component of auscultation in which the FHR is counted during several 5- to 15-second increments. Increases indicate an acceleration and decreases indicate a deceleration. The maternal radial pulse should be palpated to differentiate FHR and MHR [1,2,5]. Regardless of the method used to assess the FHR, the standard practice is to evaluate and document the FHR at specific time intervals to provide factual and accurate information [2,9].

There is a paucity of literature to recommend the optimal intervals for FHR auscultation during latent and active phase labor. Some sources recommend using a more conservative approach of assessing more frequently based on certain risk factors, though it should be noted that there are inconsistent definitions of low risk and high risk. Consequently, professional organizations have provided general guidelines for frequency of assessment for low- and high-risk patients during the intrapartum period based on existing literature [1,9]. Furthermore, recent changes regarding definitions for the latent and active phases of labor have not been reflected in all of the position statements distributed by various professional organizations (Table 3.2). In 2014, the ACOG and the Society of Maternal Fetal Medicine (SMFM) redefined the latent and active phases of labor in a consensus statement regarding the safe prevention of primary cesarean delivery, with active labor being defined as ≥6 centimeters as opposed to ≥4 centimeters [4]. The ACOG/SMFM statement did not address frequency of fetal assessment. AWHONN updated the organization's fetal monitoring position statement in 2015 to reflect auscultation assessment in accordance with these new definitions [8]. Regardless of which definition of latent and active phase is used, assessment frequency must take into account the maternal–fetal status and may need to occur more often on the basis of individual patient characteristics. Because of the scarcity of high-quality evidence regarding the optimal frequency of IA, clinicians may be best served by a multidisciplinary review of the limited evidence and formulation of consensus-based institutional protocols. Chapter 10 addresses assessment frequency versus documentation frequency in greater detail.

Documentation of Auscultated Fetal Heart Rate

Documentation of the auscultated FHR must be accompanied by other routine parameters that are assessed during labor, including UA, maternal observations and assessment, interventions, and maternal–fetal responses to these interventions. It should be noted how long the FHR was auscultated and the relationship to the uterine contraction in terms of timing (before, during, and/or immediately after a uterine contraction). The rate, rhythm, and abrupt or gradual increases or decreases of the FHR should also be described.

NOTE: It is *not* appropriate to record the descriptive terms *early, late,* and *variable decelerations* or *absent, minimal, moderate,* or *marked variability* when documenting the auscultated FHR because

TABLE 3.2   Suggested Frequency of Intermittent Auscultation

Professional Organization	Latent Phase	Active Stage Labor	Second Stage Labor
ACOG/AAP (2012)	Insufficient evidence	Low risk: q 30 minutes High risk: q 15 minutes	Low risk: q 15 minutes High risk: q 5 minutes
ACOG (2009)	Insufficient evidence	Low risk: q 15 minutes High risk: EFM	Low risk: q 5 minutes High risk: EFM
ACNM (2010)	Insufficient evidence	Low risk: q 15 minutes High risk: EFM	*Passive second stage* q 15 minutes *Active second stage* Low risk: q 5 minutes High risk: EFM
AWHONN (2015)	*<4 cm* Hourly *4–5 cm* 15–30 minutes	*≥6 cm* Low risk: q 15–30 minutes	*Passive second stage* 15 minutes *Active pushing* Low risk: q 5–15 minutes

Note: At this time, the professional organizations (AAP, ACNM, ACOG, AWHONN) have not published detailed definitions differentiating "low risk" and "high risk." Generally, continuous EFM is recommended for women who have obstetric or medical conditions (e.g., intrauterine growth restriction or chronic hypertension requiring antihypertensive medication) that place the maternal–fetal dyad at risk for adverse perinatal/neonatal outcomes or metabolic acidemia.

Adapted from: American Academy of Pediatrics (AAP), American College of Obstetricians and Gynecologists (ACOG), Guidelines for Perinatal Care, seventh ed., AAP, ACOG, Washington, DC, 2012. American College of Nurse-Midwives, Intermittent auscultation for intrapartum fetal heart rate surveillance. ACNM Ciinical Bulletin Number 13., J. Midwifery Womens Health 60 (2015) 626–632. N.F. Feinstein, A. Sprague, M.J. Trepanier, Fetal Heart Rate Auscultation, second ed., Association of Women's Health, Obstetric and Neonatal Nurses (AWHONN), Washington, DC, 2008. American College of Obstetricians and Gynecologists, Intrapartum fetal heart rate monitoring: nomenclature, interpretation, and general management principles. ACOG Practice Bulletin No. 106, Obstet. Gynecol. 114 (2009) 192–202. Association of Women's Health, Obstetric and Neonatal Nurses, Fetal heart monitoring. AWHONN Position Statement. J. Obstet. Gynecol. Neonatal Nurs. 44 (5) (2015) 683–686.

these patterns can only be interpreted with a visual assessment of a monitor tracing. However, terms that are numerically defined, such as *bradycardia* and *tachycardia*, can be used [1,2,5,10].

Interpretation of Auscultated Fetal Heart Rate

The three-tiered category system introduced by the National Institute of Child Health and Human Development [11] has been adapted by AWHONN and ACNM to a two-tier category system that reflects FHR characteristics acquired via IA. Category I auscultated FHR characteristics include an FHR BL range of 110 to 160 bpm, regular rhythm, presence or absence of FHR increases from the FHR BL, and absence of decreases from the FHR BL. Category I characteristics are strongly predictive of normal fetal acid–base status at the time of observation and do not require specific interventions other than routine management [11]. Category II auscultated FHR characteristics include everything that is not classified as Category I [1,5]. Management options for a Category II include increasing the frequency of IA, implementation of intrauterine resuscitation techniques, application of the EFM to clarify the FHR pattern visually, and notification of the primary provider (midwife or physician) [1,5].

Benefits and Limitations of Auscultation

Benefits

- Widely available and easy to use
- Less invasive
- Outcomes comparable to EFM with 1:1 nursing care
- Inexpensive
- Comfortable for the woman
- Provides freedom of movement for the woman
- 1:1 nursing care promotes "doula effect" benefits
- Allows easy FHR assessment during use of hydrotherapy

Limitations

- May be difficult to obtain the FHR in some situations, such as hydramnios and maternal obesity
- Does not provide a permanent, documented visual record of the FHR
- Counting of the FHR is intermittent
- Cannot assess visual patterns of the FHR variability or periodic changes

- Significant events may occur during periods when the FHR is not auscultated
- May not allow early detection of the FHR changes that reflect hypoxemia
- Not recommended for high-risk pregnancies

In summary, IA has been found to be effective if performed in a consistent manner by a clinician caring for a woman according to a prescribed frequency. Worldwide, auscultation is frequently and successfully employed as the first line of fetal assessment in low-risk populations. Continued research regarding auscultation, especially studies related to nurse/patient ratios, counting methods and frequency of assessments during labor, and interobserver and intraobserver reliability could prove beneficial in the acceptance of auscultation in the United States.

ELECTRONIC FETAL MONITORING

Overview

EFM may be external or internal or a combination of both. The external mode employs the use of transducers placed on the maternal abdomen to assess the FHR and UA. The internal mode uses a fetal spiral electrode (FSE) to assess the FHR and an intrauterine pressure catheter (IUPC) to assess UA and intrauterine pressure. In some countries, electronic fetal monitoring is called *cardiotocography*, or CTG. The following chart compares the external and internal modes of monitoring and gives a brief description of the equipment used for each.

External Mode	Internal Mode
Fetal Heart Rate	
Ultrasound (Doppler) transducer: High-frequency sound waves reflect mechanical action of fetal heart.	**Fetal spiral electrode:** Electrode converts fetal electrocardiogram (FECG) (as obtained from presenting part) to FHR via cardiotachometer by measuring consecutive fetal R-wave intervals. The cervix must be sufficiently dilated to allow placement. The electrode penetrates the fetal presenting part 1.5 mm, and it must be securely attached to ensure an adequate signal.

External Mode	Internal Mode
Uterine Activity	
Tocodynamometer (tocotransducer): This instrument monitors the approximate frequency and duration of contractions by means of a pressure-sensing device applied to the abdomen.	**Intrauterine pressure catheter:** This instrument quantitatively monitors frequency, duration, and intensity of contractions and resting tone. The catheter is compressed during contractions, placing pressure on a transducer tip (or the strain gauge mechanism of a fluid-filled catheter) and then converting the pressure into millimeters of mercury (mm Hg) on the UA panel of the monitor tracing. The membranes must be ruptured and the cervix sufficiently dilated for placement. Catheters are available with a second lumen that can be used for amnioinfusion.

Converting Raw Data Into a Visual Display of FHR

The FHR data collected, whether by external or internal means, must then be converted into a visual display (Figures 3.3 and 3.4). This display may be on paper, a computer screen, or often both. EFM interpretation is based on a visual assessment of data presented on a Cartesian graph. The gridlines on the horizontal (x) axis of the

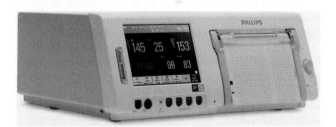

FIGURE 3.3 Philips Avalon FM 50 fetal monitor provides measurement of the FHR including noninvasive triplet monitoring, FHR high/low audible and visual alarms, and FECG. Maternal parameters include toco and intrauterine pressure, blood pressure, pulse rate, pulse oximetry, and ECG. It has cross-channel verification of maternal and fetal heart rate, displays FECG and MECG on the color display touch screen, and has a LAN interface for compatibility with hospital IT networks. (Courtesy Philips Medizin Systemes, Böblingen, Germany.)

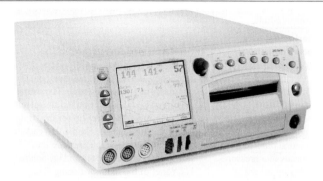

FIGURE 3.4 Corometrics 250CX fetal monitor. (Courtesy GE Healthcare, Milwaukee, WI.)

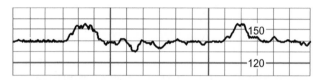

FIGURE 3.5 An FHR tracing has the appearance of an irregular horizontal line. (Courtesy David A. Miller, MD.)

graph represent time in increments of 10 seconds. The gridlines on the vertical (y) axis represent the FHR in increments of 10 bpm. As illustrated in Figure 3.5, the FHR appears on the graph as an irregular horizontal line representing the FHR over a period of time.

However, as demonstrated in Figure 3.6, closer inspection reveals that the "irregular horizontal line" is not a line at all. Instead, it is a series of individual, closely spaced points. Each point represents an individual heart rate that is calculated from the time between two successive heartbeats. This is a fundamental principle of EFM and merits a brief review.

Fetal monitoring equipment used in clinical practice detects the fetal heartbeat in one of two ways. An FSE detects the actual electrical impulses that originate in the fetal heart and make up the FECG. An external transducer uses Doppler ultrasound to detect cardiac motion. Regardless of the method of detecting the fetal heartbeat, the monitor uses the same basic principles to process the raw data for visual display. If the FHR is derived from a direct fetal electrode detecting the FECG, as illustrated in Figure 3.6, the monitor measures the distance

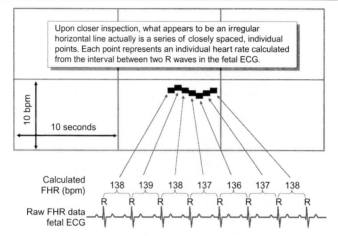

Upon closer inspection, what appears to be an irregular horizontal line actually is a series of closely spaced, individual points. Each point represents an individual heart rate calculated from the interval between two R waves in the fetal ECG.

10 bpm

10 seconds

Calculated FHR (bpm)   138   139   138   137   136   137   138

Raw FHR data fetal ECG   R   R   R   R   R   R   R   R

FIGURE 3.6 Converting raw FHR data for visual display. (Courtesy David A. Miller, MD.)

between two successive R waves and calculates a heart rate based on that single R-R interval. The individual heart rate is plotted as a single point on the FHR graph. The monitor then measures the next R-R interval, calculates a new heart rate, and plots it as a new point on the graph. This process is repeated with every subsequent R wave. If the FHR is derived from an external Doppler ultrasound transducer, the monitor uses the peak of the Doppler waveform in place of the R wave and performs the same basic calculations. A normal FHR BL rate of 140 bpm will yield approximately 140 individual graph points every minute, each representing an individual heart rate. To the eye, these individual points are spaced so closely together that they appear as a line. Variations in the FHR cause the line to appear irregular. The physiologic significance of these variations will be discussed in Chapter 5.

EXTERNAL MODE OF MONITORING

Ultrasound Transducer

Description

An ultrasound transducer is a device that is placed on the maternal abdomen and generates high-frequency ultrasound waves that are transmitted into the tissues (Figure 3.7). As the ultrasound waves

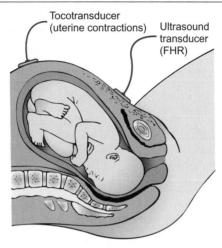

FIGURE 3.7 Placement of external transducers. The tocotransducer transmits UA. The US transducer transmits FHR. (From D.L. Lowdermilk, S.E. Perry, K. Cashion, et al., Maternity & Women's Health Care, tenth ed., Mosby, St. Louis, 2012.)

strike tissue interfaces, some of the waves are reflected back toward the transducer from which they originated. The transducer detects the returning waves and converts them into electric signals. When ultrasound waves are reflected from a moving interface, such as the fetal heart, the waves return at different frequencies. This phenomenon is known as the *Doppler effect*. The change in frequencies can be used to calculate the motion of the target. As described previously, Doppler-detected fetal heart motion is converted to a continuous graphic display of the FHR printed on the upper portion of the monitor tracing. Simultaneously, the Doppler-detected FHR is converted electronically to an audible beep and flashing light on the monitor.

The Doppler signal can be affected by changes in the position of the transducer or the fetus. Changes in the direction of the sound beam during contractions may cause a loss of signal and make the resulting tracing uninterpretable, and the transducer may need frequent repositioning due to maternal position changes. Furthermore, certain equipment errors and clinical conditions may produce artifact or data that makes interpretation confusing and difficult.

Placement of Ultrasound Transducer

A sequential procedure with rationales is provided for the application of the ultrasound transducer.

Procedure	Rationale
1. Position the woman in a comfortable sitting or side-lying position.	1. To maximize uteroplacental blood flow by avoiding supine hypotension syndrome.
2. Perform Leopold's maneuvers (see Figure 3.2).	2. To determine fetal position, lie, and presentation.
3. Align and insert the ultrasound transducer plug into the appropriate monitor port (labeled Cardio or US [for ultrasound]).	3. To provide connection without damaging connector pins (could result in a faulty signal).
4. Apply ultrasound gel to the underside of the transducer placed on the maternal abdomen.	4. To aid in the transmission of ultrasound waves.
5. Place the transducer on the abdomen, preferably over the fetal back, which is usually the point of maximum intensity.	5. To achieve the clearest signal.
6. Adjust the audio volume control while moving the transducer over the abdomen.	6. To obtain the loudest audible fetal signal.
7. Count the maternal radial pulse and compare with fetal heart rate.	7. To differentiate between maternal and fetal heart rates.
8. Secure the ultrasound transducer with the abdominal belt or other fixation device.	8. To prevent displacement of the transducer.
9. Observe the signal-quality indicator.	9. To verify clarity of input based on correct placement of the transducer.
10. Set the recorder at a paper speed of 3 cm/min and observe the FHR on the monitor strip. NOTE: A speed of 1 or 2 cm/min is used in some countries.	10. To ensure that the paper feeds correctly and that the recording is clear.
11. Reposition the transducer whenever the fetal signal becomes unclear (e.g., when the woman moves or when the fetus descends in the pelvis).	11. To ensure a clear, interpretable tracing during fetal monitoring.
12. Carefully remove the transducer from the fixation device at the completion of monitoring, and cleanse the abdomen of gel.	12. To avoid damage to the transducer and remove accumulated gel from the abdomen.
13. Box 3.1 gives guidelines for care, cleaning, and storage of external transducers.	13. To prevent damage and ensure cleanliness of equipment.

BOX 3.1   General Guidelines for Care, Cleaning, and Storage of External Transducers

---

- Exercise caution when removing and handling the US and tocotransducers so that they are not dropped or allowed to swing against any equipment to protect from damage.
- Clean transducers according to the manufacturer's operating manual, usually with a soft cloth using mild soap and water. Avoid submerging transducers or placing them beneath running water. Do not use alcohol or other cleaning solutions that may damage equipment.
- Gently and loosely coil cables for storage. Avoid tight coiling and sharp bending of the cables, which will result in damage to the wires or casing.
- Cables between monitor models and manufacturers are usually not interchangeable. Forced insertion into an incompatible monitor port is likely to result in damage.
- Dispose of disposable abdominal belts.

Tocotransducer

Description

The tocotransducer, often referred to as a *toco*, monitors UA transabdominally by means of a pressure-sensing button that is depressed by uterine contractions or fetal movement. The UA panel of the monitor paper or computer screen displays the frequency and duration of contractions. Intensity and resting tone can be assessed only with palpation or the use of an IUPC. Thus, palpation of UA to assess intensity and resting tone is mandatory when using the tocotransducer.

Placement of Tocotransducer

A sequential procedure with rationales is provided for the placement of the tocotransducer.

Procedure	Rationale
1. Position the woman in a comfortable sitting or side-lying position.	1. To maximize uteroplacental blood flow by avoiding supine hypotension syndrome.
2. Perform Leopold's maneuvers (see Figure 3.2).	2. To determine fetal position, lie, and presentation.
3. Align and insert the tocotransducer plug into the appropriate monitor port labeled Toco or UA (for uterine activity).	3. To provide connection without damaging connector pins (could result in a faulty signal).

Procedure	Rationale
4. Place the transducer on the maternal abdomen over the upper uterine segment where there is the least amount of maternal tissue between the pressure-sensing button and the uterus (where uterine contractions are best palpated).	4. To ensure that the upper uterine segment is as close as possible to the pressure-sensing button.
5. Secure the tocotransducer with the abdominal belt and ensure that there is no gel under the tocotransducer.	5. To prevent displacement of the transducer and to ensure that there is no gel accumulation that might impede function.
6. Set the recorder at a paper speed of 3 cm/min, check the printed time/date for accuracy, and observe the monitor strip or computer screen. NOTE: A speed of 1–2 cm/min is used in some countries.	6. To ensure that the paper feeds correctly, the date is accurate, and the recording is clear and received by the monitoring system.
7. Between contractions, press the UA or Toco test button for the resting baseline to print at the 20-mm Hg line on the monitor strip.	7. To prevent missing the beginning or ending of the uterine contraction (necessary for FHR pattern interpretation).
8. Monitor the frequency and duration of the contractions and palpate the strength of the contractions as well as resting tone. Document them in the woman's medical record according to facility policy.	8. The tocotransducer *cannot* measure intensity of contractions or resting tone between contractions because the depression of the pressure-sensing button varies with amount of maternal adipose tissue; therefore the information should not be relied on to assess need for analgesia in relation to perceived strength (painfulness) of contractions as registered by the monitor.
9. When monitoring is in progress, readjust abdominal belt periodically, and massage any reddened skin areas.	9. To promote comfort and maintain the proper position of the transducer.
10. Reposition the transducer periodically and secure the abdominal belt snugly.	10. To promote and ensure a good recording.

Continued

Procedure	Rationale
11. Carefully remove the transducer from the fixation device at the completion of monitoring.	11. To avoid damage to the transducer.
12. See Box 3.1 for guidelines for care, cleaning, and storage of external transducers.	12. To prevent damage and ensure cleanliness of equipment.

Advantages and Limitations of External Transducers

Advantages

- Noninvasive
- Easy to apply
- May be used during the antepartum period
- May be used with telemetry
- Does not require ruptured membranes or cervical dilation
- No known risks to woman or fetus
- Provides continuous recording of the FHR and UA

Limitations

- May limit maternal movement.
- Frequent repositioning of transducers is often needed to maintain an accurate tracing.
- Ultrasound transducer may double-count a slow FHR of less than 60 bpm, resulting in an apparently normal FHR during a bradycardia, or it may half-count an elevated FHR of more than 180 bpm, resulting in an apparently normal FHR during a tachycardia.
- MHR may be counted if the ultrasound transducer is placed over the maternal arterial vessels, such as the aorta.
- Tocotransducer provides information limited to frequency and duration of uterine contractions; it cannot accurately assess strength or intensity of uterine contractions.
- Obese women and preterm or multifetal gestations may be difficult to monitor.

INTERNAL MODE OF MONITORING

Fetal Spiral Electrode

Description

The FSE monitors the FECG from the presenting part. FSE application occurs once the amniotic membranes have been ruptured,

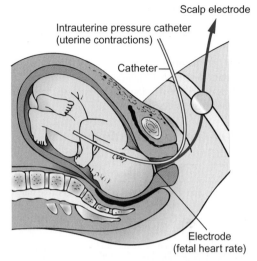

FIGURE 3.8 Diagrammatic representation of internal mode of monitoring with intrauterine pressure catheter and spiral electrode attach to fetal scalp. (From D.L. Lowdermilk, S.E. Perry, K. Cashion, et al., Maternity & Women's Health Care, tenth ed., Mosby, St. Louis, 2012.)

although it may be applied through intact membranes when necessary. Additionally, the cervix must be sufficiently dilated to allow placement, and the presenting part must be accessible and identifiable (Figure 3.8). Therefore the FSE is used only during the intrapartum period. A licensed registered nurse (RN) may place the FSE if approved by the institution policies and there is documentation of successful completion of the skills competency. The state nursing licensing board regulations for FSE placement by an RN should also be reviewed.

Contraindications

- Planned application to the fetal face, fontanels, or genitalia
- Inability to identify the portion of the fetus where application is contemplated
- Presence or suspicion of placenta previa
- Presence of active herpes lesions or human immunodeficiency virus
- Maternal infection with hepatitis B or C

Situations Requiring Caution

- Woman is positive for group B streptococcus, syphilis, or gonorrhea
- The fetus is premature

It is important to refer to the manufacturer's directions and guidelines, as well as current professional guidelines and institutional policies related to use of the FSE.

Placement of Fetal Spiral Electrode

Procedure	Rationale
1. Turn power on and insert appropriate monitor port, labeled Cardio or ECG.	1. To connect cable plug to cable into the appropriate outlet.
2a. Apply gloves and perform a sterile vaginal examination to determine presenting fetal part.	2a. To maintain aseptic technique and to avoid the fetal face, fontanels, and genitalia.
b. Retract FSE until tip is approximately 1 inch into drive handle and introduce into vagina with non-examining hand, keeping examining fingers on target area.	b. To prevent damage to the vaginal wall, glove puncture, and injury to examining fingers during placement.
c. Place the guide tube between the examining fingers and place firmly against the target area of the fetus.	c. To ensure proper placement.
d. Rotate the drive and guide tubes clockwise approximately 1½ rotations until resistance is met. Do not continue to rotate the device.	d. To ensure proper depth of placement and to avoid tissue injury from excessive placement depth.
e. Release the electrode wires from the locking device or handle notch and slide the drive and guide tubes off the electrode wires and out of the vagina.	e. To maintain proper placement and safe removal of device.
3. Discard the outer drive tube when the application procedure is completed.	3. Avoid contamination and/or exposure to blood and body fluids.
4. Connect to the leg plate cable and secure on the woman's thigh.	4. To avoid tension, pulling, or dislodging the spiral electrode. The electrode must be securely attached to ensure a good signal.

Procedure	Rationale
5. Observe the signal quality indicator.	5. To verify clear signal from electrode.
6. Set the recorder at a paper speed of 3 cm/min, and observe the FHR on the strip chart. NOTE: A paper speed of 1–2 cm/min is used in some countries.	6. To ensure that the paper feeds correctly and that the recording is clear.
7. During monitoring, check the attachment plate periodically, and reposition for comfort as needed.	7. To ensure transmission of the signal.
8. When removing the spiral electrode, turn 1½ rotations counterclockwise or until it is free from the fetal presenting part. Do not pull the electrode from the fetal skin. Do not cut wires and pull apart to remove electrode from the fetus. Disconnect the electrode from the leg plate, remove the attachment pad, and dispose of the electrode and the attachment pad according to facility policy.	8. To ensure that the electrode is removed in the opposite rotation to how it was applied; pulling the electrode straight out results in unnecessary trauma to the fetal skin, produces an observable wound, and predisposes the site to infection.
9. The electrode should be removed just before cesarean delivery, vacuum extractor use, and forceps.	9. In cesarean delivery, the electrode should not be left attached and brought up through the uterine incision. If unable to detach, cut wire at perineum and notify physician.
10. Clean the leg plate cable, if reusable, according to the facility's procedure, or follow the manufacturer's directions in the operating manual.	10. To prevent infection.
11. Loosely coil the cable and place in a secure area.	11. To prevent damage to the wires (can occur with tight coiling, resulting in loss of or an inadequate fetal signal).

Intrauterine Pressure Catheter

Description

The IUPC monitors uterine contraction frequency, duration, intensity, and resting tone (Figure 3.9). A small catheter is introduced

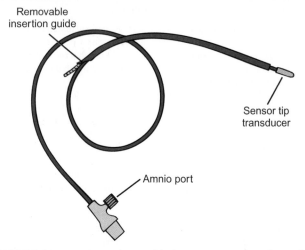

Removable
insertion guide

Sensor tip
transducer

Amnio port

FIGURE 3.9 Intrauterine catheter with the sensor transducer located in the tip of the catheter provides uninterrupted UA monitoring. Saline-filled catheters are another type of catheter in use. Note that this catheter has an amnioport that may be used for amnioinfusion. The procedure of amnioinfusion is used to treat variable decelerations in the presence of oligohydramnios. See Appendix A for more information.

through the vagina transcervically into the uterus after the amniotic membranes have been ruptured and the cervix is sufficiently dilated to identify the presenting part. The catheter is compressed during uterine contractions, placing pressure on a transducer. The pressure is then reflected on the monitor tracing in units of millimeters of mercury (mm Hg).

There are several types of IUPCs available for labor management: fluid filled, transducer tipped, and sensor tipped. Each one has specific benefits, limitations, troubleshooting procedures, and capabilities including ease of use, placement technique, ability to allow amnioinfusion, and rezeroing capability. Always refer to the manufacturer's directions and guidelines, along with the facility's policies and procedures, for information on use and insertion.

Placement of Intrauterine Pressure Catheter

The following chart shows the procedure in a sequential format for the use and insertion of the IUPC.

Procedure	Rationale
1. Turn the power on and insert the reusable cable into the appropriate monitor connector labeled UA, Toco, or Utero.	1. To activate the pressure transducer.
2. Depending on the brand of catheter, zero the monitor after connecting to the cable and before insertion. Refer to manufacturer's directions for zeroing instructions.	2. To establish a zero baseline for the catheter system based on normal atmospheric pressure.
3. If inserting a fluid-filled catheter, fill the catheter with 5 mL sterile water, leaving the syringe attached to the catheter. Maintain sterility at the maternal end of the catheter.	3. To ensure that the catheter is patent and fluid-filled before insertion; to maintain aseptic technique.
4a. Perform a sterile vaginal examination and identify the fetal presenting part.	4a. To maintain aseptic technique and to identify the optimal location for catheter insertion.
b. Insert the sterile catheter and introducer guide inside the cervix between the examining fingers; do not extend introducer guide beyond fingertips.	b. The guide is made of a hard plastic that can cause trauma if inserted farther than necessary.
c. Advance only the catheter according to the insertion depth indicator or until the blue/black or stop mark on it reaches the vaginal introitus.*	c. To ensure that enough of the catheter is inside the uterus (approximately 30–45 cm).
d. Separate and remove or slide the catheter introducer guide away from the introitus and remove; dispose of the guide appropriately.	d. To prevent the guide from sliding toward the introitus.
5. Secure the catheter to the woman's leg.	5. To ensure the woman's mobility without fear of dislodging the catheter.
6. Encourage the woman to cough or briefly perform a Valsalva maneuver. Observe the graph during this time; a sharp spike should appear when the IUPC is properly positioned.	6. To confirm placement and functioning.

Continued

Procedure	Rationale
7. Document BL resting tone in the supine position with left lateral and right lateral tilt.	7. To obtain baseline information because maternal position and IUPC position may alter measurements.
8. Rezero monitor if indicated during labor, according to manufacturer's directions.	8. To ensure that uterine activity information is correct.
9. Gently remove catheter after use and discard; store reusable cable for future use.	9. To ensure that disposable catheter is not reused.

Fluid-filled Catheters

When monitoring is in progress.

a. Flush the intrauterine catheter with sterile water every 2 hours or as necessary (the use of solutions other than sterile water can occlude and corrode the system).	a. To remove any vernix caseosa or air bubbles that may have entered the catheter and can invalidate the pressure reading.
b. Check the proper functioning of the catheter when necessary by tapping the catheter or asking the woman to cough or perform a brief Valsalva maneuver while observing the chart.	b. To ensure proper function and confirm accurate recording on the chart paper.

* Remove catheter immediately in the event of *extraovular* placement outside of the amniotic fluid space (between the chorionic membrane and endometrial lining), as evidenced by blood in the catheter.

Similar to FSE placement, a licensed RN may insert the IUPC as long as state licensing board regulations have been verified and the nurse is competency-verified according to the institution's policies.

Advantages and Limitations of Internal Monitoring

Advantages

- Capability of accurately displaying some fetal cardiac arrhythmias when linked to ECG recorder
- Accurately displays an FHR between 30 and 240 bpm
- Only truly accurate measure of all UA (e.g., frequency, duration, intensity, and resting tone)
- Allows for use of amnioinfusion

- Positional changes do not usually affect quality of FHR tracing (may affect IUPC accuracy)
- May be more comfortable than external transducer belt

Limitations

- Presenting part must be accessible and identifiable to place the FSE
- Internal electrode may record MHR in presence of fetal demise
- May not achieve adequate ECG conduction when excessive fetal hair is present
- Requires (or will result in) rupture of membranes
- Cervix must be dilated sufficiently to allow placement
- Improper insertion can cause maternal or placental trauma
- May increase risk for infection

To allay any anxiety, the woman who is electronically monitored should be given an explanation of equipment operations and the possibility of need for adjustments during labor. The care given to the electronically monitored woman is the same as that given to any woman during labor, with the additional consideration of those factors that relate directly to the monitor.

DISPLAY OF FETAL HEART RATE, UTERINE ACTIVITY, AND OTHER INFORMATION

The display on the front of the EFM shows the FHR and the uterine pressure, as well as identifies each signal source. Additional monitor options include maternal noninvasive blood pressure, MHR, maternal pulse oximetry, maternal ECG in real time, and gross fetal body movements. These parameters are also displayed on the front or face of the monitor (Figure 3.10).

In addition to the FHR and UA, other data may be printed on the monitor tracing or computer printout to include the time of day, date, and paper speed. The signal source is recorded as well as each change of parameter and mode of monitoring. Depending on the monitor's options, other maternal and fetal data may be printed on the tracing. The MHR and maternal ECG can be trended on the upper (or heart rate) section of the monitor strip. Maternal noninvasive blood pressure can also be printed as whole numbers. The manufacturer's operating manual should be available and referred to for more information, especially when assessing women with risk factors who may have concurrent monitoring of multiple parameters.

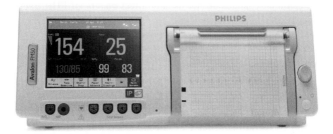

FIGURE 3.10 The monitor display shows the FHR and uterine activity and identifies the signal source for each. Other parameters may be displayed including maternal blood pressure, pulse rate, MECG, and pulse oximetry. (Courtesy Philips Medizin Systemes, Böblingen, Germany.)

Monitor Tracing Scale

The FHR and UA are printed on scaled paper (Figure 3.11). The FHR is printed on the upper section and the UA on the lower section. Monitors are preset by the manufacturers for the countries in which they are used. Note the differences in the range and scale of the FHR and UA sections, as well as in the paper/recorder speed, in Figure 3.12. The monitor strip in Figure 3.12A depicts the tracing paper that is used with monitors used in North America, with a speed of 3 cm/min. The monitor strip in Figure 3.12B depicts the tracing paper that is used in many countries outside North America, with a speed of 1 cm/min. It is imperative to use tracing paper that is designed in the correct scale to match the monitor settings.

Monitoring Multiple Gestations

Contemporary monitors have the capability of monitoring multiple gestations simultaneously. This is accomplished with two or three separate ultrasound transducers, or one fetus may be monitored via an FSE during labor, with the remaining FHRs being monitored with ultrasound transducers (Figure 3.13). Many monitors offer the unique capability of distinguishing between two or three FHRs. These features may include a distinguishing thick or dark trace for one FHR and a thin or light trace for another (Figure 3.14). The computer display may show two or three separate colors for twin or triplet gestations. Another option to distinguish the tracings in multiple gestations is a "twin offset" mechanism, which separates the

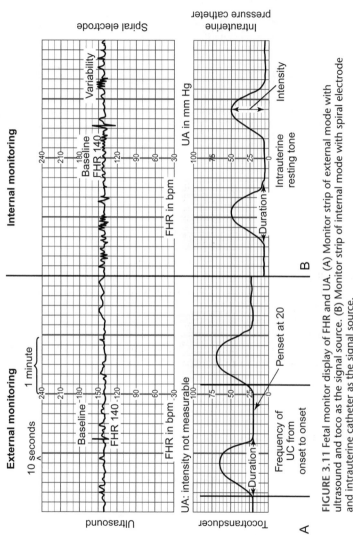

FIGURE 3.11 Fetal monitor display of FHR and UA. (A) Monitor strip of external mode with ultrasound and toco as the signal source. (B) Monitor strip of internal mode with spiral electrode and intrauterine catheter as the signal source.

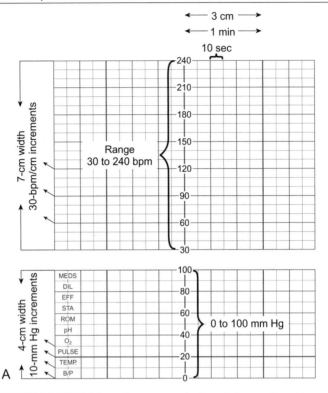

FIGURE 3.12 (A) Fetal monitor paper scale: 3-cm/min speed used in North America.

Vertical Axis
Heart Rate
    Range   30–240 bpm
    Scale   Increments of 10 bpm (30 bpm/cm)
Uterine Activity
    Range   0–100 mm Hg pressure
    Scale   Increments of 10 mm Hg
Horizontal Axis
Paper/recorder speed   3 cm/min = six 10-second subsections
                                    within 1 minute

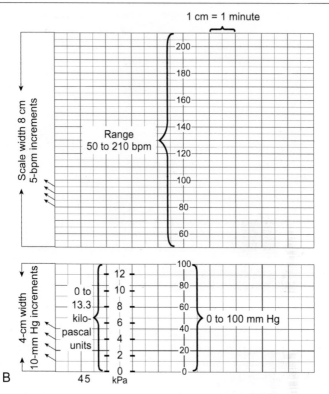

FIGURE 3.12, CONT'D (B) Fetal monitor paper scale: 1-cm/min speed used in countries outside North America, with key points identified.

Vertical Axis	
Heart Rate	
Range	50–210 bpm
Scale	Increments of 5 bpm (20 bpm/cm)
Uterine Activity	
Range	0–100 mm Hg pressure, or 0–13.3 kilopascal units (1 kPa = 7.5 mm Hg)
Scale	Increments of 10 mm Hg
Horizontal Axis	
Paper/recorder speed	1 cm/min = 2 subsections (or 2 cm/min speed = four subsections)

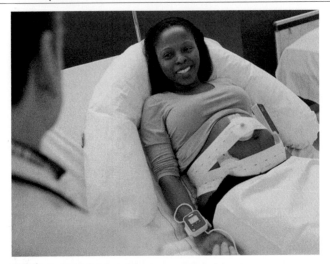

FIGURE 3.13 Monitoring of multiple gestations with separate US transducers. (Courtesy Philips Medizin Systemes, Böblingen, Germany.)

two FHRs on the tracing by a distance of about 20 bpm. Thus one fetus appears to have an FHR that is higher than the actual heart rate. The manufacturer's instruction manual should be consulted to have a clear understanding of this capability.

To clearly differentiate between twins, fetal positions in the uterus should be documented and ultrasound transducers labeled. The cross-channel verification alert may occur if both fetuses have the same/coincidental heart rates. If this occurs, relocate the ultrasound transducer(s) to detect the second FHR. In identifying twins or multiples, the presenting fetus just above the cervix is labeled A, with the remaining fetuses being identified (B, C, etc.) by their relative ascending positions [12].

Artifact Detection and Signal Ambiguity (Coincidence) with MHR

As mentioned previously, FHR misinterpretations can occur for a variety of reasons and are often referred to as *artifact*. Three leading sources of artifact include signal error, device limitations, and incorrect interpretation by the clinician or device [13]. Signal error

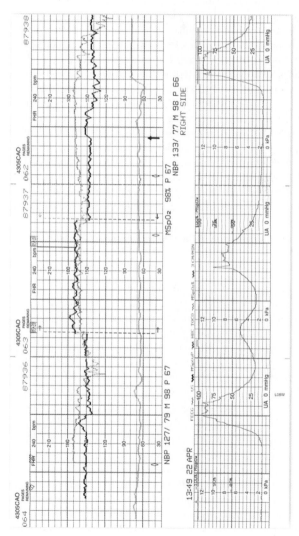

FIGURE 3.14 Dual US heart rate monitoring strip demonstrates the simultaneous external monitoring of twins. (Courtesy GE Medical Systems Information Technologies, Milwaukee, WI.)

is typically related to improper transducer placement or maternal–fetal signal interference (i.e., uterine contractions or fetal movement), which leads to a weak or undetectable FHR signal. Signal error may appear as gaps or noncontiguous marks on the tracing. Device limitations may originate from an audible FHR bradycardia or tachycardia resulting in a tracing that appears to be doubled or halved. Finally, incorrect interpretation may be caused by fetal arrhythmias, recording of the MHR, or the wrong paper speed [13–15].

Fetal monitors have built-in artifact rejection systems, which are always in operation when using the external mode of FHR monitoring. Logic circuitry rejects data when there is a greater variation than expected between successive fetal heartbeats. When repetitive variations differ by more than the accepted amount, newer monitors continue to print regardless of the extent of the excursion of the FHR. The older generation of monitors may switch from a hold mode to a non-record mode. The recorder resumes recording when the variations between successive beats fall within the predetermined parameters.

During internal monitoring, artifact is rare, and the logic system will miss only those changes that exceed the predetermined limits of the system. If there is an accessible switch to select a logic or no-logic mode, it is preferable to have the monitor in the no-logic mode when using the internal mode (FSE) to detect fetal arrhythmias.

More recently the terms *signal ambiguity* or *signal coincidence* have been highlighted in the literature. These terms refer to a circumstance where the FHR transitions to the MHR and is recorded on the tracing by the external ultrasound transducer. Despite current technology in which the external transducer detects high-frequency ultrasound waves from the fetal heart, the device may inadvertently record the MHR. This can lead to a failure to diagnose an intrauterine fetal demise or a deteriorating fetal status because of the inability to recognize a shift from the FHR to the MHR on the tracing printout or computer display [14,16] (Figure 3.15). Clinical conditions that are related to this include second-stage active pushing when the MHR may become elevated and appears as FHR accelerations, obesity, twin gestations, active fetal movement, and patient positioning during epidural placement [14,15,17–19]. Certain manufacturers offer a tocodynamometer that allows for automatic maternal pulse detection and automatic coincidence detection using cross-channel verification, allowing confirmation of both maternal and fetal signals without use of maternal pulse oximetry or manual confirmation (Figure 3.16).

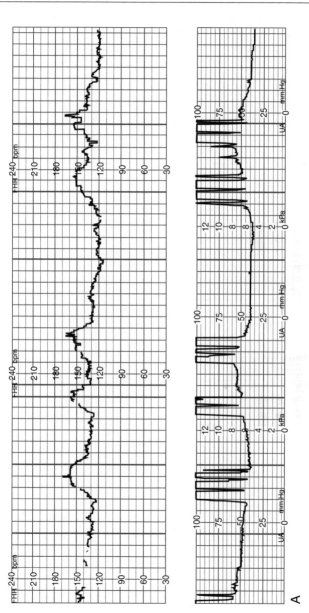

FIGURE 3.15 (A) Example of an FHR tracing showing maternal heart rate being recorded as fetal, note appearance of "accelerations" with maternal pushing efforts.

Continued

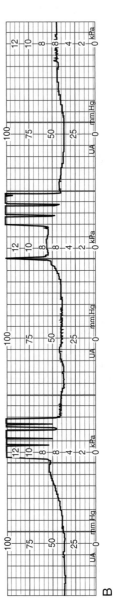

FIGURE 3.15, CONT'D (B) Now FHR tracing shows both the actual fetal heart rate (upper tracing line) concomitantly with the maternal heart rate (lower tracing line). Maternal heart rate accelerations are seen with pushing efforts.

B

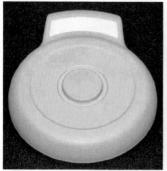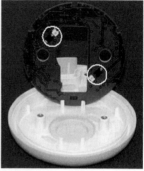

FIGURE 3.16 The modified Toco transducer M2734B, "Toco MP," allows automatic maternal pulse detection and automatic coincidence detection via cross-channel verification that confirms both maternal and fetal signals. (Courtesy Philips Medizin Systemes, Böblingen, Germany.)

Telemetry

Remote internal or external FHR monitoring via radio wave telemetry (Figure 3.17) allows women to ambulate without the loss of continuous monitoring data. A woman may feel less confined, more relaxed, and more content if she is mobile. The transducer is worn by means of an abdominal belt or other device. FHR and UA signals are continuously transmitted to a receiver that is connected to the fetal monitor. The monitor then processes and displays the data via a central display feature facilitating clinician surveillance of the telemetry-monitored patient. In addition, external watertight transducers are available for fetal surveillance via telemetry during hydrotherapy or water birth.

Troubleshooting the Monitor

The EFM is a useful tool to assess fetal well-being. As with any electronic device, problems may occur, which may require corrective actions to resolve. The following chart suggests actions for identified electromechanical problems.

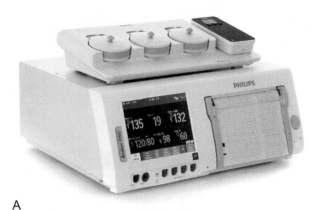

A

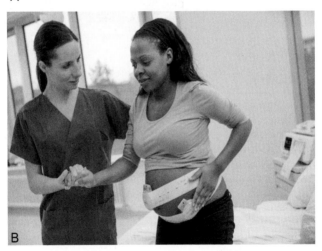

B

FIGURE 3.17 (A) The Avalon cableless solution (Avalon CL) offers a complete wireless OB area while providing all traditional fetal monitoring measurements without cables, including monitoring of twins, triplets, maternal Spo$_2$ and NiBP. The measurement device transmits information to a base station that is connected to a fetal monitor. The waterproof transducers may be used for the patient who is in bed, ambulating, or in the bath. (B) Cordless US and tocotransducer are applied to the maternal abdomen for external monitoring. (Courtesy Philips Medizin Systemes, Böblingen, Germany.)

Problem	Action
Power	■ Check power cord at wall and back of monitor.
Ultrasound	
Half or double rate	■ Assess FHR with fetoscope, stethoscope, or Doppler.
	■ Check maternal pulse to rule out maternal signal, and document maternal pulse.
	■ Reapply ultrasound gel and recheck.
	■ Move transducer to search for a better signal.
	■ Consider applying spiral electrode.
Erratic trace or display	■ Reposition transducer.
	■ Reposition woman.
	■ Tighten ultrasound belt if too loose.
	■ Check gel on transducer (if it is dry, sound waves do not penetrate the skin). Reapply gel if needed. Move transducer if fetus is out of range.
Spiral Electrode	
Erratic trace or display	■ Check attachment pad on leg for adherence to skin.
	■ Ensure that connection of FSE is secure on attachment pad and that connector is securely inserted into the leg-plate cable.
Signal quality indicator is continuously red	■ Ensure that logic switch is off to assess for fetal arrhythmia.
	■ Apply a new FSE.
Tocotransducer	
Not recording	■ Check that cable is plugged in to monitor and power is on
Numbers in high range	■ Readjust toco on abdomen; ensure that cable is fully attached to monitor.
	■ Zero monitor with toco/UA button between contractions, or replace with another toco.
Toco not picking up contractions	■ Palpate abdomen for best location to sense contractions, and reapply toco.
	■ Test toco by *lightly* depressing pressure transducer and observing readout on monitor.
	■ Tighten belt, or use another device to hold toco firmly against abdomen.
	■ Consider using an IUPC.

Continued

Problem	Action
IUPC	
Not recording	▪ Recheck cable insertion.
	▪ Flush if using a fluid-filled catheter.
Resting tone (>25 mm Hg)	▪ Palpate abdomen to identify uterine tonus before making equipment adjustments.
	▪ Adjust level of strain gauge for fluid-filled catheters to maternal xiphoid.
	▪ Zero or recalibrate non-fluid-filled catheter.
	▪ Flush if using a fluid-filled catheter.
Not recording contractions	▪ Check catheter markings at woman's introitus (catheter may have slipped out).
	▪ Replace catheter if necessary.
Elevated resting tone (*hypertonus*)	▪ Higher resting tone may be noted with multiple gestation, uterine malformation or myoma, use of oxytocin, amnioinfusion, extraovular placement.
	▪ Rezero monitor.
	▪ Replace catheter if incorrect placement.
Potential Problems	
Suspected fetal arrhythmia	▪ Auscultate FHR with fetoscope or stethoscope.
	▪ Perform fetal ECG.
Errors caused by incorrect paper speed or paper with different scale	▪ Check annotation with paper speed: it should be 3 cm/min in North America.
	▪ Check scale: it should be 30–240 bpm for FHR if paper speed is 3 cm/min or 50–210 bpm if paper speed is 1 or 2 cm/min.
Cross-channel verification alert	▪ Alert occurs with two coincidental heart rates. Verify maternal heart rate. Reposition ultrasound transducer(s) to detect second fetal heart rate.

Computerized Perinatal Data Systems

Many institutions use computerized perinatal data systems that provide central surveillance, alerts, documentation, and archiving capabilities electronically. Additionally, clinical decision support systems that include customizable tools and software technology for computer analysis of FHR and uterine activity characteristics have been introduced to inpatient obstetrical units [20,21]. Clinical decision support systems are tools or checklists that help clinicians stay within the guidelines of a specific protocol (e.g., oxytocin management) and send an electronic message or visual notification when a deviation from protocol has occurred. These tools identify developing trends (e.g., tachysystole), assist in automating repetitive tasks, and deliver decision support at the beside that simplifies and speeds the process while facilitating communication among clinicians [20,22].

A monitor display in a central position, such as the unit's main workstation, provides an opportunity to view tracings from multiple rooms concurrently (Figure 3.18). Single-screen displays of several rooms or of one patient can be accessed from remote locations such as a patient's bedside, staff locker room, clinician's office, or from home. Perinatal data systems include the capability of real-time data entry in the form of detailed notes including but not limited to vaginal examination results, medication administration, the woman's position, and vital signs. Perinatal data systems offer universal electronic health records (EHRs) that incorporate the entire perinatal and neonatal spectrum, from prenatal care through delivery, as well as postpartum and neonatal care. Reports and paper charts can be generated with a printer linked to the display or shared electronically through the healthcare institution's intranet.

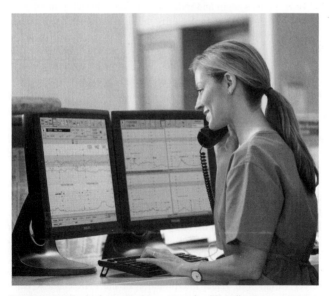

FIGURE 3.18 Central monitoring system for EFM allowing access to multiple records in a variety of formats. (Courtesy Philips Medizin Systemes, Böblingen, Germany.)

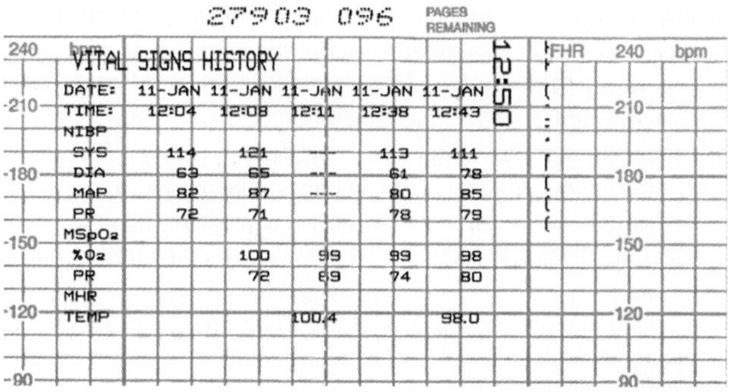

FIGURE 3.19 Clinicians can review and print trending data, such as the history of maternal blood pressure readings, and quickly determine status changes. (Courtesy GE Healthcare, Milwaukee, WI.)

The majority of central display systems provides multiple options for accessing and viewing information (Figure 3.19), including the following:

- A *system status* screen provides an instant overview of several beds on the system and indicates any alerts by room number. In addition, the system can identify the signal source of any woman on the system.
- A *trend screen* can provide the most recent few minutes of FHR and UA data on any one woman, with immediate warning of critical conditions relating to any woman in the system.
- *Scrolling* capabilities allow clinicians to review hours of FHR data in minutes, which can help identify changes over time, an important component of FHR tracing evaluation.
- An *alert screen* can provide an immediate summary of the trend analysis on any woman. The data can be made available to the staff before, during, and after an alert.

The surveillance component of a perinatal data system can be set to alert for fetal tachycardia or bradycardia, signal loss, coincidental fetal and maternal heart rates, and other maternal–fetal parameters. Ranges for the duration of, and recovery from, fetal bradycardia or tachycardia can be set at different levels for each patient. These systems are widely available from a variety of manufacturers.

One of the major limitations of EFM is the high inter- and intraobserver variation in visual interpretation of the FHR characteristics [23]. This variation among clinicians can lead to misinterpretation of the FHR tracing, which in turn can lead to poor communication and decisions that result in unnecessary intervention or delays in treatment [23,24]. Computer analysis of the FHR tracing applies artificial intelligence to the FHR tracing and assists the clinician at the bedside in complex decision-making situations concerning FHR interpretation [24,25]. Several publications investigating computer analysis against the human component of visual interpretation have been favorable, demonstrating similar agreement between the computer software and the clinician [23,25,26]. Further research is needed to determine whether this technology is a valid, objective, and reliable measure in FHR interpretation that can impact perinatal and neonatal outcomes [25].

In addition to improving the quality of care through surveillance and alert capabilities, these systems provide database access for statistical reporting for administration, research, and quality purposes, especially when integrated with other hospital or outpatient information systems. This advance allows multiple data entry points across the continuum of care and serves to link care and services provided at different sites within the healthcare/hospital network [27]. For example, if a woman presents to the birthing center in the middle of the night, the staff can readily access the entire antenatal record, the ultrasound report, and antepartum fetal surveillance notes that were completed the previous afternoon, even if performed at a different facility within the system. Additionally, some systems allow clinicians to access information and review FHR using cellular phone displays (Figure 3.20).

Electronic documentation on forms and flow sheets, together with annotated tracings and automated data acquisition of information such as maternal blood pressure and pulse, result in a complete and detailed EHR. The *archiving* and *retrieval* of the original FHR tracings has proved to be a problem for most medical record departments because the process is labor-intensive and the paper is space-consuming and subject to deterioration. Microfiche records are less bulky to store but still take time to log, sort, and file in the medical record, although some facilities continue to do this. Computer-based electronic storage systems provide secure archival and retrieval options and can help prevent loss or destruction of fetal monitoring data.

The ability to have multiple points of data entry, information retrieval, and reproduction of a woman's record and fetal monitor tracing is a significant advancement. Coupled with an interface to the hospital admission, discharge, and other hospital-based information systems, it is contributing to the trend toward comprehensive, paperless, and fully electronic information systems.

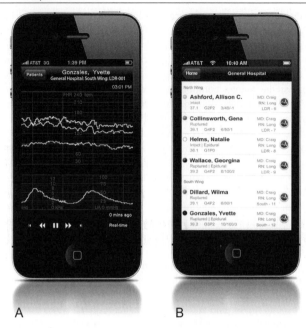

FIGURE 3.20 Providers can access near real-time FHR tracings and review patient data using their mobile phones. (A) FHR tracing, including MHR. (B) Patient listing. (Courtesy AirStrip Technologies, Inc., San Antonio, TX.)

Data-input Devices

Electronic perinatal data systems may use a variety of data-input devices, including barcode readers, keypads for data entry, light pens (Figure 3.21), touch screens, remote event markers, and standard computer keyboards. The input is subsequently printed on the tracing (Figure 3.22). The use of these options can promote accurate documentation and help eliminate the need for handwritten annotations, which are sometimes illegible. Additionally, ongoing information important to documentation such as the time, date, paper speed, and signal source is routinely entered on the monitor strip automatically. For more on documentation and health information technology, see Chapter 10.

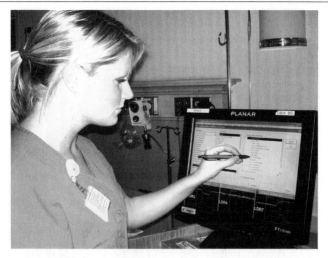

FIGURE 3.21 Data entry using drop-down menus and pen stylus for documentation directly on computer screen. (Courtesy OBIX Perinatal System, Clinical Computer Systems, Inc., Elgin, IL.)

INTEGRATED ABDOMINAL FETAL HEART RATE AND UTERINE ACTIVITY MONITORING

The pursuit to improve EFM technology that is noninvasive and accurate continues to evolve. Advances in the abdominal fetal ECG in the 1970s, followed by improved Doppler technology soon made Doppler ultrasound the standard external monitoring choice in the 1980s. Subsequently this has remained the norm in the United States. However, as discussed earlier, Doppler technology continues to suffer from reliability problems, for two principal reasons: the separation of the FHR from the MHR and the loss of signal during maternal position changes or fetal movement. Clinicians now have other solutions to the drawbacks of standard EFM. Integrated systems that incorporate MECG, FECG, and uterine electromyography (EMG) into one piece of technology are now becoming increasingly popular, especially in the obese population [27–31]. These systems provide an external monitoring solution that uses abdominally obtained electrical impulses to monitor FHR and UA. Most importantly, these

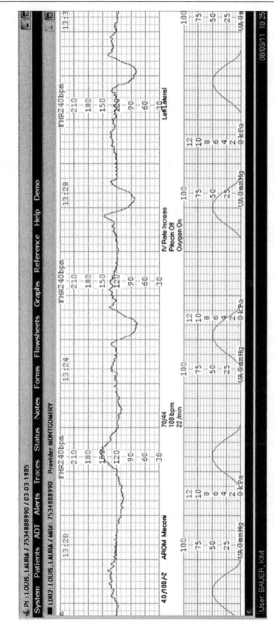

FIGURE 3.22 Documentation data is printed on monitor tracing. (Courtesy OBIX Perinatal System, Clinical Computer Systems, Inc., Elgin, IL.)

systems do not replace the need for traditional internal FHR or UA monitoring when clinically indicated.

Electrodes are placed on the pregnant abdomen to directly monitor the MHR, FHR and the EMG from the uterine muscle (Figure 3.23). Data is extracted within the device and transmitted wirelessly, via Bluetooth technology, to an interface device that allows data from the MHR, FHR, and UA to print or display on a standard commercial fetal monitor and central display [32,33].

More precisely, these devices simultaneously monitor the electrophysiologic signals on separate channels spanning the abdomen, following fetal movement changes and using a sophisticated method to uniquely identify the maternal ECG and subtract it from the signal leaving only the fetal ECG complex [27,34]. This eliminates much of the problem with fetal movement and signal interruption as well as maternal–fetal signal coincidence. Additionally, adipose tissue has less of an effect on the electrical signals monitored on the abdomen than it does on the transmission of ultrasound, so there is less signal loss in women with elevated body mass indices [28,35].

The uterine activity is a reflection of the EMG, which is electrical activity produced by uterine muscle [27]. EMG data allows increased accuracy related to frequency, occurrence of peak, and duration over traditional pressure-sensitive tocotransducers but does not provide actual intensity measurement in mm Hg as with an IUPC. Although

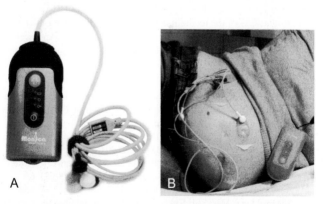

FIGURE 3.23 (A) Monica AN24 is a wireless and beltless device that can be used with existing monitors to obtain FHR via abdominal ECG. (B) Electrodes placed on maternal abdomen monitor ECG from fetal and maternal heart and the electromyogram (EMG) from the uterine muscle. (Courtesy Monica Healthcare Ltd, Nottingham, UK.)

clinicians will continue to assess contraction strength and uterine resting tone using palpation, these devices eliminate the need for belts and frequent tocotransducer readjustments common in traditional monitoring. The wireless capabilities provide similar range to those seen with cell phone Bluetooth headsets, providing patient mobility of approximately 50 feet (15 meters) from the base, allowing for a variety of maternal activities during labor.

Benefits of the abdominal fetal ECG and EMG approach include improved signal quality, elimination of maternal–fetal signal coincidence, and maternal mobility and comfort; however, the method cannot be used during hydrotherapy or water birth. Although availability of the fetal ECG noninvasively is a clear benefit, there are some fetuses that generate a poor fetal ECG as measured on the abdomen and cannot be monitored with this technology. Additionally, individual manufacturers have specific restrictions, so refer to the manufacturer's guidelines for further guidance.

SUMMARY

A variety of methods exist to safely accomplish fetal monitoring, ranging from simple auscultation and palpation to internal electronic monitoring using analysis with computerized programs. The obstetric team includes the woman and her support system. A discussion of available monitoring options, as well as patient education regarding the selection of methodology, is an important part of collaborative care. Regardless of the technique chosen, clinicians must understand the proper application, care, and use of related equipment, as well as the benefits, limitations, and specific patient selection criteria.

References

[1] American College of Nurse-Midwives, Intermittent auscultation for intrapartum fetal heart rate surveillance. ACNM Ciinical Bulletin Number 13., J. Midwifery Womens Health 60 (2015) 626–632.

[2] N.F. Feinstein, A. Sprague, M.J. Trepanier, Fetal Heart Rate Auscultation, second ed., AWHONN, Washington, DC, 2008.

[3] L. Goodwin, Intermittent auscultation of the fetal heart rate: a review of general principles, J. Perinat. Neonatal Nurs. 14 (3) (2000) 53–61.

[4] American College of Obstetricians and Gynecologists, Society for Maternal-Fetal Medicine, Safe prevention of the primary cesarean delivery: obstetric care consensus, Am. J. Obstet. Gynecol. 210 (3) (2014) 179–193.

[5] M.M. Killion, Techniques for fetal heart and uterine activity assessment, in: A. Lyndon, A.L. Usher (Eds.), Fetal Heart Monitoring Principles and Practices, fifth ed., AWHONN, Washington, DC, 2015.

[6] K. Wisner, D. Gauthier, Maternal-fetal assessment, in: A. Lyndon, L. Usher Ali (Eds.), Fetal Heart Monitoring Principles and Practices, fifth ed., AWHONN, Washington, DC, 2015.

[7] American College of Obstetricians and Gynecologists, Intrapartum fetal heart rate monitoring: nomenclature, interpretation, and general management principles. Practice Bulletin no. 106, Obstet. Gynecol. 114 (2009) 192–202.

[8] Association of Women's Health, Obstetric and Neonatal Nurses, Fetal heart monitoring. AWHONN Position Statement, J. Obstet. Gynecol. Neonatal Nurs. 44 (5) (2015) 683–686.

[9] American Academy of Pediatrics, American College of Obstetricians and Gynecologists: Guidelines for Perinatal Care, seventh ed., AAP, ACOG, Washington, DC, 2012.

[10] Documentation of fetal heart monitoring information, in: K. Wisner, L. Usher Ali (Eds.), Fetal Heart Monitoring Principles and Practices, fifth ed., AWHONN, Washington, DC, 2015.

[11] G.A. Macones, G.D. Hankins, C.Y. Spong, et al., The 2008 National Institute of Child Health and Human Development workshop report on electronic fetal monitoring: update on definitions, interpretation, and research guidelines, Obstet. Gynecol. 112 (3) (2008) 661–666.

[12] N.A. Bowers, K.K. Gromada, Care of the Multiple Birth Family: Pregnancy and Birth (Nursing Module), March of Dimes Foundation, White Plains, NY, 2006.

[13] J.T. Parer, Handbook of Fetal Heart Rate Monitoring, second ed., WB Saunders, Philadelphia, PA, 1997.

[14] D.R. Neilson, R.K. Freeman, S. Mangan, Signal ambiguity resulting in unexpected outcome with external fetal heart rate monitoring, Am. J. Obstet. Gynecol. 198 (6) (2008) 717–724.

[15] D.J. Sherman, E. Frenkel, Y. Kurzweil, A. Padua, S. Arieli, M. Bahar, Characteristics of maternal heart rate patterns during labor and delivery, Obstet. Gynecol. 99 (4) (2002) 542–547.

[16] V. Equy, S. Buisson, M. Heinen, J.P. Schaal, P. Hoffmann, F. Sergent, Confusion between maternal and fetal heart rate during the second stage of labour, Br. J. Midwifery 20 (11) (2012) 794–798.

[17] L. Hanson, Risk management in intrapartum fetal monitoring: accidental recording of the maternal heart rate, J. Perinat. Neonatal Nurs. 24 (1) (2010) 7–9.

[18] S. Paquette, F. Moretti, K. O'Reilly, Z.M. Ferraro, L. Oppenheimer, The incidence of maternal artefact during intrapartum fetal heart rate monitoring, J. Obstet. Gynaecol. Can. 36 (11) (2014) 962–968.

[19] T.R. Van Veen, M.A. Belfort, S. Kofford, Maternal heart rate patterns in the first and second stages of labor, Acta Obstet. Gynecol. Scand. 91 (5) (2012) 598–604.

[20] S.K. Hasley, Decision support and patient safety: the time has come, Am. J. Obstet. Gynecol. 204 (6) (2011) 461–465.

[21] P.R. McCartney, Computer fetal heart rate pattern analysis, MCN Am. J. Matern. Child Nurs. 36 (6) (2011) 397.

[22] S. Smith, J. Zacharias, V. Lucas, P.A. Warrick, E.F. Hamilton, Clinical associations with uterine tachysystole, J. Matern. Fetal Neonatal Med. 27 (7) (2014) 709–713.

[23] J.T. Parer, E.F. Hamilton, Comparison of 5 experts and computer analysis in rule-based fetal heart rate interpretation, Am. J. Obstet. Gynecol. 203 (5) (2010) 451.e1–451.e7.

[24] J.E. Lutomski, S. Meaney, R.A. Greene, A.C. Ryan, D. Devane, Expert systems for fetal assessment in labour. Cochrane Database Syst. Rev. (4) (2015) http://dx.doi.org/10.1002/14651858.CD010708.pub2 CD010708.

[25] I. Nunes, D. Ayres-de-Campos, C. Figueiredo, J. Bernardes, An overview of central fetal monitoring systems in labour, J. Perinat. Med. 41 (1) (2013) 93–99.

[26] S. Weiner, 753: Independent validation of a fetal heart rate pattern recognition software, Am. J. Obstet. Gynecol. 1 (208) (2013) S316–S317.

[27] B.C. Jacob, E.M. Graatsma, E. Van Hagen, G.H. Visser, A validation of electrohysterography for uterine activity monitoring during labour, J. Matern. Fetal Neonatal Med. 23 (1) (2010) 17–22.

[28] W.R. Cohen, B. Hayes-Gill, Influence of maternal body mass index on accuracy and reliability of external fetal monitoring techniques, Acta Obstet. Gynecol. Scand. 93 (6) (2014) 590–595.

[29] W.R. Cohen, S. Ommani, S. Hassan, et al., Accuracy and reliability of fetal heart rate monitoring using maternal abdominal surface electrodes, Acta Obstet. Gynecol. Scand. 91 (11) (2012) 1306–1313.

[30] J. Reinhard, B.R. Hayes-Gill, Q. Yi, H. Hatzmann, S. Schiermeier, Comparison of non-invasive fetal electrocardiogram to Doppler cardiotocogram during the 1st stage of labor, J. Perinat. Med. 38 (2) (2010) 179–185.

[31] J. Reinhard, B.R. Hayes-Gill, S. Schiermeier, W. Hatzmann, E. Herrmann, T.M. Heinrich, F. Louwen, Intrapartum signal quality with external fetal heart rate monitoring: a two way trial of external Doppler CTG ultrasound and the abdominal fetal electrocardiogram, Arch. Gynecol. Obstet. 286 (5) (2012) 1103–1107.

[32] LaborView Sensor System Products and Technology, OB Medical Systems, Available from: http://www.obmedco.com/products.html, 2015 (accessed 24.06.15).

[33] Monica AN24with IF24, Monica Healthcare. Available from: http://www.monicahealthcare.com/products/labour-and-delivery/monica-an24-with-if24 (accessed 22.06.15).

[34] E.M. Graatsma, B. Jacod, L. van Egmond, et al., Fetal electrocardiography: feasibility of long-term fetal heart rate recordings, BJOG 116 (2009) 334–338.

[35] E.M. Graatsma, J. Miller, E.J. Mulder, C. Harman, A.A. Baschat, G.H. Visser, Maternal body mass index does not affect performance of fetal electrocardiography, Am. J. Perinatol. 27 (7) (2010) 573–577.

CHAPTER 4

Uterine Activity Evaluation and Management

F etal oxygenation and acid–base status can be adversely affected by excessive uterine activity [1–6], making the assessment of uterine activity a key priority for all clinicians. Prompt response and intervention for excessive uterine activity as well as *physiologic support of normal uterine activity* in the different phases and stages of labor must be common skills for nurses, physicians, and midwives. The evaluation of uterine activity in labor, including defining clinical parameters for both normal and excessive uterine activity, is the primary focus of this chapter. Additionally, newer parameters for the diagnosis and management of abnormal labor patterns are reviewed, along with specific issues regarding the use of oxytocin.

ASSESSMENT METHODS: PALPATION AND ELECTRONIC MONITORING

Uterine activity may be assessed by manual palpation or by electronic monitoring with either an external tocotransducer or an internal intrauterine pressure catheter (IUPC). A complete assessment of uterine activity includes the identification of contraction frequency, duration, strength or intensity, and resting tone. Differences in the accuracy of uterine activity evaluation are illustrated in Figure 4.1.

Manual Palpation

Manual palpation is the traditional method of monitoring contractions. This method can measure contraction frequency, duration, and relative strength. Palpation is a learned skill that is best performed with the fingertips to feel the uterus rise upward as the contraction develops. *Mild, moderate,* and *strong* are the terms used to describe the strength of uterine contractions as determined by the examiner's hands during palpation and based on the degree of indentation of the abdomen [7,8]. For learning and for the purpose of comparison, the

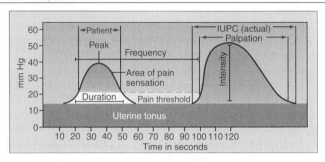

FIGURE 4.1 Comparison of relative sensitivities of assessing uterine contractions by internal monitoring (IUPC), manual palpation, and patient perception. Note that the woman does not usually perceive the contraction until the uterine pressure increases above the baseline uterine tonus. External monitor is variable. (Modified from E.J. Dickason, B.L. Silverman, J.A. Kaplan, Maternal-Infant Nursing Care, third ed., Mosby, St. Louis, MO, 1998.)

degree of indentation corresponds to the palpation sensation when feeling the parts of the adult face, as described in the following chart:

Contraction Strength	Palpation Sensation
Mild	Tense fundus but easy to indent (feels like touching finger to tip of nose)
Moderate	Firm fundus, difficult to indent with fingertips (feels like touching finger to chin)
Strong	Rigid, board-like fundus, almost impossible to indent (feels like touching finger to forehead)

Palpation of uterine activity is an important clinical skill that is used concomitantly with external electronic monitoring and as an adjunct for confirmation of uterine activity during internal electronic monitoring. With the addition of electromyography (EMG) for abdominal fetal monitoring (see Chapter 3), the need for palpation is significant because EMG signals may result in the appearance of excessive uterine activity due to increased sensitivity.

Electronic Monitoring of Uterine Activity

External uterine activity monitoring is typically achieved using a tocotransducer (to provide information about uterine contraction frequency and duration) combined with manual palpation (to evaluate relative strength). Abdominal fetal electrocardiogram (FECG) and EMG are other methods of external electronic fetal monitoring. Both methods provide continuous data and a permanent record of uterine activity. The electronic display of a contraction, when using a tocodynamometer, depends on the depression of a pressure-sensing device placed on the maternal abdomen. Factors such as placement of the transducer, belt tightness, and maternal adipose tissue result in variations of depression and will affect the graphic representation on the fetal heart rate (FHR) tracing (Figure 4.2). Thus the contractions may appear stronger (or less strong) than they truly are, making it imperative to assess strength of the uterine contraction by manual palpation when uterine activity is externally monitored.

Internal uterine activity monitoring uses an intrauterine pressure catheter (IUPC) that measures actual intrauterine pressure in millimeters of mercury (mm Hg) during both contractile and acontractile (resting) periods. As demonstrated in Figure 4.1, the intrauterine pressure catheter allows clinicians to evaluate the frequency, duration, and strength of contractions in mm Hg with improved accuracy. The following chart contrasts the data obtained with these external versus internal modes of monitoring:

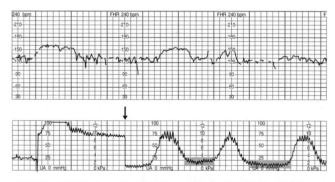

FIGURE 4.2 Adjustment of tocotransducer (arrow) to correct displacement following maternal position change. Note the tocotransducer picking up maternal breathing movements on the lower uterine activity panel as evidenced by jagged lines (highlighted). *BPM*, beats per minute. (Courtesy Lisa A. Miller, CNM, JD.)

External Mode—Tocotransducer or Abdominal EMG	Internal Mode—Intrauterine Pressure Catheter (IUPC)
Frequency of Contractions	
Measured from the onset of one contraction to the onset of the next contraction	Measured from the onset of one contraction to the onset of the next contraction
Duration of Contractions	
Measured from contraction onset to offset	Measured from contraction onset to offset
Strength/Intensity of Contractions	
The abdomen must be palpated to assess the strength of the contraction based on the degree of indentation of the fundus. The more difficult it is to indent the fundus during palpation, the stronger the contraction. *Strength* of contractions using a toco is usually documented as *mild, moderate,* or *strong* to palpation. The tracing produced using external methods will reflect contraction strength *relative* to other contractions, i.e., stronger contractions will generally produce higher waveforms.	Intrauterine pressure is measured directly and recorded on the tracing in mm Hg. *Strength* is usually documented as the numerical value at the peak of the contraction—e.g., 50 mm Hg, 70 mm Hg, etc. *Intensity* of contractions is technically a term used to identify the peak of the contraction less the resting tone, expressed in mm Hg. In clinical practice, the terms *strength* and *intensity* are often used interchangeably; it is important that whichever term is used, it is defined and used consistently.
Resting Tone	
The abdomen must be palpated to assess resting tone based on whether the fundus palpates as soft or firm (rigid). During periods of palpated resting tone the external monitor is generally set/reset to a level of 10 on the uterine activity portion of the fetal monitoring tracing.	Resting tone is measured directly and reflected on the tracing based on the intrauterine pressure in mm Hg. Resting tone is recorded as the numerical value when the uterus is completely relaxed (acontractile)—e.g., 10 mm Hg, 15 mm Hg, etc.

Electronic Display of Uterine Activity

Uterine activity is monitored and recorded on the lower section of the monitor strip (Figure 4.3). The range of the scale is from 0 to 100 mm Hg. There are five major vertical divisions of 20 mm Hg each, divided again into minor vertical representations of 10 mm Hg each. Some tracing paper manufactured in North America has four

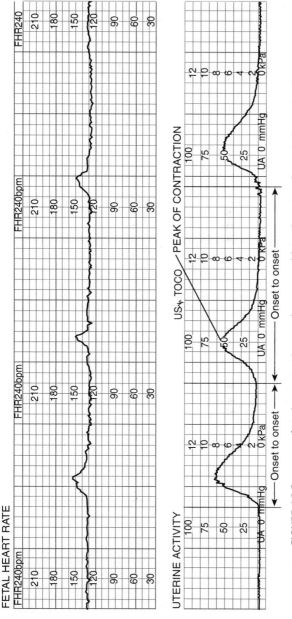

FIGURE 4.3 Frequency of uterine contractions can be measured from the onset of one uterine contraction to the onset of the next. Note other identifying information. (Courtesy Lisa A. Miller, CNM, JD.)

major vertical sections of 25 mm Hg each, with the smaller divisions representing 5 mm Hg pressure in the uterine activity section. For further information on instrumentation, please refer to Chapter 3.

REDEFINING NORMAL LABOR

New data regarding the assessment of normal labor [9] indicate that current labor patterns are different from those reported by Friedman in the 1950s [10,11]. This has led to the development of partograms (labor progress graphs) that reveal significantly slower curves, and a later onset of active labor, with a median closer to 6 cm dilation [12] (Figure 4.4). Regardless of these updated parameters, basic definitions for the stages of labor are unchanged. The first stage of labor begins with the onset of contractions and ends with complete dilation of the cervix. It is divided into two phases: latent and active. During the latent phase, irregular and infrequent uterine contractions are associated with gradual cervical softening, dilation, and effacement (thinning). During the active phase of labor, the rate of cervical dilation increases and the fetal presenting part descends. The second stage of labor begins with complete dilation of the cervix and ends with delivery of the fetus. Some clinicians differentiate the second stage into two phases, a passive phase (also called *rest and descend*,

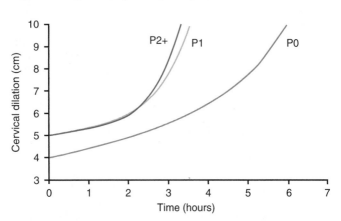

FIGURE 4.4 Average labor curves by parity in singleton term pregnancies with spontaneous onset of labor, vaginal delivery, and normal neonatal outcomes. *P0*, nulliparous women; *P1*, women of parity 1; *P2*, women of parity 2 or higher. (From J. Zhang, H.J. Landy, D. Ware Branch, et al., Contemporary patterns of spontaneous labor with normal neonatal outcomes, Obstet Gynecol 116 (2010) 1281–1287, used with permission.)

passive descent, laboring down) and an active phase, when there is spontaneous or coached pushing effort by the mother. Although a detailed review of labor management is outside the scope of this textbook, a discussion of the evaluation of uterine activity as well as labor abnormalities and oxytocin use is warranted.

DEFINING ADEQUATE UTERINE ACTIVITY

Spontaneous vaginal delivery results from the progressive dilation and effacement of the cervix and descent of the fetal presenting part, due to the work of uterine contractions. Much of the data defining the "normal" range of uterine activity was derived from the research of Caldeyro-Barcia and colleagues [13–17] in the late 1950s and the 1960s. Using intraamniotic pressure catheters, Caldeyro-Barcia and Poseiro [14] evaluated uterine activity and coined the term *Montevideo units (MVUs)* as a method of measuring uterine activity. The original formula was calculated by multiplying the average *intensity* in mm Hg (peak of contraction less resting tone) times the frequency of uterine contractions in a 10-minute period. Thus, if there are four contractions in 10 minutes with an average intensity of 40 mm Hg, the Montevideo units for that period would be 4×40, or 160 Montevideo units. Over time, it became obvious that simple *addition* of the individual contraction *intensities* over 10 minutes resulted in essentially similar numbers to the multiplication method, and since then the addition method has become common practice [7].

This early research showed that spontaneous labor began clinically when MVUs rose to between 80 and 120, with contraction strength needing to reach at least 40 mm Hg [14,15]. This would equate to two to three contractions with intensities of 40 mm Hg or more every 10 minutes for the initiation of labor. In normal labor, contractions increase in intensity and frequency as labor progresses through the first stage and into the second stage. Caldeyro-Barcia and colleagues [14–16] found that uterine activity in the first stage of normal labors generally ranged between 100 and 250 MVUs, with contractions increasing in intensity from 25 to 50 mm Hg and in frequency from three to five over 10 minutes. In the second stage, MVUs can rise to 300 to 400 [1,13–17] as contraction intensities may increase to 80 mm Hg or more and five or six contractions may be seen every 10 minutes.

Baseline uterine tone, also known as *resting tone,* averages 10 mm Hg during labor, rising from 8 to 12 mm Hg from the beginning of the first stage to the onset of the second stage. Resting tone is assessed during the time between contractions, known as *relaxation time.* Relaxation times are generally longer (60 seconds or more) in first stage labor and tend to shorten (45–60 seconds) during second stage.

Contraction duration of 60 to 80 seconds remains relatively stable from active-phase labor through the second stage [18]. These findings provide a basis for logical definitions of "adequate" uterine activity when using internal pressure catheters for assessment of uterine contractions.

Caldeyro-Barcia and Poseiro also provided crucial information related to contraction assessment when using palpation, or palpation and a tocotransducer. They found that until the intensity (peak less baseline tonus) reaches 40 mm Hg, the wall of the uterus is easily indented by palpation [15]. This correlates well with the premise that uterine contractions that palpate as moderate or stronger are likely to have peaks of 50 mm Hg or greater if they are measured by internal means, whereas palpated contractions identified as mild are likely to have peaks of less than 50 mm Hg if measured internally. These findings offer guidance for clinicians in identifying reasonable definitions of "adequate" uterine activity when using palpation (with or without a tocotransducer) for assessment of uterine contractions. Box 4.1 provides a summary of normal parameters of uterine activity in labor, and Figure 4.5 illustrates a variety of common uterine contraction patterns in normal labor.

BOX 4.1 Components of Uterine Activity during Labor

Frequency	Contraction frequency overall generally ranges from 2–5 per 10 minutes during labor, with lower frequencies seen in the first stage of labor and higher frequencies seen during the second stage of labor.
Duration	Contraction duration remains fairly stable throughout first and second stages, ranging from 45–80 seconds, not generally exceeding 90 seconds.
Strength	Uterine contractions generally range from peaking at 40–70 mm Hg in first stage of labor and may rise to over 80 mm Hg in second stage. Contractions palpated as "mild" would likely peak at <50 mm Hg if measured internally, and contractions palpated as "moderate" or greater would likely peak at 50 mm Hg or greater if measured internally.
Resting tone	Average resting tone during labor is 10 mm Hg; if using palpation, should palpate as "soft," i.e., easily indented, no palpable resistance.
Relaxation time	Relaxation time is commonly 60 seconds or more in first stage and 45 seconds or more in second stage.
Montevideo units (MVUs)	Usually range from 100 to 250 MVUs in first stage, may rise to 300–400 in second stage. Contraction intensities of ≥40 mm Hg and MVUs of 80–120 are generally sufficient to initiate spontaneous labor.

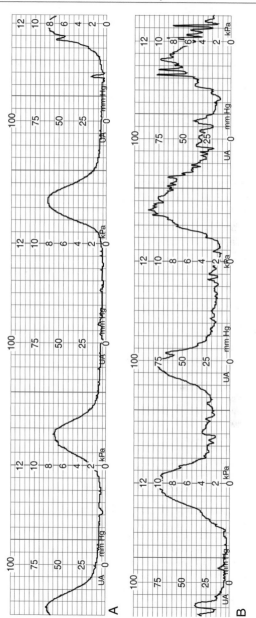

FIGURE 4.5 Examples of normal uterine activity during labor. (A) Normal contraction pattern in latent phase labor. (B) Normal contraction pattern in active-phase labor; note that contractions are more frequent but there is still adequate relaxation time.

Continued

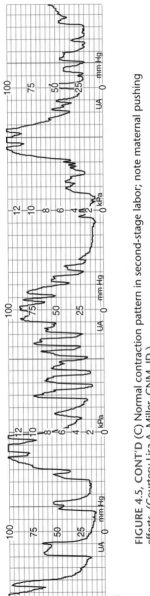

FIGURE 4.5, CONT'D (C) Normal contraction pattern in second-stage labor; note maternal pushing efforts. (Courtesy Lisa A. Miller, CNM, JD.)

In summary, applying what is known about parameters of uterine activity during normal labor:

1. allows clinicians to promote and support adequate and effective uterine activity during the different phases and stages of labor, influencing management decisions when abnormal or dysfunctional labor is diagnosed;
2. forms a basis for the safe and proper use of labor stimulants; and
3. provides a basis upon which to define excessive uterine activity by professional consensus.

DEFINING EXCESSIVE UTERINE ACTIVITY

In 2008, the National Institute of Child Health and Human Development (NICHD) issued a workshop report on fetal monitoring that included summary terms for uterine activity [19]. Prior to this report, the lack of sound, standardized definitions for uterine activity hindered both effective communication and the development of consensus-based multidisciplinary guidelines. The summary terms suggested by the NICHD are for the classification of uterine activity using *frequency of contractions averaged over a thirty-minute period* [19,20]:

Normal: less than or equal to five contractions in 10 minutes

Tachysystole: greater than five contractions in 10 minutes

Tachysystole is to be further qualified by the presence or absence of FHR decelerations and applies to spontaneous as well as stimulated labors. The workshop report stresses the *importance of other parameters* such as *duration, intensity,* and *relaxation time* in the evaluation of uterine activity, specifically stating that "frequency alone is a partial assessment of uterine activity" [19]. The report also suggests abandonment of previously used summary terms *hyperstimulation* and *hypercontractility*. Although the NICHD workshop report is clearly important progress toward the standardization of terminology, standardized terminology alone does not provide clinicians with sufficient guidance for the safe and effective management of uterine activity in labor. Tachysystole is a fairly common event and has been linked to an increase in composite neonatal morbidity [3]. Clinicians must be familiar with the normal physiology of uterine activity (described previously) as well as the relationship between excessive uterine activity and fetal acid–base status.

Excessive uterine activity has long been linked to untoward effects on FHR [2,21]. Peebles [4] noted decreased fetal cerebral oxygen saturation with shorter contraction intervals. Bakker and colleagues [1] found that fetal acidemia (umbilical artery pH ≤7.11) of all types (respiratory, metabolic, and mixed) was more prevalent in patients with excessive uterine activity during labor, both first and second stage. Specifically, a first-stage average MVU value of 261 and relaxation time of 51 seconds was noted in the acidemic group, versus average MVU value of 236 and relaxation time of 63 seconds in the nonacidemic group. In second stage, an average MVU value of 442 and relaxation time of 36 seconds were noted in the acidemic group, versus average MVU value of 402 and relaxation time of 47 seconds in the nonacidemic group [1]. Logic would therefore dictate that *avoiding* MVUs exceeding the previously discussed norm of 250 in the first stage of labor and 300 to 400 in the second stage could *decrease* the incidence of significant fetal acidemia at birth. Furthermore, in cases of external monitoring or any situation in which MVU evaluation is not feasible, *ensuring* adequate relaxation times of 60 seconds or more in first stage and 45 seconds or more in second stage could also prevent fetal acidemia at birth.

In addition to evaluating frequency, strength, and relaxation time, it is important to understand that for the fetus to be able to maintain oxygenation, *resting tone* must also be normal. *Hypertonus,* or elevated resting tone is most commonly defined as uterine resting tone greater than 20 to 25 mm Hg, or a uterus that does not return to soft if using palpation. The information in Box 4.2 can be used by clinicians and multidisciplinary committees to reach consensus on definitions for terms related to uterine activity as well as evidence-based guidelines for management of all types of excessive uterine activity. This information should serve as the starting point for the development of clear, physiologically sound, and clinically useful approaches to excessive uterine activity that include *all parameters* of uterine activity, versus focusing on frequency (tachysystole) alone.

Some clinicians contend that the management of excessive uterine activity should be based upon the presence or absence of FHR changes. This approach conflicts with what limited evidence exists regarding uterine activity and fetal oxygenation. Bakker and colleagues [1] found no difference in the occurrence of late decelerations between the acidemic and nonacidemic fetuses, suggesting that the key to avoiding acidemia is not dependent on the appearance of FHR changes but rather the presence of excessive uterine activity itself. Simpson and James [5] found that in the first stage of labor,

---

BOX 4.2   Evaluation of Uterine Activity during Labor

Preliminary Assumptions

- Normal uterine activity in first-stage labor generally does not exceed 250 MVUs
- Normal uterine activity in second-stage labor should not exceed 400 MVUs
- Normal contraction duration generally ranges from 45–90 seconds
- Normal contraction intensity (peak less resting tone) generally ranges from 25–80 mm Hg, with higher intensities common as labor progresses
- Normal uterine resting tone ranges from 8–12 mm Hg and is generally not greater than 20–25 mm Hg
- Fetal acid–base status can be affected by excessive uterine activity *before* evidenced by fetal heart rate changes

Excessive Uterine Activity

All definitions for excessive uterine activity apply to both spontaneous and/or stimulated labor; management of excessive uterine activity should be based on clinical context

- Tachysystole

Contraction frequency of greater than 5 in 10 minutes, averaged over 30 minutes; applies to spontaneous or stimulated labor

- Hypertonus

Uterine resting tone exceeding 20–25 mm Hg with an intrauterine pressure catheter or a uterus that does not return to soft by palpation during relaxation time

- Inadequate Relaxation Time

Less than 60 seconds' uterine relaxation between contractions during the first stage of labor; less than 45–50 seconds' uterine relaxation between contractions in second stage

- Excessive Contraction Duration (also known as *tetanic contractions* or *uterine tetany*)

A series of single contractions lasting 2 minutes or more

Data from references 1, 2, 4, 6, 7, 13–18, 22–26.

even five uterine contractions in 10 minutes ("normal" uterine activity by definition) over a 30-minute period resulted in a 20% decrease in fetal oxygen saturation as measured by fetal pulse oximetry. Both these studies make it clear that premising the management of uterine activity on frequency alone or basing the management of excessive uterine activity on FHR changes may lead to less than optimal fetal oxygenation and potentially the deterioration of fetal acid–base. *Waiting to respond to excessive uterine activity until there are significant changes in FHR is not appropriate.* Rather, to prevent fetal acidemia at birth, clinicians should focus on *identifying and promoting normal (adequate) uterine activity* and correcting underlying causes of any type of excessive uterine activity (Figure 4.6).

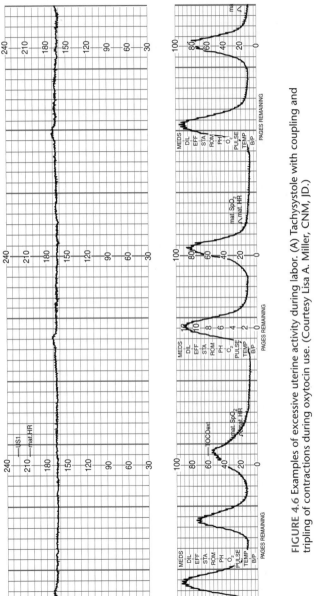

FIGURE 4.6 Examples of excessive uterine activity during labor. (A) Tachysystole with coupling and tripling of contractions during oxytocin use. (Courtesy Lisa A. Miller, CNM, JD.)

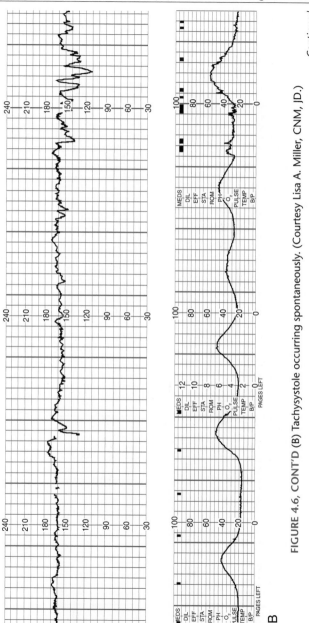

Continued

FIGURE 4.6, CONT'D (B) Tachysystole occurring spontaneously. (Courtesy Lisa A. Miller, CNM, JD.)

B

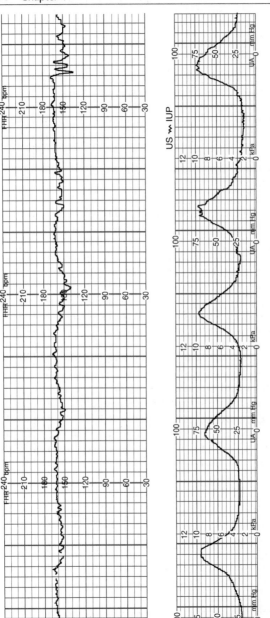

FIGURE 4.6, CONT'D (C) Normal frequency of uterine contractions but inadequate relaxation time between contractions for first-stage labor. Recommended relaxation time in first stage is 60 seconds; note possible FHR decelerations. (Courtesy Lisa A. Miller, CNM, JD.)

Common Underlying Causes of Excessive Uterine Activity

- Use of pharmacologic cervical ripening agents
- Use of synthetic oxytocin for augmentation or induction (more common with high-dose, high-frequency administration protocols)
- Abruptio placentae
- Uterine overdistention, whether iatrogenic from amnioinfusion or as a result of multiple gestation, hydramnios, or macrosomia

Interventions to Decrease Excessive Uterine Activity

1. Change maternal position to lateral side-lying.
2. Administer a bolus of intravenous (IV) fluids and/or increase the maintenance IV rate.
3. Remove cervical ripening agents or, in the case of oxytocin usage, decrease or discontinue the infusion.
4. If excessive uterine activity related to the use of cervical ripening agents or oxytocin administration is noted in association with FHR changes indicative of hypoxemia, clinicians may consider the use of a tocolytic [27].

These interventions are *specific to excessive uterine activity.* Note that the management of FHR patterns is addressed in detail in Chapter 6. It is imperative that clinicians respond appropriately to FHR changes regardless of the nature of uterine activity because uterine activity is only one of several causes of interrupted fetal oxygenation. However, FHR changes should not be a prerequisite for clinical response to excessive uterine activity. It cannot be overemphasized: Excessive uterine activity should trigger clinician response *whether or not FHR changes are observed.*

NEW TRENDS IN LABOR SUPPORT AND MANAGEMENT

With the recognition of differences in contemporary labor progression, professional organizations are working collaboratively to enhance the clinician's knowledge regarding normal labor and to provide new parameters for the approach to labor management, including recognition of the importance of individualization and shared decision making [9]. Labor abnormalities have been described historically using a variety of expressions, such as *slow progress in labor, failure to progress, dystocia, dysfunctional labor,* or *cephalopelvic disproportion* [28]. Up to 68% of unanticipated cesarean deliveries in patients with vertex presentation are reported to be due to dystocia, and given the number of repeat cesarean deliveries that follow a primary cesarean for dystocia, the diagnosis of dystocia may account for as many as 60% of all cesarean births [28].

A number of strategies have been shown to decrease the risk of dystocia. These include [28–30]:

- Avoidance of elective induction with an unripe cervix
- Avoidance of hospital admission during latent phase labor
- Upright maternal position
- Provision of continuous labor support (the "doula effect")
- Adequate maternal hydration
- Judicious use of epidural anesthesia

Because fetal monitoring includes the evaluation of the adequacy of uterine activity as well as the progress of labor, a brief overview of different labor abnormalities and possible management strategies is warranted. A clear understanding of labor progress can be helpful when interdisciplinary discussions arise regarding management of uterine activity, especially discussions regarding the utilization of oxytocin, the most common treatment for dystocia.

Latent Phase Abnormalities

Labor onset is defined as effacement and dilation of the cervix caused by regular uterine contractions. The latent phase of labor begins with the onset of labor (regular contractions, cervical change) and ends at the beginning of the active phase of first stage [28]. Latent phase is considered prolonged if it is >20 hours in nulliparous patients and >14 hours in multiparous patients [28]. Contrary to what may be seen in clinical practice, both the American College of Obstetricians and Gynecologists (ACOG) and the Society for Maternal-Fetal Medicine (SMFM) do not recommend cesarean delivery for either slow progress in latent phase or a prolonged latent phase, noting that most women will enter active phase with expectant management [9]. Considerations for the management of prolonged latent phase labor are listed next.

Management Strategies for Latent Phase Disorders[1]

1. Avoid admission to the labor unit in latent phase labor. Unless otherwise indicated, admit only if the cervix is >3 cm dilated or 100% effaced. Educate patients antenatally about the benefits of this approach, and provide instructions for comfort measures while laboring at home.
2. Assess the woman's level of fatigue, and provide appropriate labor support.
3. Encourage adequate fluid intake and small, frequent meals while the mother is at home.
4. Set specific intervals to reevaluate status, even if symptoms remain unchanged.
5. Encourage ambulation to provide comfort and increase tolerance to latent phase labor.
6. Provide adequate time for latent phase labor to progress during induction of labor. This may mean up to 18 to 20 hours of adequate uterine activity in nulliparous women.
7. Diagnose prolonged latent phase only after the presence of adequate uterine activity for >20 hours in nulliparas and >14 hours in multiparas. Use of oxytocin and/or amniotomy should be considered as opposed to cesarean delivery.
8. Unless medically indicated, avoid induction of labor, especially in the nulliparous patient with an unfavorable cervix.
9. If induction is medically indicated, evaluate patients for appropriate methods of cervical ripening.

Active-Phase Abnormalities

There are three main categories of active-phase labor abnormalities:
1. *Protraction disorders:* a slow rate of cervical dilation, defined as less than the fifth percentile statistically
2. *Arrest disorders:* where labor progresses normally initially in active phase, then stops, for a period of at least 2 hours
3. *Combined disorders:* where slow progress precedes arrest [28]

ACOG recommends that oxytocin augmentation be considered for these disorders [9]. Although traditionally the diagnosis of an arrest disorder required 2 hours without cervical change in the presence of a uterine contraction pattern that exceeded

---

[1]Adapted from references 9, 28, 29, 31–34.

200 MVUs, studies [30,35,36] now suggest that 4 hours of uterine activity exceeding 200 MVUs (or 6 hours if the average uterine activity pattern was <200 MVUs) will result in up to a 92% vaginal delivery rate with no increased risk to the newborn. The suggested management approaches for active-phase disorders are listed next.

Management Strategies for Active-Phase Disorders[2]

1. Ensure that cervix is dilated at least to 6 cm before diagnosing the active phase of labor.
2. Utilize standardized oxytocin titration to achieve adequate uterine activity while avoiding tachysystole.
3. Consider an increase in the amount of hourly IV fluids to improve uterine muscle performance.
4. Consider use of an IUPC to document adequacy of contractions; a minimum of 200 MVUs is required.
5. Consider amniotomy if membranes are intact.
6. Limit active management of labor to nulliparous patients with singleton, cephalic presentations.
7. Require a diagnosis of active-phase arrest as follows: no cervical change after at least 4 hours of adequate uterine activity or 6 hours of oxytocin administration with inadequate uterine activity.
8. Provide continuous labor support.

Second-Stage Abnormalities

Arrest of descent, failure of the fetus to rotate and descend, is the labor abnormality associated with the second stage. ACOG and SMFM now state that before confirming an arrest diagnosis in second stage, there should be at least 2 hours of active pushing in multiparous women and at least 3 hours of active pushing in the nullipara [9]. They also note that longer durations may be appropriate based on individual clinical factors. Contrary to some clinicians' practices, these time frames are not mandates for cesarean delivery but rather parameters for guiding assessment and intervention. Prolonged second stage should trigger clinical reevaluation of the three Ps: powers, passenger, and passage. Evaluation of adequacy of uterine contractions, fetal position, and pelvic diameters may provide direction regarding interventions to facilitate rotation and descent.

---

[2]Adapted from references 9, 12, 21, 22, 26, 30, 32, 35–40.

UTERINE ACTIVITY AND OXYTOCIN USE

Oxytocin, a frequent treatment choice for labor abnormalities, has been designated a high-alert medication [41], and the Association of Women's Health, Obstetric and Neonatal Nurses has published new staffing recommendations for 1:1 nursing care during intrapartum oxytocin administration [42]. Sadly, disagreements related to oxytocin management continue to be a source of conflict between nurses and physicians [34], and allegations related to oxytocin management are common in litigation [43]. There are many sound, evidence-based protocols for the administration of oxytocin, ranging from high-dose, high-frequency to low-dose, low-frequency and hybrids that combine aspects of both regimens. Because oxytocin usage can result in excessive uterine activity it is important to closely and accurately monitor uterine activity when administering oxytocin.

Several studies [38–40,44] regarding the pharmacologic characteristics of oxytocin use in relation to dysfunctional labor and dystocia show that 40 minutes are needed to achieve maximum dose level. Regarding oxytocin pharmacokinetics, reviews by Arias [45] and Sanchez Ramos [37] concluded that lower doses and less frequent increases of oxytocin are preferable because they allow time for a more physiologic approach and avoid the risk of tachysystole associated with higher doses and shorter dosing intervals. Simpson and Creehan [25,26] suggest starting doses of 0.5 to 2 mU/min with increases every 30 to 60 minutes of 1 to 2 mU/min. This approach is in keeping with one of the primary tenets of pharmacology, which is *use the lowest amount of drug needed to achieve the desired effect.* However, it should be noted that a recent systematic review of high-dose versus low-dose oxytocin for labor *augmentation* showed a decrease in cesarean delivery rate as well as a decrease in labor duration in the high-dose group. The high-dose groups did have greater incidences of tachysystole but no significant differences in neonatal outcomes. The authors noted some significant limitations of the review, including the fact that many of the reviewed trials were not blinded and decision criteria for cesarean section were not standardized [46]. Clinicians should carefully consider all the data, as well as the differences in use of oxytocin for induction versus augmentation, when deciding on oxytocin management schemes. Suggestions for the safe and effective use of oxytocin in labor are summarized in Box 4.3.

Oxytocin dosage should be titrated to uterine activity, with a goal of attaining adequate or normal uterine activity. *Coupling or tripling* of uterine contractions (Figure 4.7) is a phenomenon that may be

BOX 4.3   Suggestions for Safe and Effective Oxytocin Usage

1. Utilize isotonic intravenous fluids during oxytocin administration to avoid dilutional hyponatremia.
2. Administer oxytocin for *induction* of labor using a low-dose, low-frequency protocol to maximize pharmacologic dose response and avoid tachysystole.
3. Choose either low-dose or high-dose oxytocin for *augmentation* of labor, but increase dose using a low-frequency approach to minimize the risk of tachysystole.
4. Use standardized definitions for adequate as well as excessive uterine activity, and ensure that all team members are in accord.
5. Resolve any episodes of excessive uterine activity, regardless of whether fetal heart rate changes are present. Note that the goal of oxytocin use is *adequate* but not *excessive* uterine activity.
6. To promote optimal fetal oxygenation in first-stage labor, train team members to decrease oxytocin *before* tachysystole occurs by responding to contraction frequencies less than every 2 minutes before 30 minutes have elapsed.
7. Once an adequate pattern of uterine activity has been established, wean the oxytocin to the lowest amount necessary to maintain adequate contractions.
8. If coupling and tripling of uterine contractions occur, discontinue oxytocin for 30–60 minutes, administer an intravenous fluid bolus (isotonic), and encourage the woman to a side-lying position.

Data from references 4–6, 18, 21, 22, 25, 26, 28–30, 33–40, 43, 46, 47.

seen during oxytocin administration. Suggested treatment for this pattern is temporary discontinuation of oxytocin, lateral positioning of the mother, initiation of a fluid bolus, and a restart of oxytocin after 30 minutes or more [26].

An appropriate goal, when administering oxytocin and using internal monitoring during labor induction or augmentation, is the titration of oxytocin to establish uterine activity patterns reaching MVUs of 200 to 250. When external monitoring and palpation are being used, palpable contractions of normal duration every 2.5 to 3 minutes should correlate well with adequate Montevideo units (Figure 4.8). If labor progress is not occurring with what seems to be adequate uterine activity by palpation, the proper clinical response *is to consider internal monitoring to more accurately assess uterine activity and **not** to increase the oxytocin.*

Contraction frequency of less than every 2 minutes during oxytocin administration is a fairly common occurrence and can lead to tachysystole, even when using low-dose, low-frequency protocols.

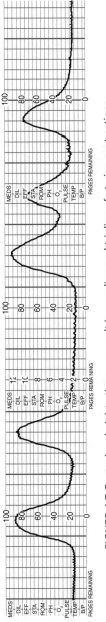

FIGURE 4.7 Oxytocin administration may result in coupling and tripling of uterine contractions. Treatment consists of discontinuation of oxytocin, maternal position change, and intravenous hydration. (Courtesy Lisa A. Miller, CNM, JD.)

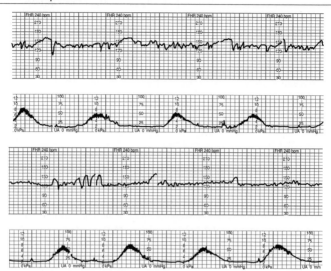

FIGURE 4.8 Example of adequate uterine activity during oxytocin augmentation using external monitoring. Note adequate relaxation time between contractions. According to nursing documentation, the contractions palpated were of moderate intensity. (Courtesy Lisa A. Miller, CNM, JD.)

Management must be based on clinical context and institutional protocol but should be geared toward returning uterine activity to adequate and appropriate for the stage of labor. In other words, clinicians should not try to achieve second-stage labor patterns in the latent or active phase of first-stage labor because this may interfere with fetal gas exchange. Continuous and ongoing evaluation of fetal status using a systematic approach can prevent fetal acidemia, improve outcomes, and also reduce medical-legal risk. Safety related to oxytocin use is achieved by avoidance of the injudicious use of oxytocin, adherence to evidence-based multidisciplinary guidelines regarding oxytocin administration, and appropriate and consistent team management of excessive uterine activity.

SUMMARY

Fetal gas exchange and acid–base status are directly affected by uterine activity during labor. Excessive uterine activity is related to fetal acidemia at birth and should be avoided by careful monitoring and cautious use of labor stimulants. Parameters for normal, or adequate, uterine activity are easily defined on the basis of normal labor physiology. Clinicians must reach consensus on definitions related to excessive uterine activity and recognize that the term *tachysystole* addresses only one aspect of uterine activity, that of frequency. Recognition of the importance of other parameters of uterine activity, such as strength, duration, resting tone, and relaxation time are equally important components of the evaluation of uterine activity during labor.

Understanding both the normal progress of labor and labor abnormalities is crucial to the promotion of improved outcomes for both mother and fetus. The availability of continuous labor support, patient education regarding appropriate admission criteria, and adequate hydration play key roles in minimizing labor abnormalities. An understanding of the pharmacologic characteristics of oxytocin, combined with a goal to attain adequate uterine activity, will lead to safe and effective use of this medication.

The evaluation of uterine activity and FHR patterns is inextricably intertwined in the care and support of the laboring mother. Focus on uterine activity assessment and management has been inconsistent in clinical practice. As Bakker [1] so aptly states, "contraction monitoring deserves full attention." It is now clear that proper and careful assessment of uterine activity deserves consideration equal to that given to FHR pattern assessment.

References

[1] P.C.A.M. Bakker, P.H.J. Kurver, D.J. Kuik, et al., Elevated uterine activity increases the risk of fetal acidosis at birth, Am. J. Obstet. Gynecol. 196 (4) (2007) 313.e1–313.e6.

[2] R. Caldeyro-Barcia, Intrauterine fetal reanimation in acute intrapartum fetal distress, Early Hum. Dev. 29 (1992) 27–33.

[3] C.C. Heuser, S. Knight, M.S. Esplin, et al., Tachysystole in term labor: incidence, risk factors, outcomes, and effect on fetal heart tracings, Am. J. Obstet. Gynecol. 209 (1) (2013) 32.e1–32.e6.

[4] D. Peebles, J. Spencer, A. Edwards, et al., Relation between frequency of uterine contractions and human fetal cerebral oxygenation saturation studied during labour by near infrared spectroscopy, Br. J. Obstet. Gynaecol. 101 (1) (1994) 44–48.

[5] K.R. Simpson, D.C. James, Effects of oxytocin-induced uterine hyperstimulation on fetal oxygen status and fetal heart rate patterns during labor, Am. J. Obstet. Gynecol. 199 (2008) 34.e1–34.e5.

[6] K.R. Simpson, L.A. Miller, Assessment and optimization of uterine activity during labor, Clin. Obstet. Gynecol. 54 (1) (2011) 40–49.

[7] Association of Women's Health, Obstetric and Neonatal Nurses, Fetal Heart Monitoring: Principles and Practices, fifth ed., Kendal Hunt, Dubuque, IA, 2015.

[8] D.L. Lowdermilk, S.E. Perry, Maternity & Women's Health Care, eleventh ed., Mosby, St. Louis, MO, 2015.

[9] American College of Obstetricians and Gynecologists, Safe prevention of the primary cesarean delivery. Obstetric Care Consensus No. 1, Obstet. Gynecol. 123 (2014) 693–711.

[10] E.A. Friedman, Labor in multiparas: a graphicostatistical analysis, Obstet. Gynecol. 8 (1956) 691–703.

[11] E.A. Friedman, Primigravid labor: a graphicostatistical analysis, Obstet. Gynecol. 6 (1955) 567–589.

[12] J. Zhang, H.J. Landy, D. Ware Branch, et al., Contemporary patterns of spontaneous labor with normal neonatal outcomes, Obstet. Gynecol. 116 (6) (2010) 1281–1287.

[13] R. Caldeyro-Barcia, Oxytocin in pregnancy and labour, Acta Endocrinol. Suppl. (Copenhagen) 34 (Suppl 50) (1960) 41–49.

[14] R. Caldeyro-Barcia, J.J. Poseiro, Physiology of uterine contractions, Clin. Obstet. Gynecol. 3 (1960) 386–408.

[15] R. Caldeyro-Barcia, J.J. Poseiro, Oxytocin and contractility of the pregnant human uterus, Ann. N.Y. Acad. Sci. 75 (1959) 813–830.

[16] R. Caldeyro-Barcia, Y. Sica-Blanco, J.J. Poseiro, et al., A quantitative study of the action of synthetic oxytocin on the pregnant human uterus, J. Pharmacol. Exp. Ther. 121 (1) (1957) 18–31.

[17] R. Caldeyro-Barcia, G. Theobald, Sensitivity of the pregnant human myometrium to oxytocin, Am. J. Obstet. Gynecol. 102 (8) (1968) 1181.

[18] G. Pontonnier, F. Puech, H. Grandjean, et al., Some physical and biochemical parameters during normal labour, Biol. Neonate 26 (3–4) (1975) 159–173.

[19] G.A. Macones, G.D. Hankins, C.Y. Spong, et al., The 2008 National Institute of Child Health and Human Development workshop report on electronic fetal monitoring: update on definitions, interpretation, and research guidelines, J. Obstet. Gynecol. Neonatal Nurs. 37 (2008) 510–515.

[20] American College of Obstetricians and Gynecologists, Intrapartum fetal heart rate monitoring: nomenclature, interpretation, and general management principles Practice Bulletin no. 106, Obstet. Gynecol. 114 (2009) 192–202.

[21] K.R. Simpson, Intrauterine resuscitation during labor: review of current methods and supportive evidence, J. Midwifery Womens Health 52 (3) (2007) 229–237.

[22] American College of Obstetricians and Gynecologists, Induction of labor, Practice Bulletin no. 107, ACOG, Washington, DC, 2009.

[23] S.B. Effer, R.P. Bértola, A. Vrettos, et al., Quantitative study of the regularity of uterine contractile rhythm in labor, Am. J. Obstet. Gynecol. 105 (6) (1969) 909–915.

[24] A.J. Krapohl, G.G. Myers, R. Caldeyro-Barcia, Uterine contractions in spontaneous labor: a quantitative study, Am. J. Obstet. Gynecol. 106 (3) (1970) 378–387.

[25] K.R. Simpson, Cervical Ripening and Induction and Augmentation of Labor, fourth ed., AWHONN, Washington, DC, 2013.

[26] K.R. Simpson, P.A. Creehan, Perinatal Nursing, fourth ed., Lippincott Williams & Wilkins, Philadelphia, PA, 2013.

[27] American College of Obstetricians and Gynecologists, Clinical management guidelines for obstetricians-gynecologists: management of intrapartum fetal heart rate tracings. Practice Bulletin no. 116, Obstet. Gynecol. 116 (2010) 1232–1240.

[28] A. Ness, J. Goldberg, V. Berghella, Abnormalities of the first and second stages of labor, Obstet. Gynecol. Clin. North Am. 32 (2) (2005) 201–220.

[29] B.M. Mercer, Induction of labor in the nulliparous gravida with an unfavorable cervix, Obstet. Gynecol. 105 (4) (2005) 688–689.

[30] S. Shields, S. Ratcliffe, P. Fontaine, et al., Dystocia in nulliparous women, Am. Fam. Physician 75 (11) (2007) 1671–1678.

[31] D.W. Dowding, H.L. Cheyne, V. Hundley, Complex interventions in midwifery care: reflections on the design and evaluation of an algorithm for the diagnosis of labor. Midwifery 27 (5) (2010) 654–659, http://dx.doi.org/10.1016/j.midw.2009.11.01.

[32] E.D. Hodnett, S. Gates, G.J. Hofmeyr, et al., Continuous support for women during childbirth. Cochrane Database Syst. Rev. 7 (2013) http://dx.doi.org/10.1002/14651858.CD003766.pub5 CD003766.

[33] C. Simon, W. Grobman, When has an induction failed? Obstet. Gynecol. 105 (4) (2005) 705–709.

[34] K.R. Simpson, D.C. James, G.E. Knox, Nurse-physician communication during labor and birth: implications for patient safety, J. Obstet. Gynecol. Neonatal Nurs. 35 (4) (2006) 547–556.

[35] D.J. Rouse, J. Owen, J.C. Hauth, Criteria for failed labor induction: prospective evaluation of a standardized protocol, Obstet. Gynecol. 96 (5 Pt 1) (2000) 671–677.

[36] D. Rouse, J. Owen, K. Savage, et al., Active phase labor arrest: revisiting the 2-hour minimum, Obstet. Gynecol. 98 (4) (2001) 550–554.

[37] L. Sanchez-Ramos, Induction of labor, Obstet. Gynecol. Clin. North Am. 32 (2) (2005) 181–200.

[38] J. Seitchik, The management of functional dystocia in the first stage of labor, Clin. Obstet. Gynecol. 30 (1) (1987) 42–49.

[39] J. Seitchik, J.A. Amico, M. Castillo, Oxytocin augmentation of dysfunctional labor. V. An alternative oxytocin regimen, Am. J. Obstet. Gynecol. 151 (6) (1985) 757–761.

[40] J. Seitchik, J. Amico, A.G. Robinson, et al., Oxytocin augmentation of dysfunctional labor. IV. Oxytocin pharmacokinetics, Am. J. Obstet. Gynecol. 150 (3) (1984) 225–228.

[41] Institute for Safe Medical Practices, High alert medications. Available from: https://www.ismp.org/tools/highalertmedications.pdf (accessed 26.08.15).

[42] Association of Women's Health, Obstetric and Neonatal Nurses, Guidelines for Professional Registered Nurse Staffing for Perinatal Units, AWHONN, Washington, DC, 2010.

[43] M. Jonsson, S.L. Nordén, U. Hanson, Analysis of malpractice claims with a focus on oxytocin use in labour, Acta Obstet. Gynecol. Scand. 86 (3) (2007) 315–319.

[44] H.D. Crall, D.R. Mattison, Oxytocin pharmacodynamics: effect of long infusions on uterine activity, Gynecol. Obstet. Invest. 31 (1) (1991) 17–22.

[45] F. Arias, Pharmacology of oxytocin and prostaglandins, Clin. Obstet. Gynecol. 43 (3) (2000) 455–468.

[46] S. Wei, Z. Luo, H. Qi, et al., High-dose vs. low-dose oxytocin for labor augmentation: a systematic review, Am. J. Obstet. Gynecol. 203 (2010) 296–304.

[47] L.A. Miller, Oxytocin, excessive uterine activity, and patient safety: time for a collaborative approach, J. Perinat. Neonatal Nurs. 23 (1) (2009) 52–58.

CHAPTER 5

Pattern Recognition and Interpretation

T he clinical application of electronic fetal heart rate (FHR) monitoring consists of three distinct, interdependent elements:
1. Definition
2. Interpretation
3. Management

This chapter focuses on standardized definitions of FHR patterns
and standard, evidence-based interpretation of FHR patterns with respect to underlying physiology. The principles developed in this chapter are used during the discussion of FHR management in Chapter 6.

THE EVOLUTION OF STANDARDIZED FHR DEFINITIONS

Electronic FHR monitoring was introduced into clinical practice almost 50 years ago before consensus was achieved regarding standardized definitions and interpretation of FHR patterns. In
1995 and 1996, the National Institute of Child Health and Human
Development (NICHD) convened a workshop to develop "standardized and unambiguous definitions for fetal heart rate tracings" [1].
These definitions have been endorsed by ACOG, the Association of
Women's Health, Obstetric and Neonatal Nurses (AWHONN), and
the American College of Nurse Midwives. In 2008, a second NICHD
consensus panel was convened to review and update the standardized
definitions published in 1997 [2]. Standardized NICHD FHR definitions are summarized in Table 5.1. Detailed discussion of individual
pattern definitions, along with evidence-based review of the underlying fetal physiology, will be presented later in this chapter.

The 2008 NICHD Consensus Report

In addition to clarifying and reiterating the FHR definitions proposed by the 1997 NICHD consensus statement, the 2008 report
recommended a simplified system for classifying FHR tracings,

TABLE 5.1   Standardized FHR Definitions

Pattern	Definition
Baseline	The mean FHR rounded to increments of 5 bpm during a 10-min segment, excluding accelerations, decelerations, and periods of marked FHR variability
	The baseline must be for a minimum of 2 min (not necessarily contiguous) in any 10-min segment, or the baseline for that segment is defined as "indeterminate"
Tachycardia	Baseline FHR >160 bpm
Bradycardia	Baseline FHR <110 bpm
Baseline variability	Fluctuations in the FHR baseline that are irregular in amplitude and frequency; variability is measured from the peak to the trough of the FHR fluctuations and is quantitated in bpm
	Variability is classified as follows:
	Absent—amplitude range undetectable
	Minimal—amplitude range detectable but ≤5 bpm
	Moderate—amplitude range 6–25 bpm
	Marked—amplitude range >25 bpm
	No distinction is made between short-term variability (or beat-to-beat variability or R-R wave period differences in the electrocardiogram) and long-term variability because in actual practice they are visually determined as a unit
Acceleration	A visually apparent abrupt increase (onset to peak <30 sec) in the FHR from the baseline
	At 32 weeks' gestation and beyond, an acceleration has a peak at least 15 bpm above baseline and a duration of at least 15 sec but <2 min
	Before 32 weeks' gestation, an acceleration has a peak at least 10 bpm above baseline and a duration of at least 10 sec but <2 min
	Prolonged acceleration lasts ≥2 min but <10 min
	If an acceleration lasts ≥10 min, it is a baseline change
Early deceleration	In association with a uterine contraction, a visually apparent, gradual (onset to nadir ≥30 sec) decrease in FHR with return to baseline
	In general, the nadir of the deceleration occurs at the same time as the peak of the contraction

Continued

TABLE 5.1   Standardized FHR Definitions—cont'd

Pattern	Definition
Late deceleration	In association with a uterine contraction, a visually apparent, gradual (onset to nadir ≥30 sec) decrease in FHR with return to baseline
	In general, the onset, nadir, and recovery of the deceleration occur after the beginning, peak, and end of the contraction, respectively
Variable deceleration	An abrupt (onset to nadir <30 sec), visually apparent decrease in the FHR below the baseline
	The decrease in FHR is at least 15 bpm and lasts at least 15 sec but <2 min
Prolonged deceleration	Visually apparent decrease in the FHR at least 15 bpm below the baseline lasting at least 2 min but <10 min from onset to return to baseline
Periodic deceleration	Accompanies a uterine contraction
Episodic deceleration	Does not accompany a uterine contraction
Sinusoidal pattern	Visually apparent, smooth, sine wave–like undulating pattern in FHR baseline with a cycle frequency of 3–5/min that persists for ≥20 min

Adapted from G.A. Macones et al. Obstet. Gynecol. 112 (2008): 661–666.

using baseline rate, variability, deceleration, and the sinusoidal pattern to group FHR tracings into one of three categories (Table 5.2). Category I includes tracings with a normal baseline rate (110–160), moderate variability, and no variable, late or prolonged decelerations. Category III includes tracings with absent variability and recurrent late decelerations, absent variability with recurrent variable decelerations, absent variability with bradycardia for at least 10 minutes, or a sinusoidal pattern for at least 20 minutes. Category II includes all tracings that do not meet criteria for classification as Category I or Category III. The proposed FHR categories represent a shorthand method of defining FHR tracings. Because Category II includes a wide range of FHR tracings, the categories alone do not provide sufficient information for FHR interpretation or management. The categories do not replace a full description of baseline rate, variability, accelerations, decelerations, sinusoidal pattern, and changes or trends over time.

TABLE 5.2   Three-tier FHR Classification System

Category I Normal	FHR tracing includes all of the following: Baseline rate: 110–160 bpm Baseline FHR variability: moderate Accelerations: present or absent Late or variable decelerations absent Early decelerations present or absent
Category II Indeterminate	Includes all FHR tracings not assigned to Categories I or III
Category III Abnormal	FHR tracing includes at least one of the following: Absent variability with recurrent late decelerations Absent variability with recurrent variable decelerations Absent variability with bradycardia for at least 10 min Sinusoidal pattern for at least 20 min

Adapted from G.A. Macones et al. Obstet. Gynecol. 112 (2008): 661–666.

Evidence-based Interpretation of FHR Patterns

This chapter reviews the relationship between FHR patterns and fetal physiology with particular emphasis on the underlying scientific evidence. Principles of FHR interpretation are stratified here by supporting evidence according to the method outlined by the U.S. Preventive Services Task Force, summarized in Box 5.1. Level I

BOX 5.1   Stratification of Scientific Evidence*

Level I	Evidence obtained from at least one properly designed randomized controlled trial.
Level II-1	Evidence obtained from well-designed controlled trials without randomization.
Level II-2	Evidence obtained from well-designed cohort or case-control analytic studies, preferably from more than one center or research group.
Level II-3	Evidence obtained from multiple time series with or without the intervention. Dramatic results in uncontrolled experiments also could be regarded as this type of evidence.
Level III	Opinions of respected authorities, based on clinical experience, descriptive studies, or reports of expert committees.

*According to method outlined by United States Preventive Services Task Force, Guide to Clinical Preventative Services. Report of the US Preventive Services Task Force, second ed., Williams and Wilkins, Baltimore, MD, 1996.

evidence is considered to be the most robust and Level III the least. Specifically, Level I and II evidence is capable of establishing statistically significant relationships. Level III evidence is descriptive. As such, level III evidence is capable of generating theories and hypotheses, but it is not capable of proving them.

As discussed previously, the primary objective of intrapartum FHR monitoring is to assess fetal oxygenation during labor. However, a number of conditions and/or exposures can influence the appearance of a FHR tracing via mechanisms unrelated to fetal oxygenation. Common maternal factors include fever, infection, medications, and thyroid disease. Common fetal factors include fever, infection, medications, prematurity, anemia, cardiac arrhythmias, anomalies, preexisting neurologic injury, and sleep cycles. Thorough assessment of an FHR tracing should take into account the factors summarized in Table 5.3. If FHR changes are thought to be related to interrupted fetal oxygenation, management is directed at assessing the oxygen pathway and improving the transfer of oxygen from the environment to the fetus, as described in Chapter 2.

TABLE 5.3   Factors Not Specifically Related to Fetal Oxygenation That May Influence FHR

Factor	Reported FHR Associations (Most Evidence Level II-3 and Level III)
Fever/infection	Increased baseline rate, decreased variability
Medications	Effects depend on specific medication and may include changes in baseline rate, frequency and amplitude of accelerations, variability, and sinusoidal pattern
Hyperthyroidism	Tachycardia, decreased variability
Prematurity	Increased baseline rate, decreased variability, reduced frequency and amplitude of accelerations
Fetal anemia	Sinusoidal pattern, tachycardia
Fetal heart block	Bradycardia, decreased variability
Fetal tachyarrhythmia	Variable degrees of tachycardia, decreased variability
Congenital anomaly	Decreased variability, decelerations
Preexisting neurologic abnormality	Decreased variability, absent accelerations
Sleep cycle	Decreased variability, reduced frequency and amplitude of accelerations

However, if an FHR abnormality is related to any of the conditions summarized in Table 5.3, individualized management is directed at the specific underlying process. During the following discussion of physiology and interpretation, FHR patterns related to interrupted fetal oxygenation are considered separately from FHR patterns caused by other mechanisms.

NICHD DEFINITIONS: GENERAL CONSIDERATIONS

The standardized definitions proposed by the NICHD in 1997 and reiterated in 2008 apply to the interpretation of FHR patterns produced by a direct fetal electrode detecting the fetal electrocardiogram (FECG) or by an external Doppler device detecting fetal cardiac motion using the autocorrelation technique. Autocorrelation is a computerized method of minimizing the artifact associated with Doppler ultrasound calculation of the FHR. This technology is built in to all modern FHR monitors. Patterns are categorized as baseline, periodic, or episodic. Baseline patterns include baseline rate and variability. Periodic and episodic patterns include FHR accelerations and decelerations. Periodic patterns are those associated with uterine contractions, and episodic patterns are those not associated with uterine contractions. Decelerations are defined as "abrupt" if the onset to nadir (lowest point) is <30 seconds and "gradual" if the onset to nadir is ≥30 seconds. Accelerations are defined as "abrupt" if the onset to peak is <30 seconds and "gradual" if the onset to peak is ≥30 seconds. Although terms such as *beat-to-beat* variability, *short-term* variability, and *long-term* variability have been used commonly in clinical practice, the 1997 and 2008 NICHD consensus reports recommended that no distinction be made among short-term, beat-to-beat, and long-term variability because in actual practice they are visually determined as a unit. A number of FHR characteristics are dependent on gestational age, so gestational age must be considered in the full description of the pattern. In addition, the FHR tracing should be evaluated in the context of maternal medical condition, prior results of fetal assessment, medications, and other factors. Finally, it is essential to recognize that FHR patterns do not occur alone and generally evolve over time. Therefore a full description of an FHR tracing requires a qualitative and quantitative description of uterine contractions and each of the FHR components.

Five Essential Components of an FHR Tracing

In addition to evaluation of uterine contractions, the five components of an FHR tracing include the following:

1. Baseline rate
2. Variability
3. Accelerations
4. Decelerations
5. Changes or trends over time

DEFINITIONS, PHYSIOLOGY, AND INTERPRETATION OF SPECIFIC FHR PATTERNS

Baseline Rate

Definition

Baseline FHR is defined as the approximate mean FHR rounded to increments of 5 bpm during a 10-minute segment, excluding accelerations, decelerations, and periods of marked variability (Figures 5.1, 5.2, and 5.3). Baseline rate is defined as a single number (for example, 145 bpm), not as a range (for example, "140–150 bpm" or "140s"), because the definitions of other FHR components, including accelerations and decelerations, are based on the degree of deviation from the

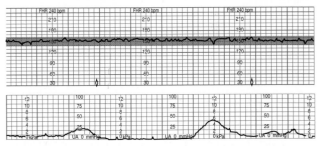

FIGURE 5.1 FHR baseline. Note that the 2-minute minimum for identifiable baseline does not require 2 contiguous or continuous minutes; rather, it is the total identifiable baseline in the 10-minute window that must add up to 2 minutes. Also, baseline may occur (and be interpreted) **during contractions,** as seen here. Baseline *(highlighted)* is identified over the entire 10-minute window, exceeding the 2-minute minimum.

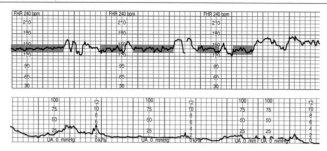

FIGURE 5.2 FHR baseline. Note that the 2-minute minimum for identifiable baseline does not require 2 contiguous or continuous minutes; rather, it is the total identifiable baseline in the 10-minute window that must add up to 2 minutes. Also, baseline may occur (and be interpreted) during contractions, as seen in Figure 5.1. Baseline *(highlighted)* is identified **between accelerations** or between segments differing by 25 bpm or more; identifiable baseline is approximately 5 minutes total (note the 2-minute minimum is met).

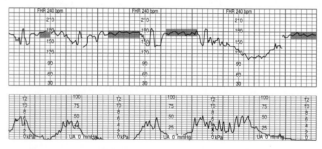

FIGURE 5.3 FHR baseline. Note that the 2-minute minimum for identifiable baseline does not require 2 contiguous or continuous minutes; rather, it is the total identifiable baseline in the 10-minute window that must add up to 2 minutes. Also, baseline may occur (and be interpreted) during contractions, as seen in Figure 5.1. Baseline *(highlighted)* is identified **between decelerations** or between segments differing by 25 bpm or more; identifiable baseline is approximately 5 minutes total (note the 2-minute minimum is met).

baseline rate. In any 10-minute window the minimum baseline duration must be at least 2 minutes (not necessarily contiguous), or the baseline for that period is deemed indeterminate (Figure 5.4). If the baseline during any 10-minute segment is deemed indeterminate, it may be necessary to refer to previous 10-minute segment(s) for determination of the baseline. A normal FHR baseline ranges from 110 to 160 bpm.

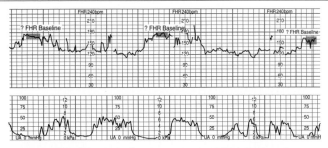

FIGURE 5.4 Indeterminate baseline. Note that there are less than 2 minutes of identifiable baseline during this 10-minute window. The baseline would be labeled *indeterminate* for this portion of the tracing, and the clinician would need to refer to previous portions of the strip to determine baseline. Prior baseline was 155 bpm.

Physiology

Baseline FHR is regulated by intrinsic cardiac pacemakers (SA node, AV node) and conduction pathways, autonomic innervation (sympathetic, parasympathetic), humoral factors (catecholamines), extrinsic factors (medications), and local factors (calcium, potassium). Sympathetic innervation and plasma catecholamines increase baseline FHR, whereas parasympathetic innervation reduces the baseline rate. Autonomic input regulates the FHR in response to fluctuations in Po_2, Pco_2, and blood pressure detected by chemoreceptors and baroreceptors located in the aortic arch and carotid arteries.

CATEGORIES OF BASELINE RATE

Tachycardia

Definition

Baseline FHR in excess of 160 bpm is defined as tachycardia (Figure 5.5).

Interpretation

Fetal oxygenation: As discussed in Chapter 2, recurrent or sustained interruption of oxygen transfer from the environment to the fetus can lead to progressive deterioration of fetal oxygenation and, eventually, to fetal metabolic acidemia. In the setting of metabolic acidemia, blunting of parasympathetic cardiac stimulation can cause the FHR to rise above the normal range. Sympathetic and humoral

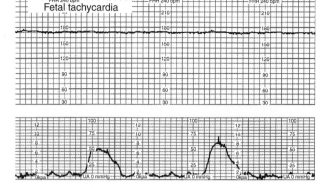

FIGURE 5.5 Fetal tachycardia: FHR >160 bpm.

factors may play roles as well. Because there are many possible causes of fetal tachycardia that are not directly related to interruption of fetal oxygenation, the association between fetal tachycardia and fetal oxygenation is nonspecific. The scientific evidence supporting a relationship between fetal tachycardia and interrupted fetal oxygenation primarily is Level III. Nevertheless, the observation of fetal tachycardia should prompt consideration of all possible causes, including interruption of oxygenation.

Other mechanisms: Many potential causes of fetal tachycardia are not directly related to fetal oxygenation. For example, abnormalities involving fetal cardiac pacemakers and/or the cardiac conduction system can result in sinus tachycardia, supraventricular tachycardia, atrial fibrillation, atrial flutter, and ventricular dysrhythmias. Maternal fever and infection and fetal anemia are well-known associations that likely act through the fetal autonomic nervous system and circulating catecholamines to cause fetal tachycardia. Maternal thyroid-stimulating antibodies can cause maternal hyperthyroidism and maternal tachycardia. Rarely, transplacental passage of thyroid-stimulating antibodies can result in fetal hyperthyroidism and tachycardia. Finally, many medications have been reported to cause fetal tachycardia. General categories include parasympatholytic drugs (atropine, hydroxyzine, phenothiazines) and sympathomimetic drugs (terbutaline, albuterol). Caffeine, theophylline, cocaine, and methamphetamine are other possible causes. Most of the scientific evidence regarding these mechanisms is Level II-3 and Level III. Potential causes of fetal tachycardia are summarized in Box 5.2.

BOX 5.2   Potential Causes of Fetal Tachycardia

Maternal fever
Infection
Medications/drugs
- Sympathomimetics
- Parasympatholytics
- Caffeine
- Theophylline
- Cocaine
- Methamphetamines
Fetal anemia
Maternal hyperthyroidism
Arrhythmias
- Sinus tachycardia
- Supraventricular tachycardia
- Atrial fibrillation
- Atrial flutter
- Ventricular arrhythmia
Metabolic acidemia

Bradycardia

Definition

Baseline FHR <110 bpm is defined as bradycardia (Figure 5.6).

Interpretation

Fetal oxygenation: In the past, the term *bradycardia* has been used interchangeably with the term *prolonged deceleration*. However, this practice is imprecise and should be avoided. According to the

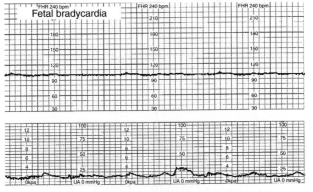

FIGURE 5.6 Fetal bradycardia: FHR <110 bpm.

definitions proposed by the NICHD, bradycardia is a baseline rate <110 bpm for at least 10 minutes, whereas a prolonged deceleration is a periodic or episodic deceleration that interrupts the baseline. Decelerations are common and can reflect interruption of fetal oxygenation. True baseline bradycardia is uncommon and is not specifically related to fetal oxygenation.

Other mechanisms: Baseline fetal bradycardia can be caused by abnormalities at the level of the cardiac pacemakers and/or conduction system. Atrioventricular dissociation or "heart block" can result from disruption of the cardiac conduction system by structural cardiac defects, viral infections (CMV), or maternal Sjögren's antibodies. Medications (adrenergic antagonists) do not commonly cause a reduction in baseline FHR <110 bpm. In descriptive studies that represent Level III evidence, fetal bradycardia has been reported in association with fetal heart failure, maternal hypoglycemia, and maternal hypothermia during cardiac surgery, urosepsis, and magnesium sulfate infusion. Potential causes of fetal bradycardia are summarized in Box 5.3.

Baseline FHR Variability

Definition

FHR variability is defined as fluctuations in the baseline FHR that are irregular in amplitude and frequency. Variability is quantitated in beats per minute and is measured from the peak to the trough in beats per minute. No distinction is made between *short-term (beat-to-beat)* variability and *long-term* variability because in actual practice they are visually determined as a unit. There is no consensus whether beat-to-beat variability alone is interpretable to the unaided eye. Variability is categorized as absent, minimal, moderate, or marked as shown in Figure 5.7.

BOX 5.3   Potential Causes of Fetal Bradycardia

Medications, including sympatholytics
Cardiac conduction abnormalities
Heart block
Heterotaxy syndrome
Structural cardiac defects
Viral infections, for example, cytomegalovirus (CMV)
Sjögren's antibodies
Fetal heart failure
Maternal hypoglycemia
Maternal hypothermia
Interruption of fetal oxygenation

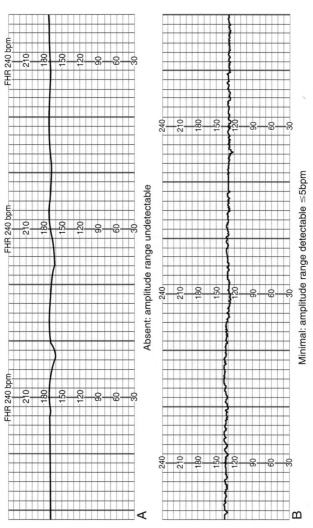

FIGURE 5.7 Classification of FHR variability. (A) Absent. (B) Minimal.

Continued

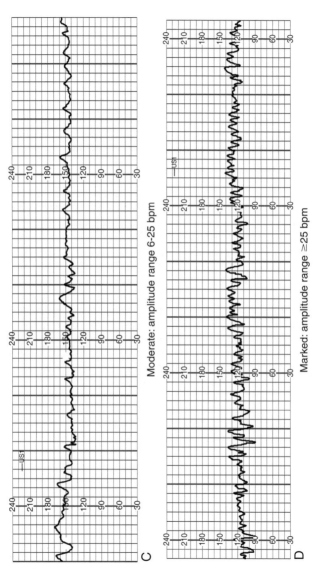

Moderate: amplitude range 6-25 bpm

Marked: amplitude range ≥25 bpm

FIGURE 5.7, CONT'D (C) Moderate. (D) Marked.

Physiology

Many factors interact to regulate FHR variability, including cardiac pacemakers (SA node, AV node) and the cardiac conduction system, autonomic innervation (sympathetic, parasympathetic), humoral factors (catecholamines), extrinsic factors (medications), and local factors (calcium, potassium). Fluctuations in Po_2, Pco_2, and blood pressure are detected by chemoreceptors and baroreceptors located in the aortic arch and carotid arteries. Signals from these receptors are processed in the medullary vasomotor center, possibly with regulatory input from higher centers in the hypothalamus and cerebral cortex. Sympathetic and parasympathetic signals from the medullary vasomotor center modulate the FHR in response to moment-to-moment changes in fetal Po_2, Pco_2, and blood pressure. With every heartbeat, slight corrections in the heart rate help to optimize fetal cardiac output and maximize the distribution of oxygenated blood to the fetal tissues. As illustrated in Figure 5.7, this variation is referred to as FHR variability and is displayed visually on the FHR graph as an irregular horizontal line. The small oscillations that represent FHR changes between each successive heartbeat have been referred to as *beat-to-beat* variability or *short-term* variability. The broader oscillations have been referred to as *long-term* variability. These terms describe two elements of FHR variability that occur together and that are evaluated as a unit. Therefore, as discussed earlier in the chapter, no distinction is made between short-term (beat-to-beat) variability and long-term variability. These terms are not included in standardized NICHD terminology. For purposes of clear and consistent communication, they should be avoided.

CATEGORIES OF BASELINE VARIABILITY

Absent Variability

Definition

As depicted in Figure 5.7, variability is defined as absent if the amplitude range of the FHR fluctuations is undetectable to the unaided eye.

Interpretation

Fetal oxygenation: Recurrent or sustained interruption of oxygen transfer from the environment to the fetus can lead to progressive deterioration of fetal oxygenation, metabolic acidemia, and blunting of parasympathetic outflow that can reduce the moment-to-moment regulation of the FHR. In the FHR tracing, these changes can be seen as minimal to absent variability. Although FHR variability ≤5 bpm is relatively common, persistently absent variability (amplitude range undetectable) is not. If variability ≤5 bpm is caused by interrupted fetal oxygenation, other FHR observations may be present, including decelerations, absent accelerations, and tachycardia. There are many possible causes of FHR variability ≤5 bpm. However, when persistent absent variability (amplitude range undetectable) is observed, careful evaluation should be undertaken to exclude fetal metabolic acidemia if possible.

Other mechanisms: Decreased FHR variability can be caused by a number of mechanisms that are unrelated to fetal oxygenation, including fetal sleep cycles, fetal tachycardia, and extreme prematurity. Congenital anomalies and preexisting neurologic injury are other possible causes. Several medications have been implicated in decreased FHR variability. General categories include central nervous system depressants (narcotics, barbiturates, phenothiazines, tranquilizers, general anesthetics) and parasympatholytics (atropine). Most of the scientific evidence regarding these mechanisms is Level III. It is important to note that most studies in the literature define "decreased" variability as ≤5 bpm and do not further stratify variability as "absent" (amplitude range undetectable) or "minimal" (amplitude range detectable but ≤5 bpm). Therefore it is not possible to draw valid distinctions regarding the relative clinical significance of these two categories. Causes of decreased FHR variability are summarized in Box 5.4.

BOX 5.4   Potential Causes of Decreased Fetal Heart Rate Variability

Fetal sleep cycle
Fetal tachycardia
Medications
- Narcotics
- Barbiturates
- Phenothiazines
- Tranquilizers
- General anesthetics
- Atropine
Prematurity
Congenital anomalies
Fetal anemia
Fetal cardiac arrhythmia
Infection
Preexisting neurologic injury
Fetal metabolic academia

Minimal Variability

Definition

Minimal variability is defined as an amplitude range that is detectable but ≤5 bpm.

Interpretation

Fetal oxygenation: Interrupted fetal oxygenation leading to metabolic acidemia and blunted autonomic regulation of the FHR can result in decreased FHR variability.

The specific relationship among minimal variability, fetal oxygenation, and fetal metabolic acidemia is not known, primarily because the literature has not consistently distinguished between minimal and absent variability. In the setting of persistently minimal variability without accelerations or moderate variability, the FHR tracing alone cannot reliably exclude metabolic acidemia.

Other mechanisms: Minimal variability may be associated with mechanisms other than interruption of fetal oxygenation, including fetal sleep cycles, fetal tachycardia, prematurity, congenital anomalies, preexisting neurologic injury, and medications, as summarized in Box 5.4. Most of the scientific evidence regarding these mechanisms is Level III.

Moderate Variability

Definition

Moderate variability (Figure 5.7) has an amplitude range of 6 to 25 bpm.

Interpretation

Fetal oxygenation: Moderate FHR variability indicates normal control of the FHR by cardiac pacemakers and conduction pathways, autonomic innervation, humoral, extrinsic, and local factors. Specifically, moderate variability indicates that autonomic regulation of the FHR is not blunted by interruption of fetal oxygenation that has progressed to the stage of metabolic acidemia. One of the central principles of electronic FHR monitoring is that moderate variability reliably predicts the absence of fetal metabolic acidemia and ongoing hypoxic injury at the time it is observed [3–8]. Supporting evidence is Level II-2, II-3, and III.

Other mechanisms: Moderate variability indicates normal neurologic regulation of the FHR at the time it is observed but does not exclude the possibility of preexisting neurologic injury [1,9–11].

Marked Variability

Definition

Marked variability is defined as FHR variability that is >25 bpm in amplitude (Figure 5.7).

Interpretation

The significance of marked variability is not known. In many cases, it likely represents a normal variant. It is plausible that marked variability reflects autonomic perturbation in the setting of early hypoxemia. Scientific evidence regarding this pattern is limited. All available evidence is Level III.

Sinusoidal Pattern

The sinusoidal pattern (Figure 5.8) is defined as a smooth, sine wave–like undulating pattern in FHR baseline with a cycle frequency of 3 to 5 per minute that persists for at least 20 minutes. It is not included in the definition of FHR variability. A practical way to distinguish FHR variability from the sinusoidal pattern is to recognize that variability is defined as fluctuations in the baseline that are irregular in amplitude and frequency, whereas the sinusoidal pattern is characterized by fluctuations in the baseline that are regular in amplitude and frequency. Sinusoidal FHR is an uncommon pattern. Although the pathophysiologic mechanism is not known, this pattern classically is associated with severe fetal anemia. Variations of the pattern have

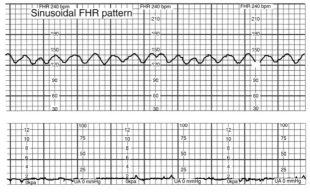

FIGURE 5.8 Sinusoidal pattern.

been described in association with chorioamnionitis, fetal sepsis, or administration of narcotic analgesics [9]. Scientific evidence regarding associated factors is Level II-2 to Level III. Evidence regarding pathophysiology is Level III.

Acceleration

Definition

Acceleration is as an abrupt (onset to peak <30 seconds) increase in FHR above baseline. The peak is at least 15 bpm above baseline, and the acceleration lasts at least 15 seconds from the onset to return to baseline (Figure 5.9). Before 32 weeks' gestation, an acceleration is defined as having a peak at least 10 bpm above baseline and a duration of at least 10 seconds. An acceleration lasting at least 2 minutes but less than 10 minutes is defined as a prolonged acceleration. An acceleration lasting 10 minutes or longer is defined as a baseline change. The amplitude of an acceleration is quantitated in bpm above the baseline excluding transient spikes or electronic artifact. The duration is quantitated in minutes and seconds.

Physiology

Accelerations in FHR frequently occur in association with fetal movement, probably as a result of stimulation of peripheral proprioceptors, increased catecholamine release, and autonomic stimulation of the heart. In the absence of spontaneous accelerations, fetal scalp stimulation or vibroacoustic stimulation can provoke fetal movement and FHR accelerations.

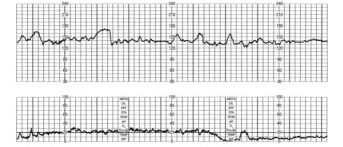

FIGURE 5.9 Accelerations of fetal heart rate in a term pregnancy. Note that the 15-bpm peak and 15-second duration criteria are met. (Courtesy Lisa A. Miller, CNM, JD.)

Interpretation

Fetal oxygenation: Accelerations, like moderate variability, reflect normal autonomic regulation of the FHR. The presence of accelerations indicates that autonomic regulation of the FHR is not blunted by interruption of oxygenation that has progressed to the stage of metabolic acidemia. A central principle of electronic FHR monitoring is that FHR accelerations are highly predictive of the absence of fetal metabolic acidemia and ongoing hypoxic injury at the time they are observed [12–15]. Supporting evidence is Level II-2, II-3, and III.

Other mechanisms: Accelerations indicate normal autonomic regulation of the FHR at the time they are observed [1,10,11,16]. However, the presence of FHR accelerations does not reliably exclude preexisting neurologic injury. Another suspected mechanism of FHR acceleration is transient compression of the umbilical vein, resulting in decreased fetal venous return and a reflex rise in heart rate. Evidence is Level III.

Decelerations

Definition

FHR decelerations are identified as early, late, variable, or prolonged. Late decelerations and early decelerations are gradual in onset and periodic in timing (associated with uterine contractions). Variable decelerations are abrupt in onset and may be periodic or episodic in timing. Prolonged decelerations may be abrupt or gradual in onset and may be periodic or episodic in timing. Decelerations are defined as recurrent if they occur with at least 50% of uterine contractions in any 20-minute segment. All decelerations are quantitated by depth in beats per minute below the baseline (excluding transient spikes or electronic artifact) and duration in minutes and seconds. Standardized NICHD terminology does not classify FHR decelerations as *mild, moderate,* or *severe* because the prognostic significance of such subclassification has not been established. The following sections review the standard definition and interpretation of each pattern.

Physiology

Early decelerations represent a reflex fetal response to fetal head compression during uterine contractions. Late, variable, and prolonged FHR decelerations represent reflex fetal responses to interruption of the oxygen pathway at one or more points.

Scientific evidence supporting these mechanisms ranges from Level II-1 to Level III.

TYPES OF DECELERATIONS

Early Deceleration

Definition

Early deceleration is defined as a gradual (onset to nadir ≤30 seconds) decrease in FHR from the baseline and subsequent return to baseline associated with a uterine contraction (Figure 5.10). In most cases the onset, nadir, and recovery of the deceleration occur at the same time as the beginning, peak, and end of the contraction, respectively. Early decelerations are defined as recurrent if they occur with at least 50% of uterine contractions in any 20-minute segment.

Interpretation

Fetal oxygenation: Early decelerations have no known relationship to fetal oxygenation.

Other mechanisms: Although the precise physiologic mechanism is not known, early decelerations are thought to represent a fetal autonomic response to changes in intracranial pressure and/or cerebral blood flow caused by intrapartum compression of the fetal head (Figure 5.11). These decelerations do not appear to be associated with poor outcome and therefore are considered clinically benign. Evidence is Level II-3 and Level III.

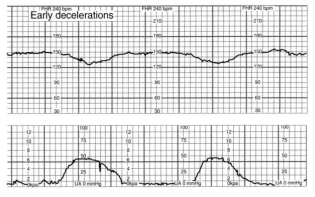

FIGURE 5.10 Early decelerations.

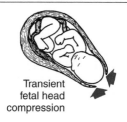

Transient
fetal head
compression

Physiologic mechanism of early deceleration

Transient fetal head compression
↓
Altered intracranial pressure and/or cerebral blood flow
↓
Reflex parasympathetic outflow
↓
Gradual slowing of the FHR
↓
Early deceleration
↓
When head compression is relieved, autonomic reflexes subside

FIGURE 5.11 Physiologic mechanism of early decelerations.

Late Deceleration

Definition

Late deceleration of the FHR is defined as a gradual (onset to nadir ≥30 seconds) decrease of the FHR from the baseline and subsequent return to the baseline associated with a uterine contraction (Figure 5.12). In most cases the onset, nadir, and recovery of the deceleration occur after the beginning, peak, and ending of the contraction, respectively. Late decelerations are defined as recurrent if they occur with at least 50% of uterine contractions in any 20-minute segment. They are defined as intermittent if they occur with <50% of contractions in any 20-minute segment.

Interpretation

Fetal oxygenation: A late deceleration is a reflex fetal response to transient hypoxemia during a uterine contraction. Myometrial contractions can compress maternal blood vessels traversing the uterine wall and disrupt maternal perfusion of the intervillous space of the

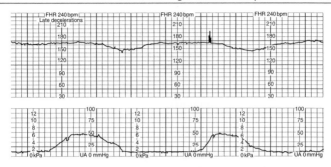

FIGURE 5.12 Late decelerations.

placenta. Reduced delivery of oxygenated blood to the intervillous space can reduce the diffusion of oxygen into the fetal capillary blood in the chorionic villi, leading to a decline in fetal Po_2 below the normal range of approximately 15 to 25 mm Hg. If the fetal Po_2 falls below a critical threshold, chemoreceptors detect the change and signal medullary vasomotor centers to initiate a protective reflex response. Sympathetic outflow causes peripheral vasoconstriction and centralization of blood volume, favoring perfusion of the brain, heart, and adrenal glands. The resulting increase in peripheral resistance causes a rise in mean arterial blood pressure and a subsequent baroreceptor-mediated reflex slowing of the heart rate to reduce cardiac output and return the blood pressure to normal. This mechanism has been elucidated elegantly in a number of animal studies [2,17–25]. It is summarized in Figure 5.13. If disruption of fetal oxygenation is recurrent or sustained, it may progress to the stage of metabolic acidemia. In the setting of metabolic acidemia, a late deceleration can reflect a direct myocardial depressant effect of hypoxia. In that event, other FHR abnormalities would be expected, such as fetal tachycardia, absent variability, and absent accelerations. For the purpose of standardized interpretation of intrapartum FHR patterns, a late deceleration reflects transient interruption of oxygen transfer from the environment to the fetus during a uterine contraction, resulting in transient fetal hypoxemia. The scientific evidence supporting the physiologic basis of a typical late deceleration is Level II-1 and II-2.

Other mechanisms: No other mechanisms are known to cause late decelerations.

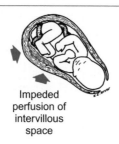

Impeded
perfusion of
intervillous
space

Physiologic mechanism of late deceleration

Uterine contraction impedes
maternal perfusion of the
placental intervillous space
↓
Transient fetal hypoxemia ——→
↓
Chemoreceptor stimulation
↓
Reflex sympathetic outflow
↓
Peripheral vasoconstriction, preferentially
shunting oxygenated blood away from the
peripheral tissues and toward central vital
organs: brain, heart, adrenal glands
↓
Increase in fetal peripheral resistance
and blood pressure
↓
Baroreceptor stimulation
↓
Reflex parasympathetic outflow
↓
Gradual slowing of the FHR
↓
Late deceleration ←——
↓
After the contraction, these reflexes subside

Note: In the presence
of fetal metabolic
acidemia, transient
hypoxemia may result
in myocardial hypoxia
and a late deceleration
secondary to direct
myocardial depression

FIGURE 5.13 Physiologic mechanism of late decelerations.

Variable Deceleration

Definition

Variable deceleration of the FHR is defined as an abrupt (onset
to nadir <30 seconds) decrease in FHR below the baseline, calculated from the most recently determined portion of the baseline
(Figure 5.14). The decrease in FHR below the baseline is at least

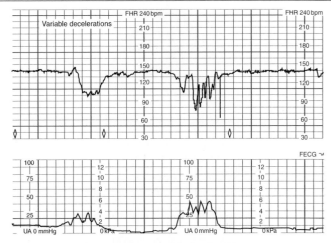

FIGURE 5.14 Variable decelerations.

15 bpm, and the deceleration lasts at least 15 seconds and <2 minutes from onset to return to baseline. Variable decelerations are not necessarily associated with uterine contractions. However, when they are, the onset, depth, and duration commonly vary with successive uterine contractions. In addition, if they are associated with uterine contractions, variable decelerations are defined as recurrent if they occur with at least 50% of uterine contractions in any 20-minute segment.

Interpretation

Fetal oxygenation: Variable decelerations result from transient mechanical compression of umbilical blood vessels within the umbilical cord (Figure 5.15) [26–35]. Initially, compression of the umbilical cord occludes the thin-walled, compliant umbilical vein, decreasing fetal venous return and triggering a baroreceptor-mediated reflex rise in FHR (commonly described as a "shoulder"). Further compression of the umbilical cord results in occlusion of the umbilical arteries, causing an abrupt increase in fetal peripheral resistance and blood pressure. Baroreceptors detect the abrupt rise in blood pressure and signal the medullary vasomotor center, which, in turn, triggers an increase in parasympathetic outflow along the vagus nerve and an abrupt decrease in heart rate. Parasympathetic stimulation of the heart may result in a junctional or idioventricular rhythm that appears as a relatively stable rate of 60 to 80 bpm at the

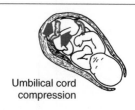

Umbilical cord
compression

Physiologic mechanism of variable deceleration

Umbilical cord compression
↓
Initial compression of umbilical vein
↓
Transient decreased fetal venous return
↓
Transient reduction in fetal cardiac output and blood pressure
↓
Baroreceptor stimulation
↓
Transient reflex rise in FHR
↓
Umbilical artery compression
↓
Abrupt rise in fetal peripheral resistance and blood pressure
↓
Baroreceptor stimulation
↓
Reflex parasympathetic outflow
↓
Abrupt slowing of the FHR
↓
Variable deceleration
↓
When umbilical cord compression is relieved, this process
occurs in reverse

FIGURE 5.15 Physiologic mechanism of variable decelerations.

base of a variable deceleration. As the cord is decompressed, this
sequence of events occurs in reverse. A *shoulder* is common after a
variable deceleration. It is important to note that the term *shoulder*
is not included in the standard NICHD definitions of FHR patterns.
This term, and others lacking standard definitions, are addressed
in a separate section of this chapter. Umbilical cord compression
results in transient disruption of normal oxygen transfer from the
environment to the fetus. During a variable deceleration, the fetal

Po$_2$ may or may not fall below the normal range of 15 to 25 mm Hg. Regardless of the effect on fetal Po$_2$, a variable deceleration is transient by definition (duration <2 min), and occasional compression of the umbilical cord usually has little clinical significance. Recurrent variable decelerations, on the other hand, can result in recurrent disruption of fetal oxygenation and lead to a cascade of progressive physiologic changes including hypoxemia, hypoxia, metabolic acidosis, and eventually metabolic acidemia. In that event, associated FHR observations may include a rising baseline rate, minimal to absent variability, absent accelerations, and slow return to baseline after decelerations. The latter has been referred to as a *variable with a late component*. This term is not defined by the NICHD and is addressed later in the chapter. For the purposes of FHR interpretation, a variable deceleration reflects transient interruption of oxygen transfer from the environment to the fetus at the level of the umbilical cord. Supporting evidence is Level II-1, II-2, II-3, and III.

Other mechanisms: Other suggested physiologic mechanisms resulting in variable deceleration include a fetal vagal response to umbilical cord stretching and reflex vagal response to head compression. The former mechanism may be similar to the mechanism underlying umbilical cord compression. The latter likely is similar to the mechanism underlying early decelerations. Supporting evidence is limited (Level III).

Prolonged Deceleration

Definition

Prolonged deceleration (Figure 5.16) of the FHR is defined as a decrease (either gradual or abrupt) in FHR at least 15 bpm below the baseline lasting at least 2 minutes from onset to return to baseline. According to NICHD terminology, a prolonged deceleration lasting 10 minutes or longer is defined as a baseline change. Under no circumstances should this statement be interpreted to suggest that a prolonged deceleration turns into a benign baseline change after 10 minutes. This statement is excluded from the ACOG endorsement of NICHD definitions in Practice Bulletin 70.

Interpretation

Fetal oxygenation: A prolonged deceleration reflects disrupted oxygen transfer from the environment to the fetus at one or more points

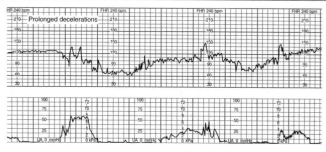

FIGURE 5.16 Prolonged decelerations.

along the oxygen pathway. As described in the introduction to FHR decelerations, there are two basic physiologic mechanisms:

1. Reflex autonomic response
2. Direct myocardial depression

A prolonged deceleration usually begins as a reflex autonomic response to disruption of the oxygen pathway. If the oxygen pathway is disrupted by mechanical compression of the umbilical cord, the FHR deceleration begins as a reflex autonomic response to fetal hypertension. Alternatively, an acute event such as placental abruption or uterine rupture can cause an abrupt fall in fetal Po_2. Reflex peripheral vasoconstriction centralizes blood volume and increases blood pressure. The resulting FHR deceleration begins as a reflex autonomic response to the rise in blood pressure triggered by falling Po_2. Regardless of the cause, sustained disruption of oxygen transfer can lead to progressive physiologic changes, including fetal hypoxemia, hypoxia, metabolic acidosis, and metabolic acidemia. Eventually, tissue hypoxia and acidosis can lead to failure of peripheral vascular smooth muscle contraction. The resultant fetal hypotension reduces diastolic blood pressure and compromises coronary blood flow, leading to myocardial hypoxia, direct myocardial depression, and slowing of the FHR. If this process is not corrected, the heart may stop beating altogether. It is likely that both mechanisms (autonomic reflex and direct myocardial depression) contribute to the underlying physiology of a prolonged FHR deceleration; however, their precise relative roles of are not known. In general, autonomic reflexes appear to predominate initially, and hypoxic myocardial depression appears to be a later mechanism. Supporting evidence is Level II-1, II-2, II-3, and III. For the purposes of standard FHR interpretation, a prolonged deceleration reflects interruption of oxygen transfer from the environment to the fetus at one or more points along the oxygen pathway.

Other mechanisms: Other proposed mechanisms of prolonged decelerations can overlap with those causing fetal bradycardia. Examples include fetal heart failure, maternal hypoglycemia, and hypothermia. Supporting evidence is Level III.

FETAL CARDIAC ARRYTHMIAS

Precise characterization of fetal cardiac arrhythmias can challenge the clinical skills of the most experienced specialist, even with the benefit of direct, magnified visualization of the fetal heart using state-of-the-art sonographic equipment with color, pulse-wave, and M-mode Doppler capability. Therefore any attempt to classify fetal cardiac arrhythmias using electronic FHR monitoring alone is destined to result in a tentative diagnosis at best. This imprecision is compounded by the fact that rates >240 bpm may be halved or not printed at all by the monitor. This severely limits the ability of the FHR monitor to distinguish between fetal conditions such as supraventricular tachycardia, atrial fibrillation, and atrial flutter, all of which can result in FHRs >240 bpm (the upper limit of the FHR graph on standard paper). Electronic FHR monitoring cannot determine whether a fetal heartbeat is initiated by an electrical impulse originating in the atrium or in the ventricle. In other words, an electronic monitor cannot reliably distinguish an atrial arrhythmia from a ventricular arrhythmia. Nevertheless, electronic FHR monitoring can offer some clues to the presence of an abnormal fetal heart rhythm. For example, dropped beats might appear on the FHR monitor as sharp downward spikes that nadir at approximately half of the baseline rate. A premature beat with a compensatory pause might appear as a sharp upward spike followed immediately by a downward spike. Bradycardia due to heart block can appear persistently or intermittently as a baseline rate that is half of the normal rate. Sinus bradycardia should be suspected if the baseline rate is <110 bpm but higher than half of the normal rate. Any FHR baseline of <110 bpm requires thorough evaluation before it can be attributed to a benign condition. If the fetal heart is not generating electrical activity, as in the case of fetal demise, a fetal scalp electrode may detect the electrical impulses from the maternal heart and record the maternal heart rate. If there is any question about the clinical significance of any unusual fetal heart rhythm that is seen on the fetal monitor or detected audibly, further evaluation with other modalities is necessary to establish an accurate diagnosis.

TERMS AND CONCEPTS NOT SUPPORTED BY EVIDENCE OR CONSENSUS

Several terms and concepts that may be encountered in practice or in the medicolegal arena are not supported by scientific evidence and are not included in standard NICHD recommendations. Some of these are discussed next.

Wandering Baseline

An FHR baseline that is within the normal range (110–160 bpm) but is not stable at a single rate for long enough to define a mean has been described as a *wandering baseline*. Absent variability and absent accelerations are prominent features. Decelerations can be present or absent. This combination of FHR findings has been suggested to indicate preexisting neurologic injury and impending fetal death. The physiologic mechanism is not known, and published data are limited (Level III). If this pattern is observed, it should be interpreted in the context of other FHR observations and clinical factors.

Lambda Pattern

The *lambda* FHR pattern is characterized by a brief acceleration followed by a small deceleration [36]. Common during early labor, this pattern has no known clinical significance. The underlying physiologic mechanism is not known (Level III).

Shoulder

As discussed earlier in the chapter, variable decelerations result from transient mechanical compression of umbilical blood vessels within the umbilical cord. Initial compression of the umbilical vein reduces fetal venous return and triggers a baroreceptor-mediated reflex rise in FHR that commonly is described as a *shoulder*. As the cord is decompressed, a second shoulder frequently follows the deceleration and likely reflects the same underlying mechanism. The precise mechanism has not been confirmed. There is no known association with adverse newborn outcome. On the other hand, there is no firm evidence that the observation reflects normal fetal oxygenation. It is considered a clinically benign observation. Supporting evidence is Level III.

Checkmark Pattern

The *checkmark pattern* is an unusual FHR pattern that has been described in association with neurologic injury, neonatal convulsions, and possible in utero fetal seizure activity. Unlike most FHR patterns described in association with neurologic injury, the checkmark pattern is not necessarily accompanied by absent baseline variability. All evidence related to the visual appearance of the pattern and the putative clinical significance is Level III.

End-stage Bradycardia and Terminal Bradycardia

Standardized NICHD FHR terminology clearly indicates that the term *bradycardia* applies to the baseline FHR. The term specifically does not apply to a "prolonged deceleration" that interrupts the baseline. The terms *end-stage bradycardia* and *terminal bradycardia* have been used to describe a prolonged deceleration observed at the end of the second stage of labor. Such decelerations are common in the course of normal vaginal delivery and usually are of little clinical significance. The precise cause is unknown; however, suggested mechanisms include umbilical cord compression, umbilical cord stretching, fetal head compression, and transient fetal hypoxemia due to excessive uterine activity and/or maternal expulsive efforts. The effect on immediate newborn outcome is variable and depends on a number of interacting factors, including but not limited to the physiologic cause of the deceleration, prior condition of the fetus, and duration of the deceleration. Consistent with NICHD terminology, end-stage bradycardia and terminal bradycardia should be discarded in favor of the more precise term *prolonged deceleration*. Evidence is Level III.

Uniform Accelerations

Various terms have been used to describe FHR accelerations. Examples include *uniform sporadic accelerations, variable sporadic accelerations, uniform periodic accelerations, sporadic periodic accelerations,* and *crown accelerations.* These terms are not included in standardized NICHD definitions, and there is no documented physiologic basis for such classification.

Atypical Variable Decelerations

Overshoot

The term *overshoot* has been used to describe a FHR pattern characterized by persistently absent variability, absent accelerations, and a variable deceleration followed by a smooth, prolonged rise in the FHR above the previous baseline with gradual return [37–41]. As with the wandering baseline, essential elements of this uncommon pattern include the persistent absence of variability and the absence of accelerations. The overshoot pattern has been attributed to a range of conditions, including "mild fetal hypoxia above the deceleration threshold," "chronic fetal distress," and "repetitive transient central nervous system ischemia." However, all of these associations are speculative and none has been substantiated by available scientific evidence. The physiologic mechanisms responsible for the overshoot pattern are not known. However, the pattern has been described in association with abnormal neurologic outcome with or without metabolic acidemia, suggesting that it might indicate preexisting neurologic injury. Because of the wide variation in reported associations and the lack of agreement regarding the definition and clinical significance of overshoot, it is best to avoid the use of this term in favor of specific terminology. All evidence regarding the overshoot pattern in humans is Level III.

Variable Deceleration with a Late Component

Variable deceleration with a late component describes a deceleration with an abrupt onset and a gradual return to baseline. The abrupt onset suggests that the deceleration begins as a reflex autonomic response to an abrupt rise in blood pressure caused by umbilical cord compression (the "variable" component of the pattern). The gradual return to baseline suggests a gradual reduction of autonomic outflow upon resolution of transient hypoxemia, as occurs in a late deceleration (the "late" component of the pattern). A plausible explanation of the pattern would be initial umbilical cord compression causing a reflex fall in FHR and a transient decline in fetal Po_2. The Po_2 probably drops below the threshold that triggers the reflex sympathetic outflow and peripheral vasoconstriction characteristic of a late deceleration. Decompression of the umbilical cord brings about rapid resolution of the variable deceleration; however, the physiologic mechanisms responsible for late deceleration resolve more slowly, causing the FHR to return slowly to the previous baseline. Although the specific physiologic mechanism has not been studied systematically, this explanation is a reasonable extrapolation from known mechanisms. Scientific evidence regarding the underlying physiologic mechanism is limited to Level III. Second-stage variable decelerations with slow recovery have been reported to increase the likelihood of operative delivery; however, no consistent effect on newborn outcome has been described [42]. In the absence of a standard definition of this pattern, its use is best avoided in favor of standard terminology—for example, *variable deceleration with gradual return to baseline*.

Mild, Moderate, and Severe Variable Decelerations

The depth and duration of variable decelerations have been suggested as predictors of newborn outcome. Kubli and colleagues proposed three categories of variable decelerations based on these characteristics [43]. According to this classification system, a mild variable deceleration was defined by a duration less than 30 seconds regardless of depth, a depth no lower than 80 bpm, or a depth of 70 to 80 bpm lasting less than 60 seconds. A moderate variable deceleration was defined by a depth <70 bpm lasting 30 to 60 seconds or a depth of 70 to 80 bpm lasting more than 60 seconds. A severe deceleration was defined as a deceleration <70 bpm lasting more than 60 seconds. There is no conclusive evidence in the literature that the depth of any type of deceleration (early, variable, late, or prolonged) is predictive of fetal metabolic acidemia or newborn outcome independent of other important FHR characteristics such as baseline rate, variability, accelerations, and frequency of decelerations. Therefore *mild, moderate,* and *severe* categories are not included in standard NICHD definitions of FHR decelerations.

Consistent with NICHD terminology, all decelerations are quantitated by depth in beats per minute and duration in minutes and seconds.

V-shaped Variables and W-shaped Variables

The visual appearance of a variable deceleration has been suggested to predict the underlying cause. For example, a *V-shaped* variable deceleration has been suggested to indicate umbilical cord compression due to oligohydramnios, whereas a *W-shaped* variable deceleration has been suggested to reflect umbilical cord compression due to a nuchal cord. There is no evidence in the literature to confirm this distinction. These terms are not included in standardized NICHD terminology.

Good Variability Within the Deceleration

At the nadir of a variable or late deceleration, the FHR frequently appears irregular, similar to the appearance of moderate variability. The visual similarity has led some to suggest that "variability" during a deceleration has the same clinical significance as baseline variability. Although the concept is physiologically plausible, it has never been studied or confirmed. In addition, it is inconsistent with standard terminology. Variability is a characteristic of the FHR baseline. The term *variability* is not used to qualify periodic or episodic decelerations that interrupt the baseline. In the absence of evidence, the safest approach is to avoid assigning undue significance to this observation.

Other Mechanisms That Lack Scientific Basis

Fetal Head Compression

Early deceleration of the FHR has long been recognized as a benign reflex response to transient compression of the fetal head during a uterine contraction. The innocuous nature of this phenomenon is underscored by the inclusion of early decelerations in NICHD Category I (2008), indicating normal fetal oxygenation. However, some have suggested that intrapartum fetal head compression can cause hypoxic-ischemic brain injury, even in a normally oxygenated fetus [44]. This notion contends that uterine contractions compress the fetal head against the maternal pelvis with such force that fetal intracranial pressure exceeds cerebral perfusion pressure, reducing intracranial blood flow to the point of regional cerebral ischemia, focal hypoxic-ischemic brain injury, and cerebral palsy (CP). Descriptive studies have reported that fetal head pressures during uterine contractions can be more than twice as high as intraamniotic pressures [45]. Other studies have demonstrated changes in fetal cerebral perfusion pressure, cerebral blood flow, and cerebral oxygen consumption during fetal head pressure [46–48]. However, no published Level I or Level II evidence has demonstrated that these changes translate to histologic or clinical evidence of neurologic injury. On the contrary, observations in fetal sheep suggest that the reflex Cushing response to head compression may be protective against such injury [49,50]. Level II evidence, in the form of case-control studies, has identified several perinatal risk factors for CP, including prematurity, infection, hemorrhage, maternal thyroid disease, and congenital malformations However, no Level I or II evidence has demonstrated a link between any measure of uterine activity and the later development of CP. The notion that localized fetal brain injury can be caused by the mechanical forces of labor is further challenged by Level II evidence from a large cohort study including more than 380,000 spontaneous vaginal deliveries and more than 33,000 cesarean deliveries without labor [51]. Neonates exposed to uterine contractions and maternal expulsive efforts of sufficient frequency, intensity, and duration to result in spontaneous vaginal delivery had no higher rates of mechanical brain injury, in the form of intracranial hemorrhage, than did neonates who were exposed to no uterine contractions. No analytic evidence in the literature has identified any objective measure of uterine activity or maternal expulsive effort as a risk factor for CP. On the contrary, analytic studies have failed to identify an association between uterine activity and CP, much less as a causal relationship. Finally, there is no evidence in the literature that this hypothetical mechanism of injury could be prevented or mitigated by any known obstetric intervention. In the absence of supporting scientific evidence, this theory should not be used as a foundation for intrapartum management decisions.

Prediction and Prevention of Fetal Stroke

An extension of the theory just described is the notion that FHR and uterine activity monitoring can be used to predict and prevent perinatal arterial ischemic stroke (PAIS). A recent meta-analysis of four studies reported a possible relationship between abnormal intrapartum FHR patterns and the later diagnosis of PAIS [52].

One of the four studies included only preterm deliveries, did not specify the FHR "abnormalities" that were observed in the control and study groups, and did not control for known confounding factors such as baseline rate; presence or absence of moderate variability; presence or absence of accelerations; or the type, number, duration, or frequency of FHR "abnormalities" [53]. The other three studies included only term deliveries, and none of these demonstrated an independent link between FHR abnormalities and PAIS [54–56]. There is no published evidence supporting a causal relationship between FHR abnormalities and PAIS at any gestational age. There is no published evidence that intrapartum electronic fetal monitoring or uterine activity monitoring is capable of detecting or predicting PAIS or that any form of obstetric intervention is capable of preventing PAIS. There is no Level I or II evidence linking PAIS independently with any measure of uterine activity or labor duration [12]. This is consistent with the 2007 consensus report of the National Institute of Neurologic Disorders and Stroke and the NICHD, which concluded that "there are no reliable predictors of perinatal ischemic stroke upon which to base prevention or treatment strategies" [19].

SUMMARY

The three basic elements of FHR monitoring are (1) terminology, (2) interpretation, and (3) management. A standardized, evidence-based approach to each element facilitates effective communication, promotes patient safety, and helps ensure optimal outcomes.

Standardized terminology has been endorsed by all major professional organizations in the United States representing providers of obstetric care. The simple agreement to adopt a common language sets the stage for the next essential step. Standardized FHR interpretation requires a critical assessment of the scientific evidence underlying the relationships between FHR patterns and fetal physiology. This chapter has reviewed in detail the relationships between specific FHR patterns and fetal physiology with particular emphasis on evidence-based interpretation. Regarding the relationship between FHR patterns and fetal oxygenation, evidence-based FHR interpretation can be distilled into two basic concepts. These concepts are illustrated in Figure 5.17.

The concepts developed in this chapter form the basis of systematic management of FHR patterns discussed in Chapter 6.

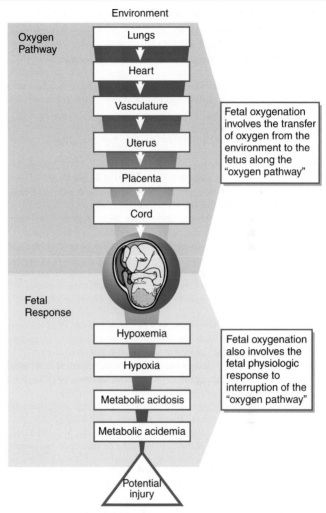

FIGURE 5.17 Two central principles of intrapartum FHR interpretation.

References

[1] Electronic fetal heart rate monitoring: research guidelines for interpretation. National Institute of Child Health and Human Development Research Planning Workshop, Am. J. Obstet. Gynecol. 177 (1997) 1385–1390.

[2] J. Itskovitz, E.F. LaGamma, A.M. Rudolph, Effect of cord compression on fetal blood flow distribution and O_2 delivery, Am. J. Physiol. 252 (1987) H100–H109.

[3] Intrapartum fetal heart rate monitoring. ACOG Practice Bulletin No.70 American College of Obstetricians and Gynecologists, Obstet. Gynecol. 106 (2005) 1453–1461.

[4] A. Fleischer, H. Schulman, N. Jagani, J. Mitchell, G. Randolph, The development of fetal acidosis in the presence of an abnormal fetal heart rate tracing. I. The average for gestational age fetus, Am. J. Obstet. Gynecol. 144 (1982) 55–60.

[5] J.A. Low, R.S. Galbraith, D.W. Muir, H.L. Killen, E.A. Pater, E.J. Karchmar, Factors associated with motor and cognitive deficits in children after intrapartum fetal hypoxia, Am. J. Obstet. Gynecol. 148 (1982) 533–539.

[6] I. Ingemarsson, A. Herbst, K. Thorgren-Jerneck, Long term outcome after umbilical artery acidemia at term birth: influence of gender and fetal heart rate abnormalities, Br. J. Obstet. Gynaecol. 104 (1997) 1123–1127.

[7] J.T. Parer, T. King, S. Flanders, M. Fox, S.J. Kilpatrick, Fetal acidemia and electronic fetal heart rate patterns. Is there evidence of an association, J. Matern. Fetal Neonatal Med. 19 (2006) 289–924.

[8] J.T. Parer, T. Ikeda, A framework for standardized management of intrapartum fetal heart rate patterns, Am. J. Obstet. Gynecol. 197 (2007) 26. e1–26.e6.

[9] C.G. Hatjis, P.J. Meis, Sinusoidal fetal heart rate pattern associated with butorphanol administration, Obstet. Gynecol. 67 (1986) 377–380.

[10] M. Hallak, J. Martinez-Poyer, M.L. Kruger, S. Hassan, S.C. Blackwell, Y. Sorokin, The effect of magnesium sulfate on fetal heart rate parameters: a randomized, placebo-controlled trial, Am. J. Obstet. Gynecol. 181 (1999) 1122–1127.

[11] G. Giannina, E.R. Guzman, Y.L. Lai, M.F. Lake, M. Cernadas, A.M. Vintzileos, Comparison of the effects of meperidine and nalbuphine on intrapartum fetal heart rate tracings, Obstet. Gynecol. 86 (1995) 441–445.

[12] S.L. Clark, M.L. Gimovski, F.C. Miller, Fetal heart rate response to scalp blood sampling, Am. J. Obstet. Gynecol. 144 (1982) 706–708.

[13] C.V. Smith, H.N. Nguyen, J.P. Phelan, R.H. Paul, Intrapartum assessment of fetal well-being: a comparison of fetal acoustic stimulation with acid base determinations, Am. J. Obstet. Gynecol. 155 (1986) 726–728.

[14] J.A. Read, F.C. Miller, Fetal heart rate aceleration in response to acoustic stimulation as a measure of fetal well-being, Am. J. Obstet. Gynecol. 129 (1997) 512–517.

[15] A. Elimian, R. Figueroa, N. Tejani, Intrapartum assessment of fetal well being: a comparison of scalp stimulation with scalp blood pH sampling, Obstet. Gynecol. 89 (1997) 373–376.

[16] E.A. Kopecky, M.L. Ryan, J.F. Barrett, P.G. Seaward, G. Ryan, G. Koren, et al., Fetal response to maternally administered morphine, Am. J. Obstet. Gynecol. 183 (2000) 424–430.

[17] C.B. Martin Jr., J. de Haan, B. van der Wildt, H.W. Jongsma, A. Dieleman, T.H. Arts, Mechanisms of late decelerations in the fetal heart rate. A study with autonomic blocking agents in fetal lambs, Eur. J. Obstet. Gynecol. Reprod. Biol. 9 (6) (1979) 361–373.

[18] H.E. Cohn, E.J. Sacks, M.A. Heymann, A.M. Rudolph, Cardiovascular response to hypoxemia and acidemia in fetal lambs, Am. J. Obstet. Gynecol. 120 (1974) 817–824.

[19] L.L. Peeters, R.D. Sheldon, M.D. Jones, E.L. Makowski, G. Meschia, Blood flow to fetal organs as a function of arterial oxygen content, Am. J. Obstet. Gynecol. 135 (1979) 637–646.

[20] B.S. Richardson, D. Rurak, J.E. Patrick, J. Homan, L. Carmichael, Cerebral oxidative metabolism during prolonged hypoxemia, J. Dev. Physiol. 11 (1989) 37–43.

[21] D.R. Field, J.T. Parer, R.A. Auslander, D.B. Cheek, W. Baker, J. Johnson, Cerebral oxygen consumption during asphyxia in fetal sheep, J. Dev. Physiol. 14 (1990) 131–137.

[22] D.L. Reid, J.T. Parer, K. Williams, D. Darr, T.M. Phermaton, J.H.H. Rankin, Effects of severe reduction in maternal placental blood flow on blood flow distribution in the sheep fetus, J. Dev. Physiol. 15 (1991) 183–188.

[23] A. Jensen, C. Roman, A.M. Rudolph, Effects of reducing uterine blood flow on fetal blood flow distribution and oxygen delivery, J. Dev. Physiol. 15 (1991) 309–323.

[24] R.H. Ball, M.I. Expinoza, J.T. Parer, Regional blood flow in asphyxiated fetuses with seizures, Am. J. Obstet. Gynecol. 170 (1994) 156–161.

[25] R.H. Ball, J.T. Parer, L.E. Caldwell, J. Johnson, Regional blood flow and metabolism in ovine fetuses during severe cord occlusion, Am. J. Obstet. Gynecol. 171 (1994) 1549–1555.

[26] J. Barcroft, Researches in Prenatal Life, Blackwell Scientific Publications, Oxford, UK, 1946.

[27] M.D. Towell, H.S. Salvador, Compression of the umbilical cord, in: P. Crasignoni, G. Pardi (Eds.), An Experimental Model in the Fetal Goat, Fetal Evaluation during Pregnancy and Labor, Academic Press, New York, 1971, pp. 143–156.

[28] S.T. Lee, E.H. Hon, Fetal hemodynamic response to umbilical cord compression, Obstet. Gynecol. 22 (1963) 553–562.

[29] M.N. Yeh, H.O. Morishima, W.E. Niemann, L.S. James, Myocardial conduction defects in association with compression of the umbilical cord. Experimental observations on fetal baboons, Am. J. Obstet. Gynecol. 121 (1975) 951–957.

[30] B. Siassi, P.Y. Wu, C. Blanco, C.B. Martin, Baroreceptor and chemoreceptor responses to umbilical cord occlusion in fetal lambs, Biol. Neonate 35 (1979) 66–73.

[31] J. Itskovitz, E.F. LaGamma, A.M. Rudolph, Heart rate and blood pressure responses to umbilical cord compression in fetal lambs with special reference to the mechanism of variable deceleration, Am. J. Obstet. Gynecol. 147 (1983) 451–457.

[32] J. Itskovitz, E.F. LaGamma, A.M. Rudolph, The effect of reducing umbilical blood flow on fetal oxygenation, Am. J. Obstet. Gynecol. 145 (1983) 813–818.

[33] L.S. James, M.N. Yeh, H.O. Morishima, S.S. Daniel, S.N. Caritis, W.H. Niemann, et al., Umbilical vein occlusion and transient acceleration of the fetal heart rate. Experimental observations in subhuman primates, Am. J. Obstet. Gynecol. 126 (1976) 276–283.

[34] E. Mueller-Heubach, A.F. Battelli, Variable heart rate decelerations and transcutaneous Po_2 during umbilical cord occlusion in fetal monkeys, Am. J. Obstet. Gynecol. 144 (1982) 796–802.

[35] C.Y. Lee, P.C. Di Loreto, J.M. O'Lane, A study of fetal heart rate acceleration patterns, Obstet. Gynecol. 45 (1975) 142–146.

[36] K. Brubaker, T.J. Garite, The lambda fetal heart rate pattern: an assessment of its significance in the intrapartum period, Obstet. Gynecol. 72 (1988) 881–885.

[37] J.A. Westgate, L. Bennet, H.H. de Haan, A.J. Gunn, Fetal heart rate overshoot during repeated umbilical cord occlusion in sheep, Obstet. Gynecol. 97 (2001) 454–459.

[38] J.R. Shields, B.S. Schifrin, Perinatal antecedents of cerebral palsy, Obstet. Gynecol. 71 (1988) 899–905.

[39] J. Saito, K. Okamura, K. Akagi, S. Tanigawara, Y. Shintaku, T. Watanabe, N., et al., Alteration of FHR pattern associated with progressively advanced fetal acidemia caused by cord compression, Nippon Sanka Fujinka Gakkai Zasshi 40 (1988) 775–780.

[40] B.S. Schifrin, T. Hamilton-Rubinstein, J.R. Shield, Fetal heart rate patterns and the timing of fetal injury, J. Perinatol. 14 (1994) 174–181.

[41] R.C. Goodlin, E.W. Lowe, A functional umbilical cord occlusion heart rate pattern. The significance of overshoot, Obstet. Gynecol. 43 (1974) 22–30.

[42] C.Y. Spong, C. Rascul, J.Y. Collea, G.S. Eglinton, A. Ghidini, Characterization and prognositic significance of variable decelerations in the second stage of labor, Am. J. Perinatol. 15 (1998) 369–374.

[43] F.W. Kubli, E.H. Hon, A.F. Khazin, H. Takemura, Observations on heart rate and pH in the human fetus during labor, Am. J. Obstet. Gynecol. 104 (1969) 1190–1206.

[44] B.S. Schifrin, S. Ater, Fetal hypoxic and ischemic injuries, Curr. Opin. Obstet. Gynecol. 18 (2006) 112–122.

[45] L. Svenningsen, R. Lindemann, K. Eidal, Measurements of fetal head compression pressure during bearing down and their relationship to the condition of the newborn, Acta Obstet. Gynecol. Scand. 67 (2) (1988) 129–133.

[46] L.I. Mann, A. Carmichael, S. Duchin, The effect of head compression on FHR, brain metabolism, and function, Obstet. Gynecol. 39 (1972) 721–726.

[47] W.F. O'Brien, S.E. Davis, M.P. Grissom, R.R. Eng, S.M. Golden, Effect of cephalic pressure on fetal cerebral blood flow, Am. J. Perinatol. 1 (1984) 223–226.

[48] C.J. Aldrich, D. D'Antona, J.A. Spencer, et al., The effect of maternal pushing on fetal cerebral oxygenation and blood volume during the second stage of labour, Br. J. Obstet. Gynaecol. 102 (1995) 448–453.

[49] A.P. Harris, R.C. Koehler, C.A. Gleason, M.D. Jones Jr., R.J. Traystman, Cerebral and peripheral circulatory responses to intracranial hypertension in fetal sheep, Circ. Res. 64 (5) (1989) 991–1000.

[50] A.P. Harris, S. Helou, R.J. Traystman, M.D. Jones Jr., R.C. Koehler, Efficacy of the Cushing response in maintaining cerebral blood flow in premature and near-term fetal sheep, Pediatr. Res. 43 (1) (1998 Jan) 50–56.

[51] D. Towner, M.A. Castro, E. Eby-Wilkens, W.M. Gilbert, Effect of mode of delivery in nulliparous women on neonatal intracranial injury, N. Engl. J. Med. 341 (1999) 1709–1714.

[52] L. Luo, D. Chen, Y. Qu, J. Wu, X. Li, D. Mu, Association between hypoxia and perinatal arterial ischemic stroke: a meta-analysis. PLoS One 9 (2) (2014), e90106. http://dx.doi.org/10.1371/journal.pone.0090106.

[53] M.J. Benders, F. Groenendaal, C.S. Uiterwaal, P.G. Nikkels, H.W. Bruinse, et al., Maternal and infant characteristics associated with perinatal arterial stroke in the preterm infant, Stroke 38 (6) (2007) 1759–1765.

[54] J. Lee, L.A. Croen, K.H. Backstrand, C.K. Yoshida, L.H. Henning, C. Lindan, D.M. Ferriero, H.J. Fullerton, A.J. Barkovich, Y.W. Wu, Maternal and infant characteristics associated with perinatal arterial stroke in the infant, JAMA 293 (6) (2005) 723–729.

[55] V. Darmency-Stamboul, C. Chantegret, C. Ferdynus, N. Mejean, C. Durand, P. Sagot, M. Giroud, Y. Bejot, J.B. Gouyon, Antenatal factors associated with perinatal arterial ischemic stroke, Stroke 43 (9) (2012) 2307–2312.

[56] J.C. Harteman, F. Groenendaal, A. Kwee, P.M. Welsing, M.J. Benders, L.S. de Vries, Risk factors for perinatal arterial ischaemic stroke in full-term infants: a case-control study, Arch. Dis. Child. Fetal Neonatal Ed. 97 (6) (2012) F411–F416.

CHAPTER 6

Intrapartum Management of the Fetal Heart Rate Tracing

Chapters 2 and 4 provided the physiologic basis for fetal heart rate (FHR) monitoring and evaluation of uterine activity. Chapter 5 reviewed the standardized National Institute of Child Health and Human Development (NICHD) definitions and introduced an evidence-based approach to the interpretation of FHR patterns. This chapter incorporates those previously developed concepts and presents a systematic, comprehensive, and multidisciplinary approach to management of intrapartum FHR tracings.

FUNDAMENTAL PRINCIPLES

As introduced at the close of Chapter 5, two central principles of evidence-based FHR interpretation provide the foundation for a systematic approach to FHR management. Figure 6.1 illustrates these principles. They are as follows:

1. Variable, late, and prolonged FHR decelerations reflect interruption of oxygen transfer from the environment to the fetus at one or more points along the oxygen pathway.
2. Moderate variability and/or accelerations reliably predict the absence of fetal hypoxic injury at the time they are observed.

A common misconception is that standardized FHR management is a "one-size-fits-all" approach that supplants individual clinical judgment and dictates the timing and method of delivery. On the contrary, standardized intrapartum FHR management is intended to encourage the timely application of individual clinical judgment and to serve as a systematic reminder of potential sources of preventable error in the effort to optimize outcomes and minimize risk. The model described in this chapter uses the standardized FHR definitions and categories proposed by the NICHD in 2008 [1]. It does not include adjunctive tests of fetal status such as fetal scalp blood sampling, fetal pulse oximetry, and fetal ST segment analysis that are currently unavailable for general clinical use in the United States. These techniques are reviewed at the end of the chapter.

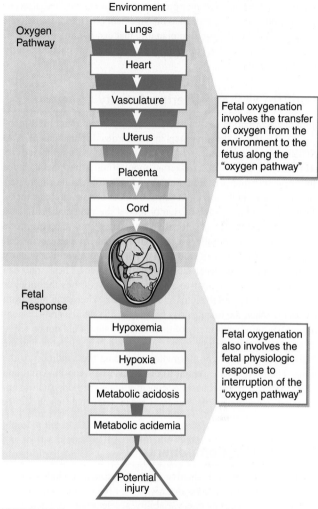

FIGURE 6.1 Two central principles of intrapartum FHR interpretation.

Standard of Care

The standard of care mandates that practitioners provide patient care that is reasonable. Reasonableness, in turn, is determined by factual accuracy and the ability to articulate a clear and understandable plan.

Standard definitions and interpretation help to ensure factual accuracy. A standardized approach to management provides a framework for organized, evidence-based planning that can minimize variation, reduce the potential for preventable error, and be articulated clearly and understandably.

Confirm FHR and Uterine Activity

Reliable information is vital to the success of intrapartum FHR monitoring. Therefore the first step in standardized management is to confirm that the monitor is recording the FHR and uterine activity accurately (Figure 6.2). If external monitoring is not adequate for definition and interpretation, a fetal scalp electrode and/or intrauterine pressure catheter might be helpful. Under certain circumstances, the FHR monitor can inadvertently record the maternal heart rate. For example, if the fetus is not alive, an internal fetal scalp electrode will record the maternal heart rate. An external Doppler device can record the maternal heart rate even if the fetus is alive. Particularly in the setting of maternal tachycardia, the maternal heart rate can appear deceptively similar to a normal FHR. At times the monitor can alternately record the fetus and the mother. When switching from one to the other, the tracing does not necessarily demonstrate discontinuity. Therefore continuity of the tracing alone should not be relied on to exclude this phenomenon. Unless the monitor is recording the FHR, it can provide no information regarding the condition of the fetus. Therefore it is essential to distinguish between maternal and FHRs. If there is any question, consider other methods such as ultrasound, palpation of the maternal pulse, fetal scalp electrode, or maternal pulse oximetry.

Evaluate FHR Components

Thorough, systematic evaluation of an FHR tracing includes assessment of uterine contractions along with the FHR components defined by the NICHD: baseline rate, variability, accelerations, decelerations, sinusoidal pattern, and changes or trends in the tracing over time. The 2008 NICHD consensus report defined three categories of FHR tracings as summarized in Table 6.1 [1]. If all FHR components are normal (Category I), the FHR tracing reliably predicts the absence of fetal metabolic acidemia and ongoing hypoxic injury. In low-risk patients, American College of Obstetrics and Gynecology (ACOG) Practice Bulletin 106 and ACOG-American Academy of Pediatrics

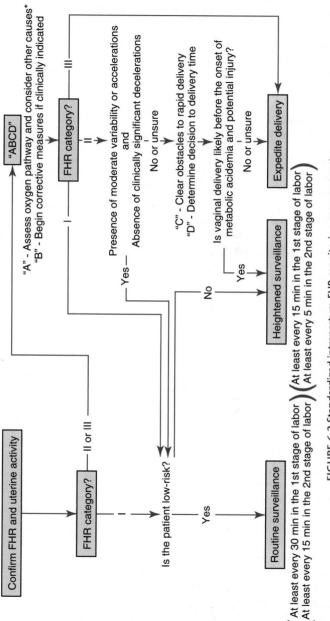

FIGURE 6.2 Standardized intrapartum FHR monitoring management.

TABLE 6.1   Three-tier FHR Classification System

Category I	
Normal	FHR tracing includes all of the following:
	Baseline rate: 110–160 bpm
	Baseline FHR variability: moderate
	Accelerations: present or absent
	Late or variable decelerations absent
	Early decelerations present or absent
Category II	
Indeterminate	Includes all FHR tracings not assigned to Categories I or III
Category III	
Abnormal	FHR tracing includes at least one of the following:
	Absent variability with recurrent late decelerations
	Absent variability with recurrent variable decelerations
	Absent variability with bradycardia for at least 10 minutes
	Sinusoidal pattern for at least 20 minutes

Adapted from G.A. Macones et al. Obstet. Gynecol. 112 (2008): 661–666.

(AAP) Guidelines for Perinatal Care recommend that the FHR tracing should be reviewed at least every 30 minutes during the active phase of the first stage of labor and at least every 15 minutes during the second stage [2,3]. In high-risk patients, the FHR tracing should be reviewed at least every 15 minutes during the active phase of the first stage of labor and at least every 5 minutes during the second stage (Figure 6.2). Nursing documentation should comply with hospital policies and procedures. Physician and midwife documentation should be performed periodically. Documentation and risk management issues are discussed in detail in Chapter 10.

A Standardized "ABCD" Approach to FHR Management

If assessment of FHR components indicates that the tracing is anything other than Category I, further evaluation is warranted. A practical, systematic "ABCD" approach to management is as follows:

A—Assess the oxygen pathway (and consider other causes of FHR changes)

B—Begin conservative corrective measures as needed

C—Clear obstacles to rapid delivery

D—Delivery plan

This approach is summarized in Table 6.2.

TABLE 6.2   ABCD FHR Management

	A Assess Oxygen Pathway	B Begin Corrective Measures If Indicated[a]		C Clear Obstacles to Rapid Delivery	D Determine Decision to Delivery Time
Lungs	Airway Breathing	Supplemental oxygen	Facility	OR availability Equipment	Response time
Heart	Heart rate and rhythm Cardiac output	IV fluid bolus Maternal position changes Correct hypotension	Staff	Consider notifying • Obstetrician • Surgical assistant • Anesthesiologist • Neonatologist • Pediatrician • Nursing staff	Consider staff • Availability • Training • Experience
Vasculature	Blood pressure Volume status		Mother	Informed consent IV access Anesthesia options Laboratory tests Blood products Urinary catheter	Surgical considerations (prior abdominal or uterine surgery) Medical considerations (obesity, hypertension, diabetes)

Continued

TABLE 6.2   ABCD FHR Management—cont'd

	A Assess Oxygen Pathway	B Begin Corrective Measures If Indicated[a]		C Clear Obstacles to Rapid Delivery	D Determine Decision to Delivery Time
Uterus	Contraction strength Contraction frequency Baseline uterine tone Uterine relaxation time Exclude uterine rupture	Stop or reduce stimulant Consider uterine relaxant	Fetus	Confirm ■ Estimated fetal weight ■ Gestational age ■ Presentation ■ Position	Consider ■ Estimated fetal weight ■ Gestational age ■ Presentation ■ Position
Placenta	Placental separation Vasa previa		Labor	Confirm ■ Accurate monitoring ■ Adequate uterine activity	Consider ■ Arrest disorder ■ Protracted labor ■ Remote from delivery ■ Poor expulsive efforts
Cord	Vaginal examination Exclude cord prolapse	Consider amnioinfusion			

Examples of clinical factors to be considered in a systematic fashion. Institutions may modify to individual circumstances. *OR,* operating room.

[a]Conservative corrective measures should be guided by clinical circumstances. For example, amnioinfusion may be appropriate in the presence of variable decelerations but would not be expected to result in resolution of late decelerations.

A: Assess the Oxygen Pathway and Consider Other Causes of FHR Changes

Rapid, systematic assessment of the pathway of oxygen transfer from the environment to the fetus can identify potential sources of interrupted oxygenation. Assessment of the maternal lungs can be as simple as checking the respiratory rate. The heart and the vasculature usually can be assessed by checking the maternal pulse and blood pressure. Uterine activity can be assessed by palpation or by review of the information obtained from a tocodynamometer or intrauterine pressure catheter. The possibility of placental separation can be assessed by checking for vaginal bleeding. Finally, the possibility of umbilical cord prolapse can be assessed by visual examination or by a vaginal examination. If rapid evaluation of these steps suggests that further investigation is warranted, it should be undertaken as deemed necessary. Chapter 5 identified a number of maternal and fetal factors that can influence the appearance of the FHR tracing by mechanisms other than interruption of fetal oxygenation (Box 6.1). If the FHR changes are thought to be due to any condition not directly related to fetal oxygenation, individualized management must be directed at the specific cause. Correction of fetal oxygenation cannot reasonably be expected to resolve FHR abnormalities that are not related to oxygenation. For example, supplemental oxygen, maternal position changes, and intravenous fluid boluses are unlikely to correct fetal tachycardia that is secondary to fetal arrhythmia or severe

---

BOX 6.1   Causes of FHR Changes Not Directly Related to Fetal Oxygenation

Maternal
- Fever
- Infection
- Medication
- Hyperthyroidism

Fetal
- Sleep cycle
- Infection
- Anemia
- Arrhythmia
- Heart block
- Congenital anomaly
- Preexisting neurologic injury
- Extreme prematurity

fetal anemia caused by parvovirus infection or Rh isoimmunization. Corrective interventions for fetal arrhythmias or severe fetal anemia can be extremely complex and usually require subspecialty consultation. Management of conditions such as these is beyond the scope of this chapter.

B: Begin Corrective Measures as Indicated

At each point along the oxygen pathway, conservative corrective measures are initiated, if indicated, to optimize fetal oxygenation (Table 6.2). Scientific evidence supporting the efficacy of each of these measures is detailed in an excellent review by Simpson and James [4]. These conservative corrective measures are summarized next.

Supplemental Oxygen

Fetal oxygenation is dependent on the oxygen content of maternal blood perfusing the intervillous space of the placenta, as discussed in Chapter 2. Administration of supplemental oxygen increase the Po_2 of inspired air, increasing both the partial pressure of oxygen dissolved in maternal blood and the amount of oxygen bound to hemoglobin. This can increase the oxygen concentration gradient across the placental blood–blood barrier and lead to increased fetal Po_2 and oxygen content. Several studies have reported resolution of FHR decelerations after administration of supplemental oxygen to the mother, providing indirect evidence of improved fetal oxygenation [4]. Direct evidence is provided by fetal pulse oximetry studies demonstrating increased fetal hemoglobin saturation after maternal administration of oxygen. Although the optimal method and duration of oxygen administration are not known, available data supports the use of a nonrebreather face mask to administer oxygen at a rate of 10 L/min for approximately 15 to 30 minutes [4].

Maternal Position Changes

There are sound physiologic reasons to avoid the supine position during labor. Supine positioning increases the likelihood that pressure on the inferior vena cava will impair venous return, cardiac output, and perfusion of the intervillous space. It also increases the likelihood that pressure on the descending aorta and/or iliac vessels will impede the delivery of oxygenated blood to the intervillous space. Prospective fetal pulse oximetry data confirm that left or right lateral positioning results in higher fetal hemoglobin saturation levels than does supine positioning [4]. In the setting of suspected umbilical cord compression, maternal position changes may result in fetal position changes and relief of pressure on the umbilical cord.

Intravenous Fluid Administration

Optimal uterine perfusion depends on optimal cardiac output and intravascular volume. Normal blood pressure does not necessarily reflect optimal intravascular volume, venous return, preload, or cardiac output. An intravascular bolus of isotonic fluid can improve cardiac output not only by increasing circulating volume but also by increasing venous return, left ventricular end diastolic pressure, ventricular preload, and, ultimately, stroke volume in accordance with the Frank-Starling mechanism. In this way, a relatively small increase in intravascular volume can have a significant effect on cardiac output and uterine perfusion. An intravenous fluid bolus of 500 to 1000 mL can result in improved fetal oxygenation even in an apparently euvolemic patient [4]. Excessive fluid administration can have serious consequences, and caution must be exercised in patients at risk for volume overload, pulmonary edema, or both. The optimal rate of intravenous fluid administration during labor is not known. Potential maternal and fetal complications argue against administering large-volume intravenous boluses of glucose-containing fluids.

Correct Maternal Blood Pressure

A number of factors predispose laboring women to transient episodes of hypotension. These include inadequate hydration, insensible fluid losses, supine position resulting in compression of the inferior vena cava, decreased venous return and reduced cardiac output, and peripheral vasodilation due to sympathetic blockade during regional anesthesia. Maternal hypotension can reduce uterine perfusion and fetal oxygenation. Hydration and lateral or Trendelenburg positioning usually correct the blood pressure. If these measures do not achieve the desired result, medication may be necessary. Ephedrine is a sympathomimetic α-amine with weak α- and β-agonist activity. The primary mechanism of action is the release of norepinephrine from presynaptic vesicles, resulting in stimulation of postsynaptic adrenergic receptors. Ephedrine has no known adverse effect on fetal outcome.

Reduce Uterine Activity

As discussed in previous chapters, excessive uterine activity is a common cause of interrupted fetal oxygenation. It is also a common source of medical-legal liability. Clinicians have used a number of terms to describe excessive uterine activity. Examples include *hyperstimulation, hypercontractility, tachysystole, hypertonus,* and *tetanic contraction.* These terms are defined inconsistently in the literature and are used inconsistently by clinicians. The 2008 NICHD consensus statement recommended using the term *tachysystole* to describe uterine contraction frequency in excess of five contractions in 10 minutes averaged over 30 minutes [1]. Normal contraction frequency is defined as five or fewer contractions in 10 minutes averaged over 30 minutes. The report specifically noted that other features of uterine activity are clinically important as well, including contraction duration, intensity, resting tone, and time between contractions. For the purposes of FHR management, if an abnormal FHR pattern is thought to be related to excessive uterine activity, options include position changes, intravenous hydration, reduction in dose or discontinuation of uterine stimulants, and/or administration of uterine relaxants. The evaluation and management of uterine activity are discussed in detail in Chapter 4.

Alter Second-stage Pushing Technique

During the second stage of labor, maternal expulsive efforts can be associated with FHR decelerations. Suggested corrective approaches include open-glottis rather than Valsalva-style pushing, fewer pushing efforts per contraction, shorter individual pushing efforts, pushing with every other or every third contraction, and, in patients with regional anesthesia, pushing only with perceived urge [4].

Amnioinfusion

Intrapartum amnioinfusion involves infusion of isotonic fluid through an intrauterine catheter into the amniotic cavity to restore the amniotic fluid volume to normal or near-normal levels. The procedure is intended to relieve intermittent umbilical cord compression, variable FHR decelerations, and transient fetal hypoxemia and to dilute thick meconium in an attempt to prevent meconium aspiration syndrome. Amnioinfusion performed for the indication of oligohydramnios and umbilical cord compression can reduce the occurrence of variable decelerations and lower the rate of cesarean delivery. It has no known effect on late decelerations. Routine amnioinfusion for meconium-stained amniotic fluid without variable decelerations is not recommended by ACOG [5]. A procedure for amnioinfusion is described in Appendix A. A systematic approach to FHR management does not require the use of all of these measures in every situation. It simply helps to ensure that important considerations are not overlooked and that decisions are made in a timely manner. In addition, it provides a framework to help clinicians articulate a thoughtful, organized plan of management, a key element of reasonableness and the standard of care.

Reevaluate the FHR Tracing

After assessing the oxygen pathway and beginning corrective measures that are deemed appropriate, the tracing is reevaluated. The time frame for reevaluation is based on clinical judgment but usually ranges from 5 to 30 minutes, in accordance with ACOG-AAP guidelines [2,3]. If the FHR tracing returns to Category I, continued surveillance is appropriate. The decision to perform routine or heightened surveillance is based on clinical judgment, taking into account the entire clinical situation. If the FHR tracing progresses to Category III despite appropriate conservative corrective measures, delivery is usually expedited. Tracings that remain in Category II warrant additional evaluation. Category II is extremely broad. It includes FHR tracings for which continued surveillance is appropriate. However, it also includes tracings that require preparations for rapid delivery. If a Category II FHR tracing reveals clinically insignificant interruption of fetal oxygenation (absent or infrequent decelerations) and excludes fetal metabolic acidemia and ongoing hypoxic injury (moderate variability and/or accelerations), continued surveillance is reasonable. Category II tracings that do not meet these criteria require further measures. If there is any question regarding the clinical significance of any decelerations, the presence of moderate variability or the presence of accelerations, the safest and easiest approach is to take the next step in the ABCD management model.

C: Clear Obstacles to Rapid Delivery

If conservative corrective measures do not result in moderate variability (and/or accelerations) and resolution of clinically significant decelerations, it is prudent to plan ahead for the possible need for rapid delivery. Planning ahead does not constitute a commitment to a particular time or method of delivery. Instead, it serves as a systematic reminder of common sources of unnecessary delay so that important factors are not overlooked and decisions are made in a timely manner. This can be accomplished by systematically gathering necessary information and communicating proactively with other members of the team. This step involves many commonsense considerations that do not necessarily require medical expertise. As a result, this step does not always receive the serious, systematic attention it warrants and is often left to the vagaries of random recall. Failure to take simple precautions to avoid unnecessary delay can jeopardize patient safety and can be a source of intense criticism in the event of an undesired outcome. Fortunately, there is an alternative to random recall. Potential sources of unnecessary delay can be grouped into five major categories. Organized in nonrandom order, from largest to smallest, these five categories include the facility, staff, mother, fetus, and labor. Table 6.2 identifies some examples of potential sources of unnecessary delay at each level. Standardized intrapartum FHR management does not mandate that each of these measures is carried out. It simply provides a practical checklist of factors to consider. The checklist approach promotes team communication, encourages timely decision making, and minimizes preventable errors.

D: Delivery Plan

After appropriate conservative measures have been implemented, it is sensible to take a moment to estimate the time needed to accomplish delivery in the event of a sudden deterioration of the FHR tracing. The anticipated decision-to-delivery time must be taken into consideration when weighing the risks and benefits of continued expectant management versus expeditious delivery. This step can be facilitated by systematically considering individual characteristics of the facility, staff, mother, fetus, and labor (Table 6.2).

Management steps A, B, C, and D are largely uncontroversial. They are readily amenable to standardization and represent the overwhelming majority of decisions that must be made during labor. However, once they are exhausted, further management decisions rely on the individual clinical judgment of the care provider who is ultimately responsible for the safety of the mother and the fetus.

Expectant Management Versus Delivery

If conservative measures are unsuccessful, the clinician must decide whether to await spontaneous vaginal delivery or to expedite delivery by other means. This decision demands individual clinical judgment, weighing the estimated time until vaginal delivery against the estimated time until the onset of metabolic acidemia and potential injury. In 2013 Clark and colleagues proposed a standardized approach to the management of persistent Category II FHR tracings [6]. The authors recommended that in the setting of moderate variability or accelerations and normal progress in the active phase or second stage of labor, expectant management with close observation is reasonable in most cases, regardless of the presence of decelerations. One exception is a prolonged deceleration, which requires immediate response. Another is the setting in which vaginal bleeding and/or previous cesarean delivery(ies) introduce the risks of placental abruption or uterine rupture. If moderate variability and accelerations are absent and recurrent significant decelerations fail to respond to corrective measures for 30 minutes, delivery should be considered regardless of the stage of labor. If moderate variability and accelerations are absent *without* recurrent decelerations, the authors recommended consideration of delivery after approximately 60 minutes. These recommendations reflect the consensus of 18 authors regarding one reasonable approach to persistent Category II FHR patterns. No single approach to such patterns has been demonstrated to be superior to all others. However, there is a growing body of evidence supporting the concept that the adoption of one appropriate management plan, by virtue of standardization alone, will yield results superior to those achieved by random application of several individually equivalent approaches [6].

One of the most common preventable errors at this point in FHR management is to postpone a difficult decision in the hope that the situation will resolve on its own. It is highly advisable during this step of FHR management to resist the urge to delay an indicated decision. Instead, the clinician should use discipline and individual clinical judgment to make and document a plan based on the best information available. If the clinician decides to expedite delivery, the rationale should be documented, and the plan should be implemented. If the clinician decides to continue to wait for vaginal delivery, the rationale and plan should be documented, and the decision should be revisited after a reasonable period of time. It is critical to recognize that, both medically and legally, "deciding to wait" is distinctly different from "waiting to decide." The former reflects the application of clinical judgment, whereas the latter can be construed as procrastination. As long as reasonable judgment is exercised, "deciding to wait" is likely to be defensible, regardless of the eventual outcome. "Waiting to decide," however, puts the clinician in the difficult position of trying to explain why he or she neglected to make a medically necessary decision in a timely fashion.

The standardized management algorithm detailed in this chapter expands the recommendations of ACOG Practice Bulletin 116 to provide an organized, systematic framework that can help clinicians at all levels of training and experience formulate a care plan that is factually accurate and articulate [7].

OTHER METHODS OF FETAL MONITORING

One of the major shortcomings of electronic fetal monitoring is a high rate of false-positive results. Even the most abnormal patterns are poorly predictive of neonatal morbidity. This has led to exploration of alternative methods of evaluating fetal status, including fetal scalp pH determination, scalp stimulation or vibroacoustic stimulation, computer analysis of FHR, fetal pulse oximetry, and ST segment analysis. In assessing the immediate condition of the newborn, umbilical cord acid–base determination is an adjunct to the Apgar score.

Intrapartum Fetal Scalp pH and Lactate Determination

Intermittent sampling of scalp blood for pH determination was described in the 1960s and studied extensively in the 1970s. However, its use has been limited by many factors, including the requirements for cervical dilation and membrane rupture, technical difficulty of the procedure, the need for serial pH determinations, and uncertainty regarding interpretation and application of results. It is used infrequently in the United States but remains a common practice in many other countries. A meta-analysis revealed that fetal scalp lactate determination was accomplished successfully more frequently than scalp pH determination. However, there were no differences in maternal, fetal, neonatal, or infant outcome [8].

Fetal Scalp Stimulation and Vibroacoustic Stimulation

A number of studies in the 1980s reported that an FHR acceleration in response to fetal scalp stimulation or vibroacoustic stimulation was highly predictive of normal scalp blood pH [9–15]. A literature review and meta-analysis by Skupski and colleagues confirmed the utility of various methods of intrapartum fetal stimulation, including scalp puncture, atraumatic stimulation with an Allis clamp, vibroacoustic stimulation, and digital stimulation [16]. It is crucial for clinicians to recognize that fetal scalp stimulation and vibroacoustic stimulation are diagnostic tools used to provoke FHR accelerations to exclude the presence of fetal metabolic acidemia. As noted previously, fetal stimulation procedures should be performed at times when the FHR is at baseline. Neither fetal scalp stimulation nor vibroacoustic stimulation is appropriate during FHR decelerations or bradycardia.

Computer Analysis of FHR

Subjective interpretation of FHR tracings by visual analysis has been hampered by inconsistency and imprecision. In an attempt to overcome this limitation, Dawes and others derived a system of numeric analysis of FHR [17]. Computer analysis of intrapartum FHR records has been reported to be more precise than visual assessment [18,19]. However, intrapartum computer analysis has not been shown to improve prediction of neonatal outcome. Keith and colleagues reported the results of a multicenter trial of an intelligent computer system using clinical data in addition to FHR data [20]. In 50 cases analyzed, the system's performance was indistinguishable from that of 17 expert clinicians. The authors reported that the system was highly consistent, recommended no unnecessary intervention, and performed better than all but two of the experts.

Fetal Pulse Oximetry

Intrapartum reflectance fetal pulse oximetry is a modification of transmission pulse oximetry that indirectly measures the oxygen saturation of hemoglobin in fetal blood. An intrauterine sensor placed in contact with fetal skin uses the differential absorption of red and infrared light by oxygenated and deoxygenated fetal hemoglobin to provide continuous estimation of fetal oxygen saturation. A number of studies have examined the utility of intrapartum fetal pulse oximetry [21–32].

Although the technology appears to reduce the incidence of cesarean delivery for fetal indications, no consistent effect on overall cesarean rates or newborn outcomes has been demonstrated. The results of a number of randomized trials led the manufacturer to announce that it would no longer distribute the sensors, effectively withdrawing the product from the market.

ST Segment Analysis

Study of the fetal electrocardiogram has produced promising initial results. In sheep, FHR decelerations that accompanied hypoxemia were associated with characteristic changes in the fetal P-R interval. In 2000, Strachan compared standard electronic fetal monitoring with electronic fetal monitoring plus P-R interval analysis in 1038 women [33]. The groups demonstrated statistically similar rates of operative intervention for presumed fetal distress and no differences in newborn outcomes. The ST segment of the fetal electrocardiogram represents myocardial repolarization. Myocardial hypoxia can lead to elevation of the ST segment and T wave secondary to catecholamine release, β-adrenoceptor activation, glycogenolysis, and tissue metabolic acidosis [34,35]. These observations have led to the development of technology to analyze the fetal electrocardiogram plus the ST waveform (STAN; Neoventa Medical, Göteborg, Sweden) [29,36]. One randomized trial in 2434 patients demonstrated a 46% reduction in operative intervention for fetal distress when ST segment analysis was added to standard electronic fetal monitoring [37]. Operative interventions for dystocia and other indications were not increased. Fewer cases of metabolic acidemia and low 5-minute Apgar scores were observed in the group with electronic fetal monitoring plus ST segment analysis; however, these differences did not reach statistical significance. Another trial using newer technology included 4966 women randomized to electronic fetal monitoring alone versus electronic fetal monitoring plus ST segment analysis [36]. When analyzed according to intention to treat, the incidence of umbilical artery acidemia was 53% lower in the electronic fetal monitoring plus ST segment analysis group. In the electronic fetal monitoring plus ST segment analysis group, the incidence of cesarean delivery for fetal distress was 8%, compared with 9% in the group monitored with electronic fetal monitoring alone ($P=0.047$). After excluding patients with inadequate FHR recordings and fetal malformations, these differences were slightly more pronounced.

A meta-analysis of four studies, including 9829 women, concluded that adjunctive ST segment analysis was associated with significantly fewer cases of severe metabolic acidemia at birth, fewer cases of neonatal encephalopathy, and fewer operative vaginal deliveries [38]. There were no significant differences in cesarean delivery rates, low 5-minute Apgar scores, or neonatal intensive care unit (NICU) admissions. One large multicenter trial randomized 5681 women to intrapartum electronic FHR monitoring alone versus electronic monitoring plus ST segment analysis [39]. No significant difference was observed in the primary outcome of metabolic acidosis, defined as an umbilical artery pH <7.05 with a base deficit of >12 mmol/L in the extracellular fluid. In the group with electronic monitoring plus ST analysis, there were statistically fewer cases of fetal blood sampling during labor (10.6% versus 20.4%, relative risk 0.52, 95% confidence interval 0.46–0.59), umbilical artery pH <7.05 and base deficit >12 mmol/L (1.6% versus 2.6%, relative risk 0.63, 95% confidence interval 0.42–0.97) and fewer cases of umbilical artery pH <7.05 (1.9% versus 2.7%, relative risk 0.67, 95% confidence interval 0.46–0.97). Total operative deliveries, cesarean deliveries, and instrumented vaginal deliveries occurred with statistically similar frequency in both groups. There were no differences in operative deliveries for fetal distress. There were no other statistically significant differences in newborn outcome. The NICHD Maternal Fetal Medicine Units Network recently completed a Phase III trial of the STAN monitor as an adjunct to electronic fetal monitoring in the United States. The multicenter trial randomized 11,108 women to undergo standard FHR monitoring with or without adjunct ST segment analysis. There were no significant differences between the two groups in the rates of operative vaginal delivery, cesarean delivery, NICU admission, meconium aspiration, or shoulder dystocia. The authors concluded that the use of STAN as an adjunct to conventional intrapartum electronic FHR monitoring did not improve perinatal outcomes or decrease operative deliveries in hospitals in the United States [40].

Umbilical Cord Blood Gas Analysis

Umbilical cord blood gas and pH assessment is a useful adjunct to the Apgar score in assessing the immediate condition of the newborn. There are no contraindications to obtaining cord gases.

ACOG [41] suggests obtaining cord gases in the following clinical situations:

- Cesarean delivery for fetal compromise
- Low 5-minute Apgar score
- Severe growth restriction
- Abnormal FHR tracing
- Maternal thyroid disease
- Intrapartum fever
- Multifetal gestations

Umbilical arterial values reflect fetal condition, whereas umbilical venous values reflect placental function. Normal findings preclude the presence of acidemia at, or immediately before, delivery.

Approximate normal values for cord blood are summarized in the following chart [42–45].

Approximate Normal Values for Cord Blood

Vessel	pH	P_{CO_2}	P_{O_2}	Base Deficit
Artery	7.2–7.3	45–55	15–25	<12
Vein	7.3–7.4	35–45	25–35	<12

The base deficit reflects utilization of buffer bases to help stabilize pH, usually in the setting of peripheral tissue hypoxia, anaerobic metabolism, and accumulation of lactic acid. An umbilical artery pH <7.20 usually is considered to define acidemia. Note that a much lower pH (7.0) is used to define the threshold of potential injury.

Acidemia is categorized as respiratory, metabolic, or mixed. Isolated respiratory acidemia is diagnosed when the umbilical artery pH is less than 7.20, the P_{CO_2} is elevated, and the base deficit is <12 mmol/L. This reflects interrupted exchange of blood gases, usually as a transient phenomenon related to umbilical cord compression. Isolated respiratory acidemia is not associated with fetal neurologic injury. Isolated metabolic acidemia is diagnosed when the pH is less than 7.20, the P_{CO_2} is normal, and the base deficit is at least 12 mmol/L. Metabolic acidemia can result from recurrent or prolonged interruption of fetal oxygenation that has progressed to the stage of peripheral tissue hypoxia, anaerobic metabolism, and lactic acid production in excess of buffering capacity. Although most cases of fetal metabolic acidemia do not result in injury, the risk is increased in the setting of significant metabolic acidemia (umbilical artery pH <7.0 and base deficit ≥12 mmol/L). Mixed (respiratory and metabolic) acidemia is diagnosed when the pH is below 7.20, the P_{CO_2} is elevated, and the base deficit is 12 mmol/L or greater. The clinical significance of mixed acidemia is similar to that of isolated metabolic acidemia. The types of acidemias (respiratory, metabolic, or mixed) are summarized in the following chart.

Types of Acidemias

Value	Respiratory	Metabolic	Mixed
pH	<7.20	<7.20	<7.20
P_{CO_2}	Elevated	Normal	Elevated
Base deficit	<12 mmol/L	≥12 mmol/L	≥12 mmol/L

The procedure for obtaining umbilical cord blood consists of double-clamping a 10- to 20-cm segment of the umbilical cord immediately after delivery. A specimen should be drawn with a 1-mL plastic syringe that has been flushed with heparin solution (1000 U/mL). Using separate syringes, draw blood from an umbilical artery first and then from the umbilical vein.

SUMMARY

Recent progress toward consensus in FHR monitoring makes it possible to construct a practical, standardized approach to FHR interpretation and management. The intrapartum FHR management model described in this chapter is not intended to dictate actions that must be taken in response to specific FHR patterns. Instead, it is intended to serve as a reminder of common sources of preventable error and an indicator of actions that should be considered to ensure that management decisions are made in a timely fashion. FHR definition, interpretation, and management should be guided by a few basic principles:

1. Simplicity is the key to consistent communication: *Unnecessary complexity predisposes to error.*
2. "Deciding to wait" is distinctly different from "waiting to decide": *The former reflects the application of clinical judgment; the latter can be construed as procrastination.*
3. The standard of care requires factual accuracy and the ability to articulate clearly and understandably: *Factual accuracy can be achieved by adhering to standardized FHR definitions and interpretation. A standardized "ABCD" approach to FHR management provides a framework that can help clinicians articulate a thorough, thoughtful, consistent plan of management.*

References

[1] G.A. Macones, G.D. Hankins, C.Y. Spong, J. Hauth, T. Moore, The 2008 National Institute of Child Health and Human Development workshop report on electronic fetal monitoring: update on definitions, interpretation, and research guidelines, Obstet. Gynecol. 112 (3) (2008) 661–666.

[2] American College of Obstetricians and Gynecologists, ACOG Practice Bulletin No. 106: Intrapartum fetal heart rate monitoring: nomenclature, interpretation, and general management principles, Obstet. Gynecol. 114 (2009) 192–202.

[3] American Academy of Pediatrics, American College of Obstetricians and Gynecologists: Guidelines for Perinatal Care (L.E. Riley, A.R. Stark, S.J. Kilpatrick, L.A. Papile, Eds.), seventh ed., Washington, DC, 2012.

[4] K.R. Simpson, D.C. James, Efficacy of intrauterine resuscitation techniques in improving fetal oxygen status during labor, Obstet. Gynecol. 105 (6) (2005) 1362–1368.

[5] American College of Obstetricians and Gynecologists, ACOG Committee Opinion No. 346. Amnioinfusion does not prevent meconium aspiration syndrome, ACOG, Washington, DC, 2006.

[6] S.L. Clark, M.P. Nageotte, T.J. Garite, R.K. Freeman, D.A. Miller, K. Rice-Simpson, et al., Intrapartum management of category II fetal heart rate tracings–towards standardization of care, Am. J. Obstet. Gynecol. 209 (2) (2013) 89–97.

[7] American College of Obstetricians and Gynecologists, ACOG Practice Bulletin No. 116. Management of intrapartum fetal heart rate tracings, Obstet. Gynecol. 116 (2010) 1232–1240.

[8] C.E. East, L.R. Leader, P. Sheehan, N.E. Henshall, P.B. Colditz, Intrapartum fetal scalp lactate sampling for fetal assessment in the presence of a non-reassuring fetal heart rate trace, Cochrane Database Syst. Rev. (3) (2010). CD006174, http://dx.doi.org/10.1002;14651858.CD006174.pub2.

[9] S.L. Clark, M.L. Gimovsky, F.C. Miller, The scalp stimulation test: a clinical alternative to fetal scalp blood sampling, Am. J. Obstet. Gynecol. 148 (3) (1984) 274–277.

[10] T.G. Edersheim, J.M. Hutson, M.L. Druzin, E.A. Kogut, Fetal heart rate response to vibratory acoustic stimulation predicts fetal pH in labor, Am. J. Obstet. Gynecol. 157 (6) (1987) 1557–1560.

[11] A. Elimian, R. Figueroa, N. Tejani, Intrapartum assessment of fetal well-being: a comparison of scalp stimulation with scalp blood pH sampling, Obstet. Gynecol. 89 (3) (1997) 373–376.

[12] I. Ingemarsson, S. Arulkumaran, Reactive fetal heart rate response to VAS in fetuses with low scalp blood pH, Br. J. Obstet. Gynaecol. 96 (5) (1989) 562–565.

[13] G.B. Polzin, K.J. Blakemore, R.H. Petrie, E. Amon, Fetal vibro-acoustic stimulation: magnitude and duration of fetal heart rate accelerations as a marker of fetal health, Obstet. Gynecol. 72 (4) (1988) 621–626.

[14] C.V. Smith, H.N. Nguyen, J.P. Phelan, R.H. Paul, Intrapartum assessment of fetal well-being: a comparison of fetal acoustic stimulation with acid-base determinations, Am. J. Obstet. Gynecol. 155 (4) (1986) 726–728.

[15] J.A. Spencer, Predictive value of a fetal heart rate acceleration at the time of fetal blood sampling in labour, J. Perinat. Med. 19 (3) (1991) 207–215.

[16] D.W. Skupski, C.R. Rosenberg, G.S. Eglington, Intrapartum fetal stimulation tests: a meta-analysis, Obstet. Gynecol. 99 (1) (2002) 129–134.

[17] G.S. Dawes, Computerised analysis of the fetal heart rate, Eur. J. Obstet. Gynecol. Reprod. Biol. 42 (Suppl.) (1991) S5–S8.

[18] G.S. Dawes, M. Moulden, O. Sheil, C.W.G. Redman, Approximate entropy, a statistic of regularity, applied to fetal heart rate data before and during labor, Obstet. Gynecol. 80 (5) (1992) 763–768.

[19] L.C. Pello, B.M. Rosevear, G.S. Dawes, M. Moulden, C.W. Redman, Computerized fetal heart rate analysis in labor, Obstet. Gynecol. 78 (4) (1991) 602–610.

[20] R.D.F. Keith, S. Beckly, J.M. Garibaldi, J.A. Westgate, E.C. Ifeachor, K.R. Greene, A multicentre comparative study of 17 experts and an intelligent computer system for managing labour using the cardiotocogram, Br. J. Obstet. Gynaecol. 102 (9) (1995) 688–700.

[21] S.L. Bloom, C.Y. Spong, E. Thom, M.W. Varner, D.J. Rouse, S. Weininger, et al., National Institute of Child Health and Human Development Maternal-Fetal Medicine Units Network: fetal pulse oximetry and cesarean delivery, N. Engl. J. Med. 355 (21) (2006) 2195–2202.

[22] G.A. Dildy, J.A. Thorp, J.D. Yeast, S.L. Clark, The relationship between oxygen saturation and pH in umbilical blood: implications for intrapartum fetal oxygen saturation monitoring, Am. J. Obstet. Gynecol. 175 (3 Pt 1) (1996) 682–687.

[23] G.A. Dildy, P.P. van den Berg, M. Katz, S.L. Clark, H.W. Jongsma, J.G. Nijhuis, et al., Intrapartum fetal pulse oximetry: fetal oxygen saturation trends during labor and relation to delivery outcome, Am. J. Obstet. Gynecol. 171 (3) (1994) 679–684.

[24] G.A. Dildy, S.L. Clark, C.A. Loucks, Preliminary experience with intrapartum fetal pulse oximetry in humans, Obstet. Gynecol. 81 (4) (1993) 630–635.

[25] G.A. Dildy, S.L. Clark, C.A. Loucks, Intrapartum fetal pulse oximetry: past, present, and future, Am. J. Obstet. Gynecol. 175 (1) (1996) 1–9.

[26] C.E. East, S.P. Brennecke, J.F. King, F.Y. Chan, P.B. Colditz, The effect of intrapartum fetal pulse oximetry, in the presence of a nonreassuring fetal heart rate pattern, on operative delivery rates: a multicenter, randomized, controlled trial (the FOREMOST trial), Am. J. Obstet. Gynecol. 194 (3) (2006) 606.e1–606.e16.

[27] T.J. Garite, G.A. Dildy, H. McNamara, M.P. Nageotte, F.H. Boehm, E.H. Dellinger, et al., A multicenter controlled trial of fetal pulse oximetry in the intrapartum management of nonreassuring fetal heart rate patterns, Am. J. Obstet. Gynecol. 183 (5) (2000) 1049–1058.

[28] C.K. Klauser, E.E. Christensen, S.P. Chauhan, L. Bufkin, E.F. Magann, J.A. Bofill, et al., Use of fetal pulse oximetry among high-risk women in labor: a randomized clinical trial, Am. J. Obstet. Gynecol. 192 (16) (2005) 1810–1819.

[29] M. Kuhnert, G. Seelbach-Goebel, M. Butterwegge, Predictive agreement between the fetal arterial oxygen saturation and fetal scalp pH: results of the German multicenter study, Am. J. Obstet. Gynecol. 178 (2) (1998) 330–335.

[30] R. Nijland, H.W. Jongsma, J.G. Nijhuis, P.P. van den Berg, B. Oeseburg, Arterial oxygen saturation in relation to metabolic acidosis in fetal lambs, Am. J. Obstet. Gynecol. 172 (3) (1995) 810–819.

[31] B. Oeseburg, B.E.M. Ringnalda, J. Crevels, H.W. Jongsma, P. Mannheimer, J. Menssen, et al., Fetal oxygenation in chronic maternal hypoxia: what's critical? Adv. Exp. Med. Biol. 317 (1992) 499–502.

[32] B. Seelbach-Gobel, M. Butterwegge, M. Kuhnert, M. Heupel, Fetal reflectance pulse oximetry. Experiences—prognostic significance and consequences—goals, Z. Geburtshilfe Perinatol 198 (1994) 67–71.

[33] B.K. Strachan, W.J. van Wijngaarden, D. Sahota, A. Chang, D.K. James, Cardiotocography only versus cardiotocography plus PR-interval analysis in intrapartum surveillance: a randomized, multicentre trial, Lancet 355 (9202) (2000) 456–459.

[34] K.H. Hökegård, B.O. Eriksson, I. Kjellemer, R. Magno, K.G. Rosén, Myocardial metabolism in relation to electrocardiographic changes and cardiac function during graded hypoxia in the fetal lamb, Acta Physiol. Scand. 113 (1) (1981) 1–7.

[35] C. Widmark, T. Jansson, K. Lindecrantz, K.G. Rosén, ECG waveform, short term heart rate variability and plasma catecholamine concentrations in response to hypoxia in intrauterine growth retarded guinea pig fetuses, J. Dev. Physiol. 15 (3) (1991) 161–168.

[36] I. Amer-Wåhlin, C. Hellsten, H. Norén, H. Hagberg, A. Herbst, I. Kjellmer, et al., Cardiotocography only versus cardiotocography plus ST analysis of fetal electrocardiogram for intrapartum fetal monitoring: a Swedish randomised controlled trial, Lancet 358 (9281) (2001) 534–538.

[37] J. Westgate, M. Harris, J.S. Curnow, K.R. Greene, Plymouth randomized trial of cardiotocogram only versus ST waveform plus cardiotogram for intrapartum monitoring in 2400 cases, Am. J. Obstet. Gynecol. 169 (5) (1993) 1151–1160.

[38] J.P. Neilson, Fetal electrocardiogram (ECG) for fetal monitoring during labour, Cochrane Database Syst. Rev. (3) (2006). CD000116.

[39] M.E.M.H. Westerhuis, G.H.A. Visser, K.G.M. Moons, E. van Beck, et al., Cardiotography plus AS analysis of fetal electrocardiogram compared with cardiotocography only for intrapartum monitoring: a randomized trial, Obstet. Gynecol. 115 (2010) 1173–1180.

[40] M.A. Belfort, G.R. Saade, E. Thom, S.C. Blackwell, U.M. Reddy, J.M. Thorp, A.T. Tita, R.S. Miller, A.M. Peaceman, D.S. McKenna, E.K. Chien, D.J. Rouse, R.S. Gibbs, Y.Y. El-Sayed, Y. Sorokin, S.N. Caritis, J.P. VanDorsten, A randomized trial of intrapartum fetal ECG ST-segment analysis, N. Engl. J. Med. 373 (7) (2015) 632–641.

[41] American College of Obstetricians, ACOG Committee Opinion. Umbilical cord blood gas and acid–base analysis, Obstet. Gynecol. 108 (5) (2006) 1319–1322.

[42] A. Nodwell, L. Carmichael, M. Ross, B. Richardson, Placental compared with umbilical cord blood to assess fetal blood gas and acid-base status, Obstet. Gynecol. 105 (1) (2005) 129–138.

[43] B. Richardson, A. Nodwell, K. Webster, M. Alshimmiri, R. Gagnon, R. Natale, Fetal oxygen saturation and fractional extraction at birth and the relationship to measures of acidosis, Am. J. Obstet. Gynecol. 178 (3) (1998) 572–579.

[44] J.T. Helwig, J.T. Parer, S.J. Kilpatrick, R.K. Laros, Umbilical cord blood acid-base state: what is normal? Am. J. Obstet. Gynecol. 174 (6) (1996) 1807–1812.

[45] R. Victory, D. Penava, O. Da Silva, R. Natale, B. Richardson, Umbilical cord pH and base excess values in relation to adverse outcome events for infants delivering at term, Am. J. Obstet. Gynecol. 191 (6) (2004) 2021–2028.

Influence of Gestational Age on Fetal Heart Rate

E lectronic fetal monitoring is a complex process in which there is significant dependence on identifying fetal heart rate (FHR) characteristics that are representative of adequate oxygenation as well as those patterns that point to a pathway of deteriorating fetal status. Gestational age plays a significant role in the process of pattern interpretation as gestational age can influence FHR characteristics including baseline rate, variability, accelerations, and the appearance of periodic and episodic changes. In order to have a more standardized approach to interpreting FHR characteristics, healthcare providers should have an understanding of gestational age terminology as specific definitions have been implemented for communication and research purposes. Refer to Table 7.1 for definitions [1]. Prematurity subcategories incorporating gestational age ranges have also been used, but these terms are not consistently defined and lack standardization [2]. Physiologic characteristics along the gestational age continuum change as the pregnancy advances, making monitoring a challenge in terms of collecting and interpreting data especially in the broad extremes of gestational age. This chapter reviews available data regarding the physiologic characteristics noted along the gestational age ranges, with emphasis on interpretation of fetal monitoring data and assessment of fetal status.

THE PRETERM FETUS

Worldwide every year, preterm birth accounts for approximately 15 million infants being born before 37 weeks and 1.1 million infants succumbing to prematurity complications. Compared with other countries, prematurity rates in the United States persistently remain in the top 10, although in recent years, the preterm birth rate in the United States has gradually decreased over 11% when the peak preterm birth rate was 12.8% in 2006 [3–5]. The birth rate in gestations between 34 and 36 weeks has decreased the most, whereas less than 34 weeks remains relatively consistent in numbers [5,6].

TABLE 7.1   Gestational Age Classifications

Preterm	<37 0/7 weeks
Early term	37 0/7 weeks to 38 6/7 weeks
Full term	39 0/7 weeks to 40 6/7 weeks
Late term	41 0/7 weeks to 41 6/7 weeks
Postterm	≥42 0/7 weeks

Adapted from American College of Obstetricians and Gynecologists, Definition of term pregnancy (ACOG Committee Opinion No. 579), Author, Washington, DC, 2013.

An appreciation of the complexity of preterm FHR interpretation is necessary in terms of determining a plan of care and avoiding unnecessary interventions. Many preterm births compared with term births are associated with medical or maternal-fetal complications as well as underlying placental dysfunction, leading to higher rates of perinatal and neonatal morbidity and mortality [7–9]. Data suggest that changes in preterm FHR patterns, specifically tachycardia, recurrent decelerations, and loss of variability, are typically consistent with an interruption of oxygenation related to pregnancy complications (i.e., fetal growth restriction), making preterm fetuses more susceptible to hypoxia and acidosis [10–14]. In addition, progression of FHR tracing characteristics exhibiting the absence of metabolic acidemia may progress more rapidly to indeterminate or abnormal FHR characteristics in the compromised preterm fetus compared with the term fetus [15]. These findings underscore the importance of clinical acumen regarding the FHR patterns of preterm fetuses. Quantitative data is limited concerning preterm FHR characteristics compared with the term fetus. In general, preterm FHR characteristics in the antepartum period include:

- Baseline rate frequently at the higher end of the normal FHR range
- Minimal variability may be observed in extremely preterm fetuses
- Lower frequency and amplitude of accelerations with a peak of at least 10 bpm above the baseline and a duration of at least 10 seconds until approximately 32 weeks' gestation
- Variable decelerations with shorter depth and duration often unrelated to uterine contractions or periods of hypoxemia

During the intrapartum period, preterm FHR characteristics, such as baseline and variability, are similar to those in the antepartum period, although the appearance and progression to indeterminate and abnormal patterns may occur more rapidly.

Baseline Fetal Heart Rate in the Preterm Fetus

The baseline FHR decreases as gestational age increases [16,17]. In a preterm fetus, a baseline rate close to 155 to 160 bpm can be normal because of an immature fetal autonomic nervous system in which the baseline FHR is the result of resistance between the parasympathetic and sympathetic systems [13]. With advancing gestation, the parasympathetic system becomes more dominant, resulting in a gradual decrease of the baseline [15]. The higher baseline rate must be interpreted with caution because this may indicate progressive fetal hypoxia, infection, or maternal pyrexia. Preterm fetal tachycardia is more prognostic of acidemia, low Apgar scores, and adverse neonatal outcomes including neonatal death compared with the term fetus [13,18]. Tachycardia (FHR baseline >160) should always be evaluated using a systematic approach (described in Chapter 6) regardless of gestational age.

Baseline Variability in the Preterm Fetus

Similar to FHR baseline, variability within the baseline rate changes with advancing gestational age [19]. In the preterm fetus, variability may be less than the term fetus based on the immature vagal and sympathetic branches of the autonomic nervous system [20,21]. The baseline variability typically increases with fetal growth though the exact amount has not been quantified in the literature.

Periodic and Episodic Heart Rate Changes in the Preterm Fetus

Accelerations

Accelerations of the FHR in association with fetal movement begin in the second trimester of pregnancy. These accelerations are a result of the fetal somatic nervous system, which connects the central nervous system to muscle, allowing the fetus to perform specific movements and behaviors [9,15]. An FHR acceleration before 32 weeks' gestation is defined by a peak of ≥10 bpm above the baseline and a duration of ≥10 seconds from onset to offset [22] (Figure 7.1). Prior to 32 weeks' gestation, the preterm fetus may not have the physiologic maturity to generate accelerations that meet these criteria [23,24].

Similar to FHR baseline and variability, there is an increase in the number, amplitude, and duration of FHR accelerations, especially between 26 and 28 weeks' gestation and 30 to 32 weeks'

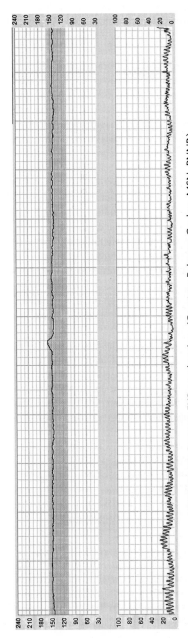

FIGURE 7.1 Preterm FHR acceleration. (Courtesy Rebecca Cypher, MSN, PNNP.)

gestation as the physiologic mechanisms responsible for FHR accelerations mature [17,25]. After 32 weeks' gestation, FHR accelerations are defined as abrupt increases from the baseline of at least ≥15 bpm, lasting ≥15 seconds from onset to offset [26]. However, a number of fetuses with gestations <32 weeks, particularly those after 24 to 26 weeks' gestation, may meet the criteria for ≥15 bpm lasting ≥15 seconds [27,28]. Many providers require that future tracings in these fetuses continue to reflect the peak ≥15 bpm, duration ≥15-second parameters on the basis of the premise that maturational development does not normally regress.

Decelerations

Between 20 and 30 weeks' gestation, spontaneous decelerations occur, typically variable decelerations, which are characteristically in association with fetal activity and the absence of uterine contractions. These decelerations are generally minimal in depth and short in duration [9,24] (Figure 7.2). Throughout labor in the preterm population, roughly 70% of patients between 28 and 33 weeks' gestation and 55% between 34 and 36 weeks' gestation will have variable decelerations [13] compared with an occurrence rate of 20% to 30% in the term pregnancy [29]. Experts speculate that preterm variable decelerations are related to decreased amounts of Wharton's jelly around the umbilical cord, oligohydramnios, or an immature fetal myocardium leading to reduced contractility of the heart [15]. Early decelerations are rarely observed, with the majority occurring in gestations over 35 weeks [13]. Late decelerations do not occur more or less frequently in preterm birth, but clinical conditions that are associated with late decelerations (i.e., fetal growth restriction) are more likely to occur in the preterm fetus. This has the potential to cause adverse perinatal and neonatal outcomes, including acidosis and long-term neurologic deficits [13,29].

If additional information is needed regarding fetal status in the antepartum period, testing methods such as a biophysical profiles, contraction stress tests, or Doppler flow studies may be utilized. Refer to Chapter 9 for additional information.

Behavioral States in the Preterm Fetus

Certain types of fetal behaviors, such as the presence of fetal movement, have been associated with a nonacidotic fetus. Spontaneous fetal movement takes place by 7 to 8 weeks' gestation, with maternal perception occurring between 16 and 18 weeks' gestation [30,31].

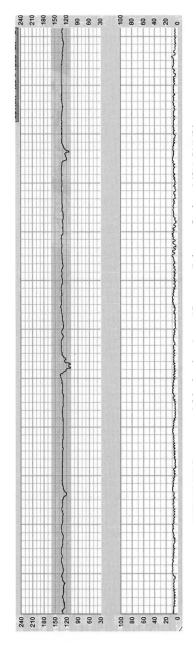

FIGURE 7.2 Preterm variable decelerations. (Courtesy Rebecca Cypher, MSN, PNNP.)

Fetal activity becomes more coordinated and defined by the third trimester as the central nervous system matures. Four fetal behavioral states have been defined and verified by ultrasound. They are quiet sleep, active sleep, quiet awake, and active awake. The behavior and associated FHR patterns of each of these four states are described in Table 7.2. The fetus may cycle among these states.

Quiet sleep and active sleep are the dominant patterns. As the fetus matures, the length of time in quiet sleep is extended from a mean of 4 minutes in midtrimester to as long as 2 hours by 40 weeks'

TABLE 7.2 Fetal Behavioral States

State	Behavior	Associated FHR Pattern
1 F: Quiet sleep or quiescence	<ul><li>Absence of rapid eye movement (REM)</li><li>Infrequent body and startle movement</li><li>Rhythmic fetal breathing and mouthing movement</li></ul>	<ul><li>Regular/stable FHR baseline</li><li>Minimal to absent variability</li><li>Rare accelerations with fetal movement (FM)</li></ul>
2 F: Active sleep	<ul><li>Frequent body movement</li><li>Abrupt head and limb movement</li><li>REM</li><li>Irregular fetal breathing and mouthing movement</li></ul>	<ul><li>Wider variation in FHR baseline</li><li>Minimal to moderate variability</li><li>Frequent accelerations with FM</li></ul>
3 F: Quiet awake	<ul><li>Infrequent to absent body movement</li><li>REM</li><li>Irregular mouthing movement</li></ul>	<ul><li>Stable FHR baseline</li><li>Moderate variability</li><li>Absent accelerations</li></ul>
4 F: Active awake	<ul><li>Continuous and vigorous movement</li><li>REM</li><li>Irregular fetal breathing and mouthing movement</li></ul>	<ul><li>Unstable FHR baseline</li><li>Moderate to marked variability</li><li>Frequent prolonged accelerations fusing into tachycardic rate</li></ul>

Adapted from J.I. de Vries, G.H. Visser, E.J. Mulder, et al., Diurnal and other variations in fetal movement and heart rate patterns at 20-22 weeks, Early Hum. Dev. 15 (6) (1987) 333–348.

C.B. Martin, Behavioral states in the human fetus. J. Reprod. Med. 26(8) (1981) 425–432.

gestation [30,32]. Clinically, fetuses in fetal behavioral state 1 F, quiet sleep, may have a reduction in variability and absence of accelerations that coincide with movement [32]. Pathologic causes must be excluded before these FHR observations can safely be attributed to benign changes in a behavioral state. Alternatively, frequent accelerations during 4 F, active awake state can be confusing in clearly identifying the baseline rate. In that event, simultaneous evaluation of the FHR tracing and fetal movement can help differentiate baseline rate (between fetal movements) from accelerations (during fetal movements).

Preterm Uterine Activity

Preterm uterine activity monitoring may be technically challenging. The smaller uterus may not accommodate effective placement of both toco- and ultrasound transducers. Low-amplitude, high-frequency (LAHF) uterine contractions, frequently called *uterine irritability*, are not uncommon before term. LAHF contractions have been defined as measuring <5 mm on the tocotransducer and occurring at 1- to 2-minute intervals [33] (Figure 7.3). In most cases, these contractions are clinically benign; however, occasionally they may progress to preterm labor, causing cervical dilation and effacement [34] or may signal evolving placental abruption. Contractions that do not resolve must be evaluated and treated in the context of the clinical presentation and FHR observations.

Tocolytic Therapy and Effect on Fetal Heart Rate

There is no evidence to support that long-term or maintenance tocolytic therapy prevents preterm birth or has a favorable impact on neonatal outcomes [35]. These medications often temporarily reduce or eliminate uterine activity for a brief time but do not remove or reverse the underlying etiology. Additionally, no tocolytic agent is 100% efficacious and safe [36]. Evidence does support a short course of a first-line tocolytic agent, such as prostaglandin synthase inhibitors, calcium channel blockers, and beta-sympathomimetic, to patients experiencing preterm labor [35]. Delaying delivery for up to 48 hours with a first-line tocolytic agent allows for administration of antenatal corticosteroids to accelerate fetal lung maturation, magnesium sulfate for fetal neuroprotection, and transport to a higher level of maternal–fetal care [36–38].

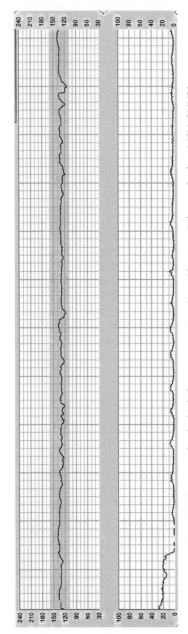

FIGURE 7.3 Low-amplitude, high-frequency contractions. (Courtesy Rebecca Cypher, MSN, PNNP.)

Indomethacin

Indomethacin is the main prostaglandin synthase inhibitor (also known as a cyclooxygenase [COX] inhibitor) used for preterm labor. Usual dosing is 50 to 100 mg followed by 25 to 50 mg every 6 hours. Therapy is often limited to 48 hours and is not recommended after 32 weeks' gestation. Amniotic fluid volume (AFV) and fetal renal anatomy should be assessed before initiating therapy due to the fetal risk of constriction of the ductus arteriosus and decreased renal function, resulting in oligohydramnios. Treatment beyond 48 hours requires intensive surveillance of amniotic fluid volume and ductal flow [39–41]. If oligohydramnios develops, the FHR tracing may demonstrate variable decelerations, reflecting transient umbilical cord compression [42,43].

Nifedipine

Calcium channel blockers such as nifedipine (Procardia) may be used as a first-line tocolytic agent. A variety of dosing regimens using oral capsules have been described in the literature. One protocol includes an initial loading dose of 10 to 40 mg followed by 10 to 20 mg every 4 to 6 hours, with titration based on the contraction pattern. Maternal side effects are related to smooth muscle relaxation, resulting in peripheral vasodilation, which causes maternal hypotension as well as a compensatory rise in heart rate and stroke volume. Peripheral dilation and maternal hypotension can lead to hypoperfusion of the uterus and placenta [44]. Any medication that reduces maternal blood pressure has the potential to interfere with normal maternal perfusion of the intervillous space. As discussed in Chapter 5, recurrent or sustained disruption of fetal oxygenation can result in FHR changes ranging from decelerations to loss of variability, loss of accelerations, and changes in baseline rate.

Beta mimetics

Beta mimetics such as terbutaline (Brethine) were frequently administered in the past using a variety of dosing regimens and routes. This agent quickly became unpopular secondary to side effects (cardiac toxicity and death) and a U.S. Food and Drug Administration safety announcement stating that injectable terbutaline should not be used beyond 48 to 72 hours due to potential adverse outcomes [44,45]. Generally, 0.25 mg is given subcutaneously and repeated in 15 to 30 minutes if there is inadequate uterine response and no significant side effects. Total dosing in 4 hours should not exceed 0.5 mg [44]. Oral terbutaline is not advised because of similar safety concerns and lack of evidence to support a role in preterm labor prevention [35,44,45]. The most common maternal side effect is tachycardia, which may be associated with increased oxygen consumption. Beta mimetics cross the placental barrier and may result in fetal tachycardia [44]. Fetal tachycardia may be associated with loss of variability, and with prolonged use fetal arrhythmias may develop.

Magnesium Sulfate

Despite systematic reviews and comparative trials indicating that intravenous magnesium sulfate is neither more nor less successful than other tocolytic agents in delaying delivery, preventing preterm birth, or improving neonatal and maternal outcomes, magnesium sulfate continues to be administered on a regular basis. Magnesium sulfate has been given in the context of preterm labor, but contemporary literature has demonstrated a link in the medication's role in providing neuroprotective benefits to the fetus [35,46,47]. Several neuroprotection treatment regimens have been described in the literature including a 6-gram loading dose followed by 2 grams/hour for up to 12 hours with resumption of the protocol when preterm delivery is imminent [46]. Magnesium sulfate crosses the placenta, and fetal serum magnesium concentrations often correlate with maternal serum levels [48]. The use of magnesium sulfate has been associated with decreasing baseline, decreased rate of variability, and loss of accelerations [48–51] (Figure 7.4). Pathologic causes should be excluded before these changes are attributed to magnesium sulfate therapy. Exposure to magnesium sulfate does not increase the incidence of bradycardia or category change [52]. As discussed in Chapters 6 and 9, vibroacoustic stimulation can provoke accelerations and may improve variability though a blunted response may be elicited when magnesium sulfate is infusing [53]. Biophysical profiles and Doppler flow studies may also provide useful information regarding interpretation and management of the FHR tracing [54–56].

Antenatal Corticosteroid Therapy

Current guidelines recommend a single course of antenatal corticosteroids (betamethasone or dexamethasone) to be administered between 23 and 34 weeks' gestation to enhance fetal lung maturity, reduce the risks of respiratory distress syndrome, and lower neonatal morbidity and mortality rates in those pregnancies at risk for preterm delivery. Single-course therapy consists of betamethasone two doses

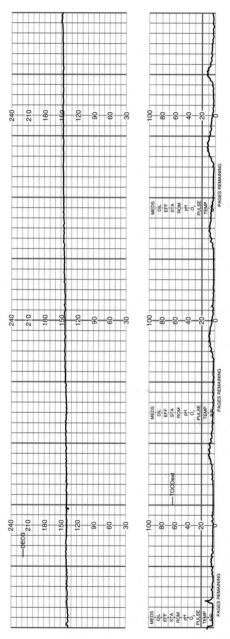

FIGURE 7.4 Preterm fetus and FHR during therapy with magnesium sulfate. (Courtesy Rebecca Cypher, MSN, PNNP.)

of 12 mg given intramuscularly 24 hours apart or dexamethasone four doses of 6 mg given intramuscularly 12 hours apart [35].

No long-term negative effects from a single course of cortico-steroids have been reported. There are direct, transient effects on fetal movement, FHR, and variability that typically return to base-line within 4 days of administration [57,58]. Betamethasone has been associated with an increase in FHR baseline, decreasing variability, and loss of accelerations. There is limited data on dexamethasone, which has concluded that the effect on FHR characteristics is similar to betamethasone, although other experts argue there is no significant change [35,57,58]. Neither of these medications has been associated with altered Doppler flow in the fetal middle cerebral artery and um-bilical artery.

Transient periods of suppression of biophysical characteristics (movement, fetal breathing, and reactivity) may be noted in pa-tients receiving betamethasone. By 48 hours, the biophysical pro-file (BPP) score (see Chapter 9) may be as low as 6 of 10 when the maximum peak of the steroid has been reached [58,59]. These observations may be misinterpreted as a deteriorating fetal oxygen-ation status. Knowledge of these changes should be considered to avoid an iatrogenic preterm delivery. In these situations, Doppler flow studies in conjunction with biophysical profiles may assist with interpretation and management of the FHR following steroid administration.

Monitoring the Preterm Fetus

Antepartum Fetal Assessment

Antepartum fetal assessment is an integral part of assessing fetuses at risk for an injury that is a result of a disrupted oxygenation pathway. The goal is to improve perinatal outcomes, specifically stillbirth and long-term neurologic impairments, while avoiding unnecessary in-terventions and unwarranted preterm delivery [60,61]. Fetal assess-ment is reviewed in Chapter 9.

Triage and Inpatient Antepartum Monitoring

Continuous FHR monitoring, although frequently performed during the antepartum period for patient evaluation or treatment of preterm labor, preterm premature rupture of membranes, or preeclampsia, can cause a clinical dilemma for healthcare providers [15]. There is a risk that a false-positive, indeterminate, or abnormal FHR tracing will prompt unnecessary delivery of an uncompromised fetus when

FHR monitoring is performed prior to term. The earlier in gestation this occurs, the higher the likelihood of serious iatrogenic sequelae of prematurity. This risk must be balanced against the anticipated benefits of the information obtained from the monitor. Fetal monitoring may offer the benefit of early detection of disrupted fetal oxygenation so that corrective measures or operative intervention can be performed in a timely fashion [14,15,33]. Corrective measures, such as position changes, might benefit the preterm fetus and are discussed in Chapter 6. The decision to initiate or discontinue fetal monitoring or to perform continuous versus intermittent monitoring in the preterm patient is made on an individual basis after an objective assessment of the anticipated risks, benefits, limitations, and alternatives. The patient must be an active participant in the decision-making process.

Intrapartum Monitoring

Except in cases of life-limiting anomalies or obstetric complications leading to preterm birth prior to viability, intrapartum management typically includes continuous monitoring with regular review of the FHR tracing, as outlined in Chapter 6. As mentioned earlier, disrupted oxygenation in the preterm fetus may progress more rapidly to metabolic acidemia and potential injury [14,29]. In addition, the possibility of infection must be considered in cases of preterm labor and/or preterm premature membrane rupture. The effects of infection and/or inflammation on the FHR tracing are not completely understood, but limited evidence supports the observations that inflammation results in abnormal fetal cardiac function [3,62]. In preterm gestations, the FHR tracing may be less reliable in excluding metabolic acidemia and predicting outcome because of the differences in FHR characteristics between preterm and term fetuses. All these factors must be taken into consideration when planning intrapartum management of the preterm fetus.

THE LATE TERM AND POSTTERM FETUS

As mentioned previously, universal definitions for term pregnancy have been implemented that allow for delivery of quality healthcare [1]. The precise incidence of late term and postterm pregnancy is unknown because of the variety of definitions used in the past in research and data collection. However, induction rates for late term and postterm pregnancies appear to be decreasing because there is an increasing number of inductions for medical and obstetric reasons at earlier gestational ages [6,63]. Although the precise magnitude of risk is not known, fetal and neonatal morbidity and mortality increase as pregnancy advances beyond 39 to 40 weeks' gestation [64].

Fetal Assessment

Antepartum fetal assessment is reviewed in Chapter 9. The definition, interpretation, and management of intrapartum FHR patterns in this population is no different from those in the preterm fetus except for accelerations.

Risks Associated with Postterm Pregnancy

Postmaturity or Dysmaturity Syndrome

At the time of initial newborn assessment, the postterm fetus may have features associated with *postmaturity* or *dysmaturity* syndrome. Clinical signs include reduced subcutaneous tissue; dry, wrinkled, peeling skin; meconium staining; hypothermia; and hypoglycemia, polycythemia, and hyperviscosity [65,66]. These findings are thought to reflect disruption of normal placental transfer of oxygen and nutrients due to altered surface area and inadequate exchange within the placenta leading to decreased blood flow, which results in nutritional deprivation, fetal wasting, decreased fat and glycogen stores, oligohydramnios, and chronic hypoxemia with compensatory hematopoiesis [63,67,68].

Oligohydramnios

Oligohydramnios is observed with increased frequency in the late term and postterm gestation. This is related to reduced placental function leading to selective fetal perfusion of the brain, heart, and adrenal glands, with less blood flow being distributed to the kidneys, the main source of amniotic fluid [63]. The term pregnancy has an estimated amniotic fluid volume of 700 to 800 mL, which declines at a rate of 8% per week after 40 weeks' gestation [69]. Sonographic descriptions of decreased fluid volume are outlined in Chapter 9. The morbidity associated with oligohydramnios is well documented and includes increased incidences of intrauterine fetal death, meconium-stained amniotic fluid, meconium aspiration syndrome, umbilical cord compression resulting in variable decelerations, cesarean delivery for fetal indications, and low Apgar scores and umbilical artery pH values [64,70,71]. Intrapartum amnioinfusion may reduce the frequency of decelerations and improve Apgar scores and cord pH values, as well as decrease the incidence of cesarean birth for fetal indications [26,72,73].

Meconium

The literature on advancing pregnancy supports that there is a higher incidence of meconium-stained fluid after 36 weeks' gestation [74,75]. However, meconium passage alone is not a reliable indicator of fetal compromise. In many cases, meconium passage may simply reflect a maturing fetus. Alternatively, it may reflect stimulation of the vagal system by umbilical cord compression, and stress related to hypoxia or infection [76,77]. Even when meconium passage is not secondary to these causes, there is the risk of meconium aspiration syndrome. The risk is compounded by low amniotic fluid volume, resulting in thick, undiluted meconium that is more likely to obstruct the fetal airway. As discussed in Chapter 6, routine amnioinfusion for meconium-stained amniotic fluid is not recommended.

Management of Postterm Pregnancy

The optimal management for postterm pregnancies, including the type of intervention and timing of delivery, remains controversial. Most agree that some form of surveillance is indicated and induction of labor after 42 0/7 weeks and by 42 6/7 weeks' gestation is recommended because of the increased perinatal morbidity and mortality [64]. The decision for induction of labor versus expectant management is dependent on a variety of factors, such as the gestational age, fetal surveillance results, Bishop score of the cervix, and maternal preference. At a minimum, fetal surveillance, including fetal movement counting and antenatal testing, should be conducted [63,64]. The presence of clinically significant decelerations or oligohydramnios warrants consideration of induction.

SUMMARY

Maturation of the physiologic mechanisms responsible for regulation of the FHR is associated with characteristic changes in the FHR tracing. In addition, many factors associated with preterm and late term or postterm pregnancy can influence the appearance of the FHR tracing, including medications, infection, placental function, and oligohydramnios. All these factors must be taken into consideration when interpreting the FHR tracing and planning management of pregnancies before and after term.

References

[1] American College of Obstetricians and Gynecologists, Definition of term pregnancy. Committee Opinion No. 579, Obstet. Gynecol. 122 (2013) 1139–1140.

[2] T.N. Raju, B.M. Mercer, D.J. Burchfield, G.F. Joseph, Periviable birth: executive summary of a Joint Workshop by the Eunice Kennedy Shriver National Institute of Child Health and Human Development, Society for Maternal-Fetal Medicine, American Academy of Pediatrics, and American College of Obstetricians and Gynecologists, Am. J. Obstet. Gynecol. 210 (5) (2014) 406–417.

[3] R. Galinsky, G.R. Polglase, S.B. Hooper, M.J. Black, T.J. Moss, The consequences of chorioamnionitis: preterm birth and effects on development, J. Pregnancy 2013 (2013) 1–11.

[4] C.P. Howson, M.V. Kinney, L. McDougall, J.E. Lawn, Born too soon: the global action report on preterm birth, Reprod. Health 10 (Suppl. 1) (2012) S1–S9.

[5] J.A. Martin, B.E. Hamilton, M.J.K. Osterman, et al., Births: final data for 2013, Natl. Vital Stat. Rep. 64 (1) (2015).

[6] C. Gyamfi-Bannerman, C.V. Ananth, Trends in spontaneous and indicated preterm delivery among singleton gestations in the United States, 2005–2012, Obstet. Gynecol. 124 (6) (2014) 1069–1074.

[7] C.V. Ananth, A.M. Vintzileos, Maternal-fetal conditions necessitating a medical intervention resulting in preterm birth, Am. J. Obstet. Gynecol. 195 (6) (2006) 1557–1563.

[8] H.-Y. Chen, S.P. Chauhan, C.V. Ananth, et al., Electronic fetal heart rate monitoring and its relationship to neonatal and infant mortality in the United States, Am. J. Obstet. Gynecol. 204 (6) (2011) 491.e1–491.e10.

[9] Y. Sorokin, L.J. Kierker, S. Pillay, et al., The association between fetal heart rate patterns and fetal movements in pregnancies between 20 and 30 weeks' gestation, Am. J. Obstet. Gynecol. 143 (3) (1982) 243–249.

[10] J.M. Ayoubi, F. Audibert, C. Boithias, et al., Perinatal factors affecting survival and survival without disability of extreme premature infants at two years of age, Eur. J. Obstet. Gynecol. Reprod. Biol. 105 (2) (2002) 124–131.

[11] J.M. Ayoubi, F. Audibert, M. Vial, et al., Fetal heart rate and survival of the very premature newborn, Am. J. Obstet. Gynecol. 187 (4) (2002) 1026–1030.

[12] P. Holmes, L.W. Oppenheimer, A. Gravelle, M. Walker, M. Blayney, The effect of variable heart rate decelerations on intraventricular hemorrhage and other perinatal outcomes in preterm infants, J. Matern. Fetal Med. 10 (4) (2001) 264–268.

[13] M. Westgren, S. Holmquist, N.W. Venningsen, I. Ingemarsson, Intrapartum fetal monitoring in preterm deliveries: prospective study, Obstet. Gynecol. 60 (1) (1982) 99–106.

[14] M. Westgren, P. Hormquist, I. Ingemarsson, N. Svenningsen, Intrapartum fetal acidosis in preterm infants: fetal monitoring and long-term morbidity, Obstet. Gynecol. 63 (3) (1984) 355–359.

[15] K. Afors, E. Chandraharan, Use of continuous electronic fetal monitoring in a preterm fetus: clinical dilemmas and recommendations for practice, J. Pregnancy 2011 (2011) 1–7.

[16] R.D. Eden, L.S. Seifert, J. Frese-Gallo, et al., Effect of gestational age on baseline fetal heart rate during the third trimester of pregnancy, J. Reprod. Med. 32 (4) (1987) 285–286.

[17] T. Wheeler, A. Murrills, Patterns of fetal heart rate during normal pregnancy, Br. J. Obstet. 85 (1) (1978) 18–27.

[18] D.R. Burrus, T.M. O'Shea, J.C. Veille, E. Mueller-Heubach, The predictive value of intrapartum fetal heart rate abnormalities in the extremely premature infant, Am. J. Obstet. Gynecol. 171 (4) (1994) 1128–1132.

[19] G.H. Visser, G.S. Dawes, C.W. Redman, Numerical analysis of the normal human antenatal fetal heart rate, Br. J. Obstet. Gynaecol. 88 (8) (1981) 792–802.

[20] U. Schneider, E. Schleussner, A. Fiedler, et al., Fetal heart rate variability reveals differential dynamics in the intrauterine development of the sympathetic and parasympathetic branches of the autonomic nervous system, Physiol. Meas. 30 (2) (2009) 215–226.

[21] P. Van Leeuwen, D. Cysarz, F. Edelhäuser, D. Grönemeyer, Heart rate variability in the individual fetus, Auton. Neurosci. 178 (1) (2013) 24–28.

[22] G.A. Macones, G.D. Hankins, C.Y. Spong, et al., The 2008 National Institute of Child Health and Human Development workshop report on electronic fetal monitoring: update on definitions, interpretation, and research guidelines, Obstet. Gynecol. 112 (3) (2008) 661–666.

[23] R.A. Castillo, L.D. Devoe, M. Arthur, et al., The preterm nonstress test: effects of gestational age and length of study, Am. J. Obstet. Gynecol. 160 (1) (1989) 172–175.

[24] M. Pillai, D. James, The development of fetal heart rate patterns during normal pregnancy, Obstet. Gynecol. 76 (5) (1990) 812–816.

[25] R. Gagnon, K. Campbell, C. Hunse, J. Patrick, Patterns of human fetal heart rate accelerations from 26 weeks to term, Am. J. Obstet. Gynecol. 157 (3) (1987) 743–748.

[26] F.S. Miyazaki, N.A. Taylor, Saline amnioinfusion for relief of variable or prolonged decelerations. A preliminary report, Am. J. Obstet. Gynecol. 146 (6) (1983) 670–678.

[27] L.D. Devoe, Antepartum fetal heart rate testing in preterm pregnancy, Obstet. Gynecol. 60 (4) (1982) 431–436.

[28] J.P. Lavin, M. Miodovnik, T.P. Barden, Relationship of nonstress test reactivity and gestational age, Obstet. Gynecol. 63 (3) (1984) 338–344.

[29] B. Zanini, R.H. Paul, J.R. Huey, Intrapartum fetal heart rate: correlation with scalp pH in the preterm fetus, Am. J. Obstet. Gynecol. 136 (1) (1980) 43–47.

[30] J.I. de Vries, G.H. Visser, E.J. Mulder, et al., Diurnal and other variations in fetal movement and heart rate patterns at 20–22 weeks, Early Hum. Dev. 15 (6) (1987) 33–348.

[31] S.T. Blackburn (Ed.), Neurologic, muscular, and sensory systems, in: Maternal, Fetal & Neonatal Physiology, fourth ed., Elsevier, Philadelphia, PA, 2013, pp. 509–559.

[32] M. Pillai, D. James, Human fetal mouthing movements: a potential biophysical variable for distinguishing state 1F from abnormal fetal behavior; report of 4 cases, Eur. J. Obstet. Gynecol. Reprod. Biol. 38 (2) (1991) 151–156.

[33] R.B. Newman, P.J. Gill, S. Campion, et al., Antepartum ambulatory tocodynamometry: the significance of low-amplitude, high-frequency contractions, Obstet. Gynecol. 70 (5) (1987) 701–705.

[34] M. Katz, R.B. Newman, P.J. Gill, Assessment of uterine activity in ambulatory patients at high risk of preterm labor and delivery, Am. J. Obstet. Gynecol. 154 (1) (1986) 44–47.

[35] American College of Obstetricians and Gynecologists, Management of preterm labor. Practice Bulletin No. 127, Obstet. Gynecol. 119 (2012) 1308–1317.

[36] J.S. Jørgensen, L.K.K. Weile, R.F. Lamont, Preterm labor: current tocolytic options for the treatment of preterm labor, Expert Opin. Pharmacother. 15 (5) (2014) 585–588.

[37] American College of Obstetricians and Gynecologists, Magnesium sulfate use in obstetrics. Committee Opinion No. 573, Obstet. Gynecol. 122 (2013) 727–728.

[38] E.O. Van Vliet, E. Schuit, K.Y. Heida, et al., Nifedipine versus atosiban in the treatment of threatened preterm labour (Assessment of Perinatal Outcome after Specific Tocolysis in Early Labour: APOSTEL III-Trial), BMC Pregnancy Childbirth 14 (1) (2014) 93.

[39] J. King, V. Flenady, S. Cole, et al., Cyclo-oxygenase (COX) inhibitors for treating preterm labour, Cochrane Database Syst. Rev. (2) (2005). CD001992.

[40] J.R. Niebyl, D.A. Blake, R.D. White, et al., The inhibition of premature labor with indomethacin, Am. J. Obstet. Gynecol. 136 (8) (1980) 1014–1019.

[41] I.B. Van den Veyver, K.J. Moise Jr., Prostaglandin synthetase inhibitors in pregnancy, Obstet. Gynecol. Surv. 48 (1993) 493–502.

[42] D.M. Clive, J.S. Stoff, Renal syndromes associated with nonsteroidal antiinflammatory drugs, N. Engl. J. Med. 310 (9) (1984) 563–572.

[43] M.C. Gordon, P. Samuels, Indomethacin, Clin. Obstet. Gynecol. 38 (4) (1995) 697–705.

[44] A. Abramovici, J. Cantu, S.M. Jenkins, Tocolytic therapy for acute preterm labor, Obstet. Gynecol. Clin. North Am. 39 (1) (2012) 77–87.

[45] Food Drug Administration, FDA drug safety communication: new warnings against use of terbutaline to treat preterm labor. Available from: http://www.fda.gov/drugs/drugsafety/ucm243539.htm (accessed 11.16.15).

[46] American College of Obstetricians and Gynecologists, Magnesium sulfate before anticipated preterm birth for neuroprotection. Committee Opinion No. 455, Obstet. Gynecol. 115 (2010) 669–671.

[47] D.J. Rouse, D.G. Hirtz, E. Thom, et al., A randomized, controlled trial of magnesium sulfate for the prevention of cerebral palsy, N. Engl. J. Med. 359 (9) (2008) 895–905.

[48] C.R. Duffy, A.O. Odibo, K.A. Roehl, G.A. Macones, A.G. Cahill, Effect of magnesium sulfate on fetal heart rate patterns in the second stage of labor, Obstet. Gynecol. 119 (6) (2012) 1129–1136.

[49] M.W. Atkinson, M.A. Belfort, G. Saade, K.J. Moise, The relation between magnesium sulfate therapy and fetal heart rate variability, Obstet. Gynecol. 83 (6) (1984) 967–970.

[50] M. Hallack, J. Martinez-Poyer, M.L. Kruger, et al., The effect of magnesium sulfate on fetal heart rate parameters: a randomized, placebo-controlled trial, Am. J. Obstet. Gynecol. 181 (5) (1999) 1122–1127.

[51] A. Nensi, D. De Silva, P. von Dadelszen, et al., Effect of magnesium sulphate on fetal heart rate parameters: a systematic review, J. Obstet. Gynaecol. Can. 36 (12) (2014) 1055–1064.

[52] A.M. Stewart, G.A. Macones, A.O. Odibo, R. Colvin, A.G. Cahill, Changes in fetal heart tracing characteristics after magnesium exposure, Am. J. Perinatol. 31 (10) (2014) 869–874.

[53] D.M. Sherer, Blunted fetal response to vibroacoustic stimulation associated with maternal intravenous magnesium sulfate therapy, Am. J. Perinatol. 11 (6) (1994) 401–403.

[54] S. Carlan, W. O'Brien, The effect of magnesium sulfate on the biophysical profile of normal term fetuses, Obstet. Gynecol. 77 (5) (1991) 681–684.

[55] P.S. Ramsey, D.J. Rouse, Magnesium sulfate as a tocolytic agent, Semin. Perinatol. 25 (4) (2001) 236–247.

[56] D.M. Twickler, D.D. McIntire, J.M. Alexander, et al., Effects of magnesium sulfate on preterm fetal cerebral blood flow using doppler analysis, Obstet. Gynecol. 115 (1) (2010) 21–25.

[57] V. Mariotti, A.M. Marconi, G. Pardi, Undesired effects of steroids during pregnancy, J. Matern. Fetal Neonatal Med. 16 (2) (2004) 5–7.

[58] K.M. Verdurmen, J. Renckens, J.O. van Laar, S.G. Oei, The influence of corticosteroids on fetal heart rate variability: a systematic review of the literature, Obstet. Gynecol. Surv. 68 (12) (2013) 811–824.

[59] O. Deren, C. Karaer, L. Onderoglu, et al., The effect of steroids on the biophysical profile and Doppler indices of umbilical and middle cerebral arteries in healthy preterm fetuses, Eur. J. Obstet. Gynecol. Reprod. Biol. 99 (1) (2001) 72–76.

[60] American College of Obstetricians and Gynecologists, Antepartum fetal surveillance. Practice Bulletin No. 146, Obstet. Gynecol. 124 (2014) 182–192.

[61] C. Signore, R.K. Freeman, C.Y. Spong, Antenatal testing: a reevaluation, Obstet. Gynecol. 113 (3) (2009) 687–701.

[62] R. Romero, J. Espinoza, L.F. Goncalves, et al., Fetal cardiac dysfunction in preterm premature rupture of membranes, J. Matern. Fetal Neonatal Med. 16 (3) (2004) 146–157.

[63] N. Walker, J.H. Gan, Prolonged pregnancy, Obstet. Gynaecol. Reprod. Med. 25 (3) (2015) 83–87.

[64] American College of Obstetricians and Gynecologists, Management of late-term and postterm pregnancies. Practice Bulletin No. 146, Obstet. Gynecol. 124 (2014) 390–396.

[65] L. Ballard, K.K. Novak, M. Driver, A simplified score for assessment of fetal maturation of newly born infants, J. Pediatr. 95 (5) (1979) 769–774.

[66] S.H. Clifford, Postmaturity, with placental dysfunction: clinical syndromes and pathologic findings, J. Pediatr. 44 (1) (1954) 1–13.

[67] F. Mannino, Neonatal complications of postterm gestation, J. Reprod. Med. 33 (3) (1988) 271–276.

[68] H. Vorherr, Placental insufficiency in relation to postterm pregnancy and fetal postmaturity: evaluation of fetoplacental function; management of the postterm gravida, Am. J. Obstet. Gynecol. 123 (1) (1975) 67–103.

[69] T.R. Moore, Amniotic fluid dynamics reflect fetal and maternal health and disease, Obstet. Gynecol. 116 (3) (2010) 759–765.

[70] C.J. Bochner, A.L. Medearis, J. Davis, et al., Antepartum predictors of fetal distress in postterm pregnancy, Am. J. Obstet. Gynecol. 157 (2) (1987) 353–358.

[71] P.F. Chamberlain, F.A. Manning, I. Morrison, C.R. Harman, I.R. Lange, Ultrasound evaluation of amniotic fluid volume: I. The relationship of marginal and decreased amniotic fluid volumes to perinatal outcome, Am. J. Obstet. Gynecol. 150 (3) (1984) 245–249.

[72] F.S. Miyazaki, F. Nevarez, Saline amnioinfusion for relief of repetitive variable decelerations: a prospective randomized study, Am. J. Obstet. Gynecol. 153 (3) (1985) 301–306.

[73] M.P. Nageotte, L. Bertucci, C.V. Towers, et al., Prophylactic amnioinfusion in pregnancies complicated by oligohydramnios: a prospective study, Obstet. Gynecol. 77 (5) (1991) 677–680.

[74] I. Balchin, J.C. Whittaker, R.F. Lamont, P.J. Steer, Maternal and fetal characteristics associated with meconium-stained amniotic fluid, Obstet. Gynecol. 117 (4) (2011) 828–835.

[75] Y. Oyelese, A. Culin, C.V. Ananth, L.M. Kaminsky, A. Vintzileos, J.C. Smulian, Meconium-stained amniotic fluid across gestation and neonatal acid–base status, Obstet. Gynecol. 108 (2) (2006) 345–349.

[76] S.N. Ahanya, J. Lakshmanan, B.L. Morgan, M.G. Ross, Meconium passage in utero: mechanisms, consequences, and management, Obstet. Gynecol. Surv. 60 (1) (2005) 45–56.

[77] J. Lakshmanan, M.G. Ross, Mechanism (s) of in utero meconium passage, J. Perinatol. 28 (Suppl. 3) (2008) S8–S13.

CHAPTER 8

Fetal Assessment in Non-obstetric Settings

etal assessment and care of the pregnant woman can occur in a variety of locations, including the surgical setting, critical care units, emergency departments, and separate obstetric triage units that are gaining hold as a critical access area for obstetric patients. These units function similarly to emergency departments in that the unit is able to evaluate and treat presenting symptoms, prioritize care, improve utilization of staffing and patient services, as well as create a plan that incorporates maternal–fetal well-being [1]. When the patient receives care outside of the obstetric setting, it is often because the pregnancy is below the limits of viability or requires surgical or medical expertise.

The focus of this chapter is maternal–fetal assessment and management in the non-obstetric setting. Collaboration among the multidisciplinary team members in these settings is essential when the pregnant woman is cared for because patients need the *right* providers at the *right* time and in the *right* setting. Evaluation of the pregnant patient brings a unique set of dilemmas, but a systematic approach to patient evaluations should be conducted in the same manner as with the nonpregnant patient, beginning with a comprehensive history and physical [2]. Regardless of the setting, the needs of the fetus should not be overlooked. The healthcare team must have the requisite skills and be qualified to evaluate the fetus based on their education, experience, and performance standards. It is imperative that communication between services and healthcare team members are clear and timely to ensure that the maternal–fetal dyad receives appropriate care by the most appropriate staff member.

PREGNANCY ANATOMY AND PHYSIOLOGY

Knowledge of the physiologic and anatomic adaptations of pregnancy is crucial because pregnancy alters anatomy and physiology to such an extent that the recognition of clinical symptoms and non-obstetric emergencies may be distorted and normal discomforts may

BOX 8.1 Physiologic Adaptations to Pregnancy

Cardiovascular
- Physiologic anemia, hypervolemia (expansion of plasma volume greater than expansion of red cell mass)
- Blood volume increases by 30%–40% (1200–1500 mL higher than prepregnant state)
- Plasma increases 70%, cells 30%
- Hematocrit of 32%–34% is not unusual
- Cardiac output increases 30%–50% (a result of increased blood volume)
- Heart rate and stroke volume increase
- Systemic vascular resistance decreases, with resultant decrease in blood pressure and mean arterial pressure
- Uteroplacental vascular bed is dilated; passive low resistance system
- Uterofetoplacental unit receives 20% of cardiac output
- Peripheral edema; dyspnea; presence of third heart sound
- Pelvic venous congestion

Hematologic
- Increased clotting factors VII, VIII, IX, and X, and fibrinogen (hypercoagulable)
- Decreased serum albumin may lower colloid osmotic pressure (predisposing to pulmonary edema)

Renal
- Smooth muscle relaxation, increased urinary stasis, hydronephrosis, hydroureter; increased susceptibility to urinary tract infection
- Increased creatinine clearance
- Decrease in serum creatinine and urea nitrogen (BUN)

Respiratory
- Tidal volume increases by 30%–40%; respiratory rate unchanged
- Oxygen consumption increases by 20%
- Diaphragm elevated by the growing fetus
- Arterial P_{CO_2} decreases as a result of hyperventilation, resulting in a "compensated" respiratory alkalosis

Gastrointestinal
- Smooth muscle relaxes, increasing gastric emptying time
- Gastric motility decreases, sphincters relax, higher likelihood of aspiration

Musculoskeletal
- Increased risk of ligament injury secondary to relaxin and progesterone
- Shifting center of gravity with growth of fetus, diastasis of the rectus abdominus
- Symphyseal separation

Adapted from references 2 and 6–9.

contribute to a puzzling picture [3–5]. Some changes are dramatic enough that they would be considered pathologic in the nonpregnant woman (Box 8.1). For example, the symphysis pubis protects the bladder, but in pregnancy the bladder shifts to an intraabdominal position, making this area more susceptible to injury [4]. Laboratory values may be altered in the pregnant patient versus the nonpregnant patient because of the adaptations required by the body to support the pregnancy [2,4]. Not only does the pregnant woman present with unique challenges; the fetus also requires assessment and possible intervention. Fetal stability depends on maternal stability. If caregivers do not understand and support the adaptations of the pregnancy, there is potential for adverse maternal and fetal outcomes.

EMERGENCY DEPARTMENT ASSESSMENT AND CARE

Pregnant women may seek care through emergency departments for a variety of reasons including emergency or trauma situations, lack of access to primary or obstetric care, inability to schedule an appointment, and convenience [1,10]. Initially a *primary* survey occurs when the patient first presents and is asked, "Why are you here?" so that a quick assessment can be completed, which is crucial to determining triage and treatment priorities. A *secondary* survey includes obtaining detailed information about signs, symptoms, the mechanism of injury if applicable, as well as a thorough head-to-toe physical assessment [4,10]. This is, of course, predicated on the woman's ability to communicate.

Findings from the primary survey and establishing the gestational age are usually the best indicators for identifying the department in which the woman's care would be most appropriately managed. Special attention to the pregnancy is a part of the assessment and not merely an afterthought.

Pregnant women may present for a variety of nonpregnancy and pregnancy-related reasons. A decision tree algorithm is useful for triage of the maternal–fetal dyad to determine whether the woman should remain in the emergency department or be transferred to surgery, critical care, or the obstetric unit [1,11]. Emergency department staff members generally have algorithms to follow for nonpregnant patients; however, standard obstetric algorithms are not as common. Each institution should have a written guideline or triage decision tree that is developed jointly with the emergency department and obstetric staff that addresses at which gestational age care will be managed in the emergency department versus the labor and delivery unit, which conditions prompt obstetric consultations, situations in which an obstetric nurse is present in the emergency department, and guidelines for discharge or transfer to another care setting [1]. Several useful references about caring for the maternal–fetal dyad in the non-obstetric setting are available for creating or updating institutional guidelines [11–14]. Before discharge or transfer to another area or facility, an assessment is required to confirm both maternal *and* fetal well-being [15].

Patients at 20 weeks' gestation or greater are typically referred to an obstetric setting, but this gestational age is not absolute. The criteria for an internal transfer from the emergency department to the obstetric setting are dependent on institutional policies, procedures, and resources. It is important to remember that specific diagnoses are limited to certain gestational ages, such as preeclampsia in the second and third trimester, and should be included in the treatment algorithms when addressing assessment of the pregnant patient in the emergency department. Women who present to the emergency department complaining of well-recognized obstetric concerns (e.g., vaginal bleeding, contractions, rupture of membranes, increased or watery vaginal discharge, abdominal pain, pelvic pressure, decreased fetal movement) may be transferred immediately to the obstetric unit for further assessment and management. For those women with vague symptoms, such as headache, edema, nausea and vomiting, or "just not feeling well," the decision about where to evaluate is not always so clear unless a policy or guideline is in place. Well-meaning care in a non-obstetric setting for the woman with a complicated disorder only found in pregnancy has the potential of being detrimental to both the woman and the fetus. Discussion between the emergency department and the obstetric setting may be the best method of determining whose expertise is most needed for the evaluation and care of the maternal–fetal dyad.

When a woman presents to the emergency department with cardiovascular or respiratory complaints, the maternal vital signs should be assessed and documented without delay. There are certain abnormalities or "triggers" in the patient's vital signs and condition that point to an emergency that requires immediate activation of diagnostic and intervention resources. Recognition of these events through a warning system such as the Modified Early Obstetric Warning System (MEOWS) can be utilized in emergency departments and protocols. In the MEOWS system, a physician or other qualified clinician is called for prompt bedside evaluation when the pregnant patient exhibits any one warning sign in the red area or two warning signs in the yellow at any one time [14,16] (Table 8.1). Additional emergency department screening questions, regardless of the presenting problem, include but are not limited to:

- Presence or absence of fetal movement (if appropriate for gestational age, usually ≥18–20 weeks)

TABLE 8.1   MEOWS Color-coded Trigger Parameters

	Trigger: Red	Trigger: Yellow
Temperature, °C	<35 or >38	35–36
Systolic blood pressure, mm Hg	<90 or >160	150–160 or 90–100
Diastolic blood pressure, mm Hg	>100	90–100
Heart rate, beats per minute	<40 or >120	100–120 or 40–50
Respiratory rate, breaths per minute	<10 or >30	21–30
Oxygen saturation, %	<95	—
Pain score	—	2–3
Neurologic response	Unresponsive, pain	Voice

From S. Singh, A. McGlennan, A. England, R. Simons R, A validation study of the CEMACH recommended modified early obstetric warning system (MEOWS), Anaesthesia 67 (1) (2012) 12–18.

- Presence or absence of cramping, pelvic pressure, backache, or contractions
- Presence or absence of vaginal bleeding or leaking of fluid

PREGNANT TRAUMA VICTIM ASSESSMENT AND CARE

Trauma during pregnancy is a leading contributor to maternal mortality in the United States [7,8,17]. Motor vehicle accidents are the most common mechanism of trauma mostly due to improper or lack of seatbelt placement. Another major cause of trauma is related to falls [8,17–19], but it is important to understand that even the most minor situation can be life threatening to the patient and fetus due to the anatomic and physiologic changes that occur in pregnancy [6,7]. Certain injuries are unique to the pregnant trauma patient: uterine rupture, placental abruption, preterm labor and delivery, and intrauterine fetal demise. Consideration of gestational age is an important factor because a decision may need to be made about an operative intervention on behalf of the fetus. Trauma concerns specific to pregnancy are in Table 8.2.

Maternal–Fetal Transport, Assessment, and Care

In trauma situations, first responders will provide the initial evaluation and management of the pregnant trauma patient, which should be maternally focused and consistent with advanced trauma life support (ATLS) protocols [17,20]. Alerting the emergency

TABLE 8.2   Trauma Concerns Specific to Pregnancy

Abruption	
Result of "shearing" effect when uterus is deformed by external forces, causing separation from placenta	Can trigger diffuse intravascular coagulation because of high concentration of thromboplastin in placenta
	Electronic fetal monitoring is most sensitive means of detecting abruption
	Ultrasound most specific but lacks sensitivity
Vaginal bleeding poor predictor of abruption	May be a later sign; watch for increasing fundal height, increased uterine activity, increased pain
Uterine Rupture	
Blunt trauma	Use ultrasound, x-ray; palpate fetal parts outside uterus; assess pain
Maternal–Fetal Hemorrhage	
Four to five times more common in injured woman than in noninjured woman	Fetal anemia, death, or isoimmunization
Fetal Compromise	
Nonspecific complication but most common	Late decelerations, tachycardia, loss of variability
Preterm Contractions	
Common after blunt trauma	Abruption with potential for fetal hypoxia
Fetal Injuries	
Skull fractures, intracranial hemorrhage	More common in third trimester

department early during transport allows the staff to inform the obstetric department of the need for collaborative care immediately upon arrival. First responders must promote maternal circulation and oxygenation and consider occult hemorrhage and shock in the pregnant trauma victim. Modifications of ATLS guidelines to be provided without delay before transport include supplementary oxygen, intravenous access, and lateral positioning on the patient's side or with a backboard tilt of 15 degrees in pregnancies greater than 20 weeks' gestation to prevent supine hypotension [20,21]. Vital signs should be assessed at the same frequency as for the nonpregnant woman, and fetal status should only be considered once maternal stability has been established [20]. Once maternal stabilization has been confirmed, the FHR may be evaluated with a Doppler if available. If the patient is conscious, information regarding fetal activity and the presence or absence of contractions should be obtained. Determination of the gestational age may be of great benefit in determining fetal age and the need for prompt obstetric intervention on arrival to the emergency department because fetal viability is more probable if the uterine fundal height is between the umbilicus and xiphoid process [7,20] (Figure 8.1). Simply noting the height of the uterus as above or below the maternal umbilicus may help determine whether the pregnancy is more than or less than 20 weeks' gestation.

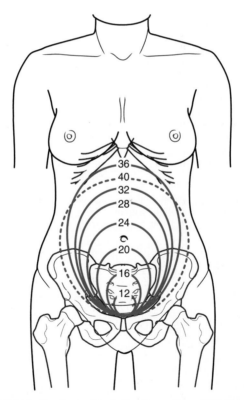

FIGURE 8.1 Uterine size and gestational age. (From M.V. Muench, J.C. Canterino, Trauma in pregnancy, Obstet. Gynecol. Clin. North Am. 34 (3) (2007) 555–583.)

Primary and Secondary Survey in the Emergency Department

Primary Survey

Similar to the first responders, the emergency department will complete a *primary survey* of a pregnant trauma patient on arrival, which again will encompass the immediate evaluation of the patient, not the fetus. Initial management of the pregnant patient is no different from that of the nonpregnant patient, so maternal health will take priority over fetal health unless the patient is undergoing cardiopulmonary resuscitation and requires a perimortem cesarean delivery.

The primary survey of the patient with trauma is an assessment based on the letters A-B-C-D-E.

The components are [4,21–23]:

Airway

Breathing

Circulation

Disability (neurologic—alert, voice, pain, unresponsive)

Exposure (examine)

Foremost in the primary survey is to assess the establishment of *airway* (A) stabilization. Adequate respirations (B, *breathing*) must be established, with supplemental oxygen being given to prevent maternal hypoxia and desaturation, which in turn can lead to fetal hypoxemia [20]. Pulse oximetry and arterial blood gases will verify that the patient is adequately oxygenated when necessary.

Blood pressure, pulse, and capillary refill (C, *circulation*) will typically verify how well the patient is being perfused. Uterine blood flow represents 10% to 15% of maternal cardiac output, or approximately 700 to 800 mL per minute. Significant blood loss, especially if blunt or penetrating injury has occurred, may set off a cascade of maternal blood flow being shunted away from the uterus to permit maternal self-preservation at the expense of the fetus. The fetus acts as an early warning system for the woman so the fetal heart rate (FHR) is frequently considered the "fifth" vital sign because adequate uterine perfusion can correlate with normal FHR characteristics, whereas abnormal FHR characteristics may reflect inadequate maternal oxygenation and circulation [7,17,20]. This can manifest into FHR characteristics that reflect fetal hypoxemia secondary to maternal hypovolemia and reduced uteroplacental perfusion, including fetal tachycardia, decreasing variability, and recurrent decelerations *even before* there are changes in maternal vital signs [4,7,8]. Compared with the nonpregnant patient, average blood volume expansion in the pregnant woman is approximately 40% to 50%, but when maternal hypotension occurs relatively late in the progression of hypovolemic shock, more than 30% of the maternal circulating volume has been lost [6,8,24]. Catecholamines are released as a result of volume loss, leading to vasoconstriction of blood vessels that facilitate maternal perfusion to the vital organs at the expense of uteroplacental blood flow and an intact oxygenation pathway. Thus aggressive volume resuscitation through two large-bore intravenous catheters is encouraged even when the hypovolemic woman is normotensive to maintain maternal–fetal hemodynamics [24]. As discussed previously, attention should continue to focus on keeping the patient's position at a 15-degree angle with a trauma backboard or wedge and not a supine position. Supine positioning results in decreased stroke volume secondary to decreased blood return to the heart [6]. This is critical to maintaining preload and cardiac output because supine positioning results in compression of the inferior vena cava in pregnant women after 20 weeks' gestation, which produces an up to 30% reduction in cardiac output [7,22].

The neurologic evaluation (D, *disability assessment*) is performed by using the A-V-P-U method (alert, voice, pain, and unresponsive) of the Glasgow Coma Scale. By following steps A to D, cardiovascular or central nervous system trauma can be identified. The patient can then be *exposed* (E) to examine for other obvious signs of physical trauma [21,22].

Secondary Survey

The *secondary survey* becomes the priority at the conclusion of the primary survey once the patient is stabilized. A detailed pregnancy history and head-to-toe physical examination is performed in an effort to gather pertinent pregnancy information and identify all injuries that may have been overlooked in the primary survey [7,8]. During the secondary survey, as long as appropriate trained personnel are available, an extensive maternal-fetal assessment should include [7,17,20] the following:

- Past and current pregnancy history
- Estimated gestational age (fundal height or ultrasound)
- Marking the top of the fundus to observe for an increasing fundal height
- Sterile speculum examination if vaginal bleeding is present or there is evidence of ruptured membranes

- Focused assessment sonographic trauma (FAST) ultrasound for potential intraabdominal hemorrhage; may be incorporated with obstetric ultrasound
- Obstetric ultrasound with capable personnel: fetal number; cardiac activity; fetal position; biometrics; placental location; visualization of possible streaming vessels or placental hematoma indicating placental injury; amniotic fluid volume; biophysical profile
- Doppler ultrasound of middle cerebral artery identifying possible acute fetal anemia
- Kleihauer-Betke test to evaluate for maternal–fetal hemorrhage

The Kleihauer-Betke test may be performed to detect the degree of maternal–fetal hemorrhage in which fetal cells are circulating in the maternal circulation in excess of what can be treated with a standard dose of Rho(D) immune globulin. This test determines the amount of Rho(D) immune globulin that is needed in the unsensitized Rh-negative pregnant trauma patient as additional fetal cells may come in contact with maternal circulation. The Kleihauer-Betke is not used to determine the need for RhoGAM [7,20,25]. In trauma, maternal–fetal hemorrhage is more common with an anterior placenta [26]. Changes in the FHR combined with a positive Kleihauer-Betke may signal hypoxemia, fetal anemia, and potential fetal compromise. If significant fetal hemorrhage has occurred, it may manifest into tachycardia or a sinusoidal pattern on the FHR tracing [25,27,28]. Doppler ultrasound of the middle cerebral artery may also demonstrate a compensatory response to hemorrhage.

Electronic fetal monitoring is a valuable adjunct tool for fetal evaluation in the pregnant trauma victim with a viable fetus as long as it does not interfere with vital maternal treatment [19]. Continuous fetal monitoring versus intermittent auscultation is preferred, because auscultation is limited in detecting specific FHR characteristics, such as variability and deceleration type [29]. Loss of variability and late or prolonged decelerations are the most sensitive findings in the detection of abruption though other FHR characteristics such as tachycardia, bradycardia, and a sinusoidal pattern may be observed [29,30]. It is imperative to establish a baseline FHR. Similar to the laboring patient, any FHR tachycardia should be regarded with suspicion and managed as outlined in Chapter 6.

Although there is a general consensus that electronic fetal monitoring is an integral part of the ongoing assessment of the maternal–fetal dyad, there are no established standards for the duration of monitoring [19,31]. Experts advocate for a minimum of 2 to 6 hours, although monitoring time should be extended in those patients experiencing a Category II FHR tracing, contractions, vaginal bleeding, abdominal pain, or significant maternal injury [7,19,20,32]. Uterine irritability or contractions may provide clues to placental abruption. Ultrasound has limited usefulness and low sensitivity in distinguishing a placental abruption, so a negative result does not exclude the possibility [20,26,33]. At greater than 20 weeks' gestation, 90% of pregnant trauma patients will demonstrate some type of uterine activity in the first 4 hours. Data shows that within the first hour, 64% of women will contract every 5 minutes or less, declining to 29% of women by the fourth hour. Patients without contractions or with less than one contraction every 10 minutes may be removed from electronic fetal monitor and discharged as long as there is evidence of fetal movement, normal FHR characteristics, and absence of vaginal bleeding or ruptured membranes [31]. Women who continue to contract with more than four to six contractions per hour, women who have a Category II or III FHR tracing, or who have sustained blunt abdominal trauma require longer assessment, preferably a minimum of 24 hours due to a reported increased abruption rate [26,29,33]. Increased abruption rates are even more increased in those patients having greater than eight contractions in the initial 4 hours [26]. At discharge, labor instructions, how to perform fetal kick counts, and when to notify the healthcare provider should be reviewed with the patient.

Emergent and Perimortem Cesarean Birth

As mentioned previously, the gravid uterus in the supine position compresses the inferior vena cava, resulting in reduced cardiac output [6,24]. If cesarean birth is performed, compression of the inferior vena cava is relieved, which results in blood volume being shunted back into the systemic system, helping to restore or improve maternal hemodynamics [3,23]. Emergency cesarean birth in the patient with a viable gestational age is distinguished from perimortem cesarean birth by the fact that emergency cesarean birth is performed for variety of maternal or fetal indications, such as a Category II or III FHR tracing, whereas perimortem cesarean birth is carried out at the time of maternal death [32].

A perimortem cesarean birth in the pregnant trauma patient may be performed when cardiopulmonary resuscitation is unsuccessful, ideally within 4 to 5 minutes, though this is being questioned as some experts advocate for a maternal resuscitative hysterotomy based on the type of rhythm (shockable versus non-shockable) [34–36]. The indication for performing a perimortem cesarean birth is less clear when times reach beyond this timeframe [32]. Nonpregnant patients suffer irreversible brain damage from anoxia within 3 to 4 minutes, but pregnant women become hypoxic more quickly. The neonatal outcome may be more favorable if a perimortem cesarean birth occurs [23]. The optimal location for a perimortem cesarean birth is at the current location of the trauma patient to avoid delay between cardiopulmonary resuscitation and perimortem cesarean birth [3]. Delivery of the fetus may allow for fetal resuscitation and perhaps a successful maternal resuscitation. A decision tree for the unstable pregnant trauma patient may be a useful resource (Figure 8.2).

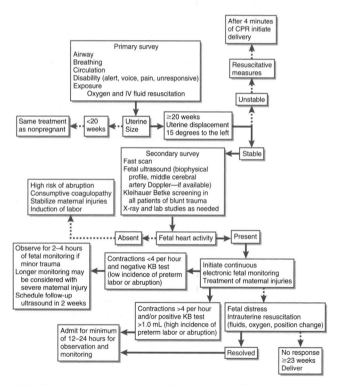

FIGURE 8.2 Maternal trauma algorithm. (From M.V. Muench, J.C. Canterino, Trauma in pregnancy, Obstet. Gynecol. Clin. North Am. 34 (3) (2007) 555–583.)

Stabilization and Discharge

If the patient is unstable, transfer from the emergency department to the operating room or a critical care unit may occur. Once stabilized, the complex pregnant trauma patient may be transferred to the perinatal unit for continued care and monitoring. A collaborative approach among the obstetric, surgical, and critical care staff needs to be comprehensive, accurate, timely, and direct in order to promote an optimal environment for maternal–fetal well-being [37]. Once a pregnant patient is ready to be discharged, education concerning safety during pregnancy should be completed. Counseling pregnant patients on appropriate seatbelt use is an important aspect of discharge teaching. The lap belt and shoulder harness are both worn simultaneously, with the lap belt being securely placed below the abdomen and over the anterior superior iliac spine and symphysis pubis. The shoulder harness should cross between the patient's breasts and below the neck [18,29]. Anatomic adaptations in pregnancy, such as joint laxity and an altered center of gravity can lead to coordination and balance issues, which in turn results in patient falls [6,19]. Reviewing key risk factors, such walking on slippery or icy walkways or carrying heavy objects, utilizing safety features such as staircase handrails, and use of proper body mechanics, including the proper way to lift objects, may help the pregnant woman avoid accidents.

NON-OBSTETRIC SURGICAL PROCEDURES: MATERNAL–FETAL ASSESSMENT AND CARE

Typically, elective surgery is best delayed until after delivery. Nonurgent but indicated non-obstetric surgical procedures are preferably delayed until 14 to 22 weeks' gestation, although if the surgery cannot wait, the procedure is generally reserved for the periviable timeframe and beyond. Urgent or emergency procedures should be performed regardless of the gestation age [5,38–40]. Quantifying the types and management of non-obstetric surgical procedures, incidence, and pregnancy outcomes is difficult because data on surgical conditions in pregnancy as well as surgical and anesthetic techniques is limited and outdated [39]. The most extensive review of data demonstrated a 0.75% incidence of non-obstetric surgical procedures, although this number may be higher because of the increasing rate of comorbidities in the patient population [41]. Major presenting conditions requiring surgical intervention include trauma, appendicitis, biliary diseases (i.e., cholecystitis and pancreatitis), bowel obstructions, adnexal masses, and breast or cervical cancers [2,4,40,42–45]. Key points in coordinating care for the maternal–fetal dyad include collaboration within a multidisciplinary team comprised of the obstetrician, surgical staff, anesthesia, neonatology, and nursing personnel as adjustments in management may be required during the procedure [2,37,38]. Formulating a perioperative plan of care enhances the outcome for the maternal–fetal dyad.

Intraoperative Maternal–Fetal Assessment

The cascading effects of interrupted maternal–fetal oxygen transfer may be related to events that occur intraoperatively to include decreased uterine blood flow, maternal hypotension, and depression of the fetal cardiovascular system from anesthetic agents [46]. The advantage of intraoperative fetal assessment is that it allows for optimization of the maternal condition if the fetus is showing signs of compromise [9]. Indeterminate or abnormal FHR patterns would most likely occur because of these maternal–fetal physiologic changes. Therefore, prompt assessment and treatment may help avoid intraoperative adverse events. Goals for intact fetal survival consist of [2,46,47]

- Maintaining maternal blood pressure and intravascular volume with adequate hemodynamic and fluid management
- Maintaining maternal oxygenation with adequate respiratory support and ventilation

An accepted standard of care linked to fetal assessment during non-obstetric surgical procedures or intervening on behalf of the viable fetus is nonexistent at this time. In fact, conflicting expert opinions exist regarding the necessity of intraoperative monitoring, although it appears most healthcare providers record the FHR pre- and postoperatively instead of intraoperatively [46,48,49]. The American College of Obstetricians and Gynecologists states: "The decision to use fetal monitoring should be individualized and if used, may be based on gestational age, type of surgery, and facilities available" [38]. Collaboration is requisite among the surgeon, anesthesiologist, and obstetrician to determine whether intraoperative fetal assessment is necessary. The advantage of fetal assessment for surgical procedures includes enhanced communication among disciplines related to altered maternal anatomy and physiology; patient positioning to optimize blood flow and oxygenation to the fetus; the safety of medications utilized during the procedure; and prompt identification of an FHR pattern requiring emergent cesarean birth [38]. Furthermore, fetal assessment during the surgical procedure demonstrates that the healthcare team acknowledges a second patient [50].

If fetal monitoring is utilized, the following guidelines should be followed [38]:

- Doppler FHR pre- and postprocedure for the previable fetus
- A healthcare provider with cesarean delivery privileges should be readily available
- Neonatal and pediatric service must be available in the institution performing the surgery
- A qualified individual adept at both performing fetal assessment and interpreting the status of uterine activity and FHR characteristics should be readily available
- At a minimum, simultaneous FHR and uterine contraction monitoring in the viable fetus should be performed pre- and postprocedure to assess fetal status and uterine quiescence
- Continuous intraoperative fetal monitoring may be appropriate when all of the following can be accomplished:
  - Viable fetus
  - External application of ultrasound and tocotransducer, if feasible
  - Informed consent for emergency cesarean birth, if possible
  - Type of surgical procedure allows for safe interruption or alteration to provide access for emergency cesarean birth

Depending on the type of surgery, intraoperative monitoring can be done with a Doppler or an ultrasound and tocotransducer that may need to be covered with a sterile sleeve when sterility is required. In cases in which transabdominal monitoring is not practical, transvaginal Doppler ultrasound may be utilized in selected cases [2,9,46].

The FHR characteristically demonstrates a decreasing baseline that remains in the lower limits of normal and decreasing variability with induction of general anesthesia (Figure 8.3). This may be related to a portion of the fetal brainstem that regulates FHR being anesthetized [9,51]. Baseline FHR and variability changes caused by intraoperative medication administration must be differentiated from FHR alterations that result from fetal hypoxia such as recurrent decelerations, tachycardia, or bradycardia. Spontaneous decelerations are usually not found in these patients [46,47]. Postoperative monitoring of uterine activity and fetal assessment are continued as appropriate for gestational age, type of surgery performed, physician orders, and presence or absence of uterine contractions. Interpretation and management of intraoperative and postoperative FHR changes should be guided by the principles outlined in Chapters 2, 5, and 6.

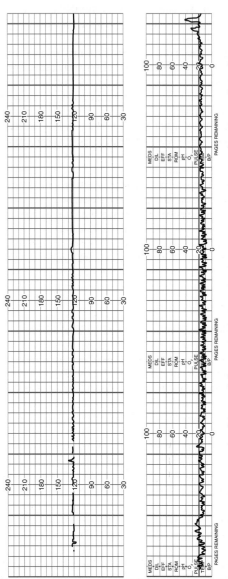

FIGURE 8.3 Example of 34 weeks' gestation FHR tracing in a pregnant patient undergoing unilateral mastectomy under general anesthesia. Note the normal range baseline, minimal to absent variability, and lack of periodic and nonperiodic changes. (Courtesy Rebecca Cypher, MSN, PNNP.)

Tocolytic Agents and Antenatal Corticosteroids

Studies that included pregnant patients having non-obstetric surgical procedures have demonstrated a higher incidence of miscarriage and preterm birth, but this may be related to the surgical procedure, uterine manipulation, or the underlying condition requiring surgery [9]. Therefore reducing the risk of uterine contractions and subsequent preterm labor may be best accomplished by minimizing uterine manipulation [2,43]. Routine administration of prophylactic tocolytic agents has not been shown to be beneficial because these agents are not indicated for preterm labor prevention [2,52]. Evaluation using methods such as fetal fibronectin or transvaginal cervical length may be more useful before determining whether tocolytic agents are required [52].

A prophylactic course of antenatal corticosteroids may be considered between 23 and 34 weeks' gestation to enhance fetal lung maturity given that there may be a potential increased risk for preterm delivery. The decision to administer antenatal corticosteroids prophylactically or to wait for uterine contractions should be individualized to the patient, the clinical situation, and risk factors [42]. Refer to Chapter 7 for dosing and impact on the FHR tracing.

Surgery When Gestation Is Greater Than 24 Weeks

When surgery is needed by a woman whose gestation is more than 23 to 24 weeks' gestation, the following points should be kept in mind:

- Preoperative cervical examination provides baseline information.
- Preoperative medications are indicated to assist with gastric emptying and neutralizing gastric contents because of decreased gastric motility and relaxed gastric sphincters.
- Left uterine displacement after 20 weeks' gestation assists in avoiding hypotension and providing improved uteroplacental perfusion.
- Maintaining maternal oxygen saturation above 95% and maternal mean arterial pressure greater than 65 mm Hg helps keep the uterus perfused.
- If the surgery is performed outside the labor and delivery unit, neonatal equipment such as a radiant warmer, incubator, and resuscitation equipment must be immediately available in the room.

FEDERAL LAW AND TRIAGE

Triage incorporates a rapid assessment of the woman, identification of the concerns, determination of the acuity of the problem, and arrangement for the appropriate personnel and equipment to meet the woman's needs. Triage of pregnant patients is regulated by federal law via the Emergency Medical Treatment and Active Labor Act [15]. This act ensures public access to emergency services regardless of insurance or capacity to pay. Hospitals must triage and provide a medical screening examination (MSE) to determine whether an emergency medical condition exists, including labor. The MSE is performed by a licensed provider on the basis of the history and physical and consists of procedures and tests that will identify medical and obstetric conditions [53]. Triage and an MSE must be performed in a timely manner, with appropriate treatment and stabilization based on the clinical situation. The patient may require transfer, once stabilized, when a higher level of care is necessary, there are capacity limitations in bed management at the transferring facility, or the patient requests transfer [53]. The Emergency Nurses Association and Association of Women's Health, Obstetric and Neonatal Nurses state that a pregnant woman's care should take place in the area best prepared to handle her needs and support the development of hospital policies and procedures that specifically outline triage, care, and disposition of the patient [11].

SUMMARY

The initial emergent event and the physiologic challenges of pregnant women require exceptional teamwork and communication, combined with workable institutional protocols. Caregivers in the emergency department should understand fetal and maternal physiology to provide safe care to pregnant women. Collaboration between the emergency department and the labor and delivery staff is essential for developing guidelines and protocols.

References

[1] D.J. Angelini, Overview of obstetric triage and potential pitfalls, in: D.J. Angelini, D. LaFontaine (Eds.), Obstetric Triage and Emergency Care Protocols, Springer, New York, 2013, pp. 1–9.

[2] M.K. Stewart, K.P. Terhune, Management of pregnant patients undergoing general surgical procedures, Surg. Clin. North Am. 95 (2) (2015) 429–442.

[3] E.J. Lavonas, I.R. Drennan, A. Gabrielli, A.C. Heffner, C.O. Hoyte, A.M. Orkin, K.N. Sawyer, M.W. Donnino, Part 10: special circumstances

of resuscitation: 2015 American Heart Association Guidelines Update for Cardiopulmonary Resuscitation and Emergency Cardiovascular Care, Circulation 132 (Suppl. 2) (2015) S501–S518.

[4] M.T. Coleman, V.A. Trianfo, D.A. Rund, Nonobstetric emergencies in pregnancy: trauma and surgical conditions, Am. J. Obstet. Gynecol. 177 (3) (1997) 497–502.

[5] M. Inturrisi, Perioperative assessment of fetal heart rate and uterine activity, J. Obstet. Gynecol. Neonatal Nurs. 29 (3) (2000) 331–336.

[6] M.C. Gordon, Maternal physiology, in: S.G. Gabbe, J.R. Niebyl, J.L. Simpson, M.B. Landon, H.L. Gala, E. Jauniaux, D.A. Driscoll (Eds.), Obstetrics: Normal and Problem Pregnancies, sixth ed., Elsevier, Philadelphia, PA, 2012, pp. 42–65.

[7] M.V. Muench, J.C. Canterino, Trauma in pregnancy, Obstet. Gynecol. Clin. North Am. 34 (3) (2007) 555–583.

[8] D.C. Ruffolo, Trauma care and managing the injured pregnant patient, J. Obstet. Gynecol. Neonatal Nurs. 38 (6) (2009) 704–714.

[9] M. Van De Velde, F. De Buck, Anesthesia for non-obstetric surgery in the pregnant patient, Minerva Anestesiol. 73 (4) (2007) 235–240.

[10] V. Bacidore, N. Warren, C. Chaput, V.A. Keough, A collaborative framework for managing pregnancy loss in the emergency department, J. Obstet. Gynecol. Neonatal Nurs. 38 (6) (2009) 730–738.

[11] Emergency Nurses Association, Association of Women's Health, Obstetric and Neonatal Nurses, Joint Position Statement: The Obstetrical Patient in the ED, ENA, Des Plaines, IL, 2011. Available from: http://www.ena.org/SiteCollectionDocuments/Position%20Statements/OBPatientED.pdf.

[12] American College of Obstetricians and Gynecologists, Nonobstetric surgery in pregnancy. ACOG Committee Opinion no. 474, Obstet. Gynecol. 117 (2) (2011) 420–421.

[13] American College of Obstetricians and Gynecologists, Levels of maternal care. ACOG Obstetric Care Consensus no. 2, Obstet. Gynecol. 125 (2) (2015) 502–515.

[14] American College of Obstetricians and Gynecologists, Preparing for clinical emergencies in obstetrics and gynecology. ACOG Committee Opinion no. 590, Obstet. Gynecol. 123 (2) (2014) 722–725.

[15] Centers for Medicare and Medicaid Services, Emergency Medical Treatment and Labor Act, Available from: http://www.cms.gov/Regulations-and-Guidance/Legislation/EMTALA/index.html?redirect=/EMTALA/, 2012 (accessed 19.03.15).

[16] S. Singh, A. McGlennan, A. England, R. Simons, A validation study of the CEMACH recommended modified early obstetric warning system (MEOWS), Anaesthesia 67 (1) (2012) 12–18.

[17] J. Foroutan, G.G. Ashmead, Trauma in pregnancy, Postgrad. Obstet. Gynecol. 34 (14) (2014) 1–5.

[18] T. Luley, C.B. Fitzpatrick, C.A. Grotegut, et al., Perinatal implications of motor vehicle accident trauma during pregnancy: identifying populations at risk, Am. J. Obstet. Gynecol. 208 (6) (2013) 466.e1–466.e5.

[19] H. Mendez-Figueroa, J.D. Dahlke, R.A. Vrees, D.J. Rouse, Trauma in pregnancy: an updated systematic review, Am. J. Obstet. Gynecol. 209 (1) (2013) 1–10.

[20] S. Einav, H.Y. Sela, C.F. Weiniger, Management and outcomes of trauma during pregnancy, Anesthesiol. Clin. 31 (1) (2013) 141–156.

[21] J.P. Lavery, M. Staten-McCormick, Management of moderate to severe trauma in pregnancy, Obstet. Gynecol. Clin. North Am. 22 (1) (1999) 69–90.

[22] American College of Surgeons Committee on Trauma, Advanced Trauma Life Support, ninth ed., American College of Surgeons, Chicago, IL, 2012.

[23] S. Morris, M. Stacey, ABC of resuscitation: resuscitation in pregnancy, BMJ 327 (7426) (2003) 1277–1279.

[24] J. Bonnar, Massive obstetric haemorrhage, Baillieres Best Pract. Res. Clin. Obstet. Gynaecol. 14 (1) (2000) 1–18.

[25] B.J. Wylie, M.E. D'Alton, Fetomaternal hemorrhage, Obstet. Gynecol. 115 (5) (2010) 1039–1051.

[26] M.D. Pearlman, J.E. Tintinalli, R.P. Lorenz, A prospective controlled study of outcome after trauma during pregnancy, Am. J. Obstet. Gynecol. 162 (6) (1990) 1502–1507.

[27] H.D. Modanlou, R.K. Freeman, Sinusoidal fetal heart rate pattern: its definition and clinical significance, Am. J. Obstet. Gynecol. 142 (8) (1982) 1033–1038.

[28] H.D. Modanlou, Y. Murata, Sinusoidal heart rate pattern: reappraisal of its definition and clinical significance, J. Obstet. Gynaecol. Res. 30 (3) (2004) 169–180.

[29] M.C. Chames, M.D. Pearlman, Trauma during pregnancy: outcomes and clinical management, Clin. Obstet. Gynecol. 51 (2) (2008) 398–408.

[30] J.K. Williams, L. McClain, A.S. Rosemurgy, et al., Evaluation of blunt abdominal trauma in the third trimester of pregnancy: maternal and fetal considerations, Obstet. Gynecol. 75 (1) (1990) 33–37.

[31] M. Curet, C.R. Schermer, G.B. Demarest, et al., Predictors of outcome in trauma during pregnancy: identification of patients who can be monitored for less than 6 hours, J. Trauma 49 (1) (2000) 18–25.

[32] R.D. Barraco, W.C. Chiu, T.V. Clancy, et al., Practice management guidelines for the diagnosis and management of injury in the pregnant patient: the EAST Practice Management Guidelines Work Group, J. Trauma 69 (1) (2010) 211–214.

[33] M.A. Dahmus, B.M. Sibai, Blunt abdominal trauma: are there any predictive factors for abruptio placentae or maternal-fetal distress? Am. J. Obstet. Gynecol. 169 (4) (1993) 1054–1059.

[34] M. Lavecchia, H.A. Abenhaim, Cardiopulmonary resuscitation of pregnant women in the emergency department, Resuscitation 91 (2015) 104–107.

[35] C.H. Rose, A. Faksh, K.D. Traynor, D. Cabrera, K.W. Arendt, B.C. Brost, Challenging the 4- to 5-minute rule: from perimortem cesarean to resuscitative hysterotomy, Am. J. Obstet. Gynecol. 213 (5) (2015) 653–656.

[36] V.L. Katz, D.J. Dotters, W. Droegemueller, Perimortem cesarean delivery, Obstet. Gynecol. 68 (4) (1986) 571–576.

[37] K.L. Torgersen, Communication to facilitate care of the obstetric surgical patient in a postanesthesia care setting, J. Perianesth. Nurs. 20 (3) (2005) 177–184.

[38] American College of Obstetricians and Gynecologists, Critical care in pregnancy. ACOG Practice Bulletin no. 100, Obstet. Gynecol. 113 (2) (2009) 443–450.

[39] E.A. Baldwin, K.S. Borowski, B.C. Brost, C.H. Rose, Antepartum non-obstetrical surgery at ≥23 weeks' gestation and risk for preterm delivery, Am. J. Obstet. Gynecol. 212 (2) (2014) e1–e5.

[40] C. Caren, D.A. Edmonson, Common general surgical emergencies in pregnancy, in: D.J. Angelini, D. LaFontaine (Eds.), Obstetric Triage and Emergency Care Protocols, Springer, New York, 2013, pp. 197–216.

[41] R.I. Mazze, B. Kallén, Reproductive outcome after anesthesia and operation during pregnancy: a registry study of 5405 cases, Am. J. Obstet. Gynecol. 161 (5) (1989) 1178–1185.

[42] M. Naqvi, A. Kaimal, Adnexal masses in pregnancy, Clin. Obstet. Gynecol. 58 (1) (2015) 93–101.

[43] H.T. Sharp, The acute abdomen during pregnancy, Clin. Obstet. Gynecol. 45 (2) (2002) 405–413.

[44] S. Viswanathan, B. Ramaswamy, Pregnancy-associated breast cancer, Clin. Obstet. Gynecol. 54 (4) (2011) 546–555.

[45] K.Y. Yang, Abnormal pap smear and cervical cancer in pregnancy, Clin. Obstet. Gynecol. 55 (3) (2012) 838–848.

[46] M.A. Rosen, Management of anesthesia for the pregnant surgical patient, Anesthesiology 91 (4) (1999) 1159–1163.

[47] M. Balki, P.H. Manninen, Craniotomy for suprasellar meningioma in a 28-week pregnant woman without fetal heart rate monitoring, Can. J. Anaesth. 51 (6) (2004) 573–576.

[48] T. Horrigan, R. Villareal, L. Weinstein, Are obstetrical personnel required for intraoperative fetal monitoring during non-obstetrical surgery? J. Perinatol. 19 (2) (1999) 124–126.

[49] C.C. Kilpatrick, C. Puig, L. Chohan, et al., Intraoperative fetal heart rate monitoring during nonobstetric surgery in pregnancy: a practice survey, South. Med. J. 103 (3) (2010) 212–215.

[50] R.M. Denaro, Expecting the best: considerations for the pregnant patient, OR Nurse 2014 2 (8) (2008) 45–48.

[51] P.L. Liu, T.M. Warren, G.W. Ostheimer, J.B. Weiss, L.M. Liu, Fetal monitoring in parturients undergoing surgery unrelated to pregnancy, Obstet. Anesth. Digest. 6 (1) (1986) 185.

[52] K.M. Groom, Pharmacological prevention of prematurity, Best Pract. Res. Clin. Obstet. Gynaecol. 21 (5) (2007) 843–856.

[53] J.M. Kriebs, Legal considerations in obstetric triage: EMTALA and HIPPA, in: D.J. Angelini, D. LaFontaine (Eds.), Obstetric Triage and Emergency Care Protocols, Springer, New York, 2013, pp. 11–18.

Antepartum Fetal Assessment

When electronic fetal heart rate (FHR) monitoring was initially developed and studied, it required direct access to the fetus and was therefore limited to the intrapartum period. The development of Doppler ultrasound technology made it possible to monitor the FHR externally and in situations outside of the intrapartum setting. Observations and experience gained from early intrapartum monitoring was applied to the antepartum period and led to the development of antepartum testing.

The goals of antepartum testing are the following:

1. Identify fetuses at risk for injury due to interrupted oxygenation so that permanent injury or death might be prevented.
2. Identify appropriately oxygenated fetuses so that unnecessary intervention can be avoided.

COMPARING ANTEPARTUM TESTING METHODS

The *false-negative rate* is the key measure of effectiveness of any antepartum test. It is most often defined in the literature as the incidence of fetal death within 1 week of a normal antepartum test (Box 9.1). Reported false-negative rates range from 0.4 to more than 6 per 1000 with current testing methods. The *false-positive rate* is another important feature in antepartum testing. A false-positive test usually is defined as an abnormal test that prompts delivery but that is not associated with evidence of acute interruption of fetal oxygenation (meconium-stained amniotic fluid, intrapartum FHR abnormalities, abnormal umbilical artery blood gas results, low Apgar scores), or chronic interruption of fetal oxygenation (fetal growth restriction under the 10th percentile for gestational age). False-positive rates range from 30% to 90% with current testing methods.

In August 2007, the Eunice Kennedy Shriver National Institute of Child Health and Human Development (NICHD), the National Institutes of Health Office of Rare Diseases, the American College of Obstetricians and Gynecologists (ACOG), and the American Academy of Pediatrics jointly sponsored a 2-day workshop to evaluate

BOX 9.1   Key Measures of the Effectiveness of Antepartum Testing

False negative: Fetal death within 1 week of a normal antepartum test
False positive: Abnormal test that prompts delivery but is not associated with acute or chronic interruption of fetal oxygenation

and summarize the scientific evidence supporting the use of antepartum assessment of fetal condition [1].

Antepartum testing is used primarily in patients who are considered to be at *increased risk for interruption of fetal oxygenation* by any of the mechanisms described in Chapter 2. The participants of the 2007 NICHD workshop reviewed the evidence regarding indications for antepartum testing, the reported gestational ages at which to initiate testing for various conditions, and the recommended options for testing mode and schedule and published their findings in 2009 [1]. Table 9.1 provides a summary of the available evidence regarding testing indication, initiation, and mode and schedule of testing from the 2009 report.

The panel concluded that data were insufficient to support recommendations for the following conditions:

- Advanced maternal age (≥35 years)
- Advanced maternal age (≥40 years)
- Black race
- Maternal age <20 years
- Nulliparity
- Parity >10
- Assisted reproductive technology
- Abnormal serum markers
- Obesity (body mass index ≥25)
- Less than 12 years of education
- Smoking >10 cigarettes per day
- Thrombophilia
- Thyroid disorders

If testing is to be used in these conditions, it should be initiated in general no earlier than 32–34 weeks [2]. Possible exceptions include conditions such as chronic hypertension with fetal growth restriction [2]. Earlier initiation is likely to result in false-positive tests, possible unnecessary intervention, and potential iatrogenic prematurity. The relative capabilities and limitations of various methods of antepartum testing, including test indications, timing of initiation,

TABLE 9.1   Recommendations for Initiation of Antepartum Testing

Maternal and Fetal Indications	Reported Gestational Age at Initiation	Reported Options for Testing Mode and Schedule
Diabetes—diet controlled	Not indicated	Not applicable
Diabetes—insulin controlled Class A2, B, C, D without hypertension, renal disease, or fetal growth restriction	32 weeks	Weekly CST with midweek NST
Diabetes—insulin controlled Class A2, B, C, D without hypertension, renal disease, or fetal growth restriction	32 weeks	Twice-weekly NST or Twice-weekly BPP
Diabetes—insulin controlled Class A2, B, C, D without hypertension, renal disease, or fetal growth restriction	34 weeks	Twice-weekly NST with weekly AFI
Diabetes—insulin controlled Class R or F	26 weeks	Weekly CST with midweek NST
Diabetes—insulin controlled Any class with hypertension, renal disease, or fetal growth restriction	26 weeks	Weekly CST with midweek NST
Diabetes—insulin controlled Any class with hypertension, renal disease, or fetal growth restriction	28 weeks	Twice-weekly NST or Twice-weekly BPP
Chronic hypertension	26 weeks	Twice-weekly NST plus AFI
Chronic hypertension	33 weeks	Twice-weekly MBPP
Chronic hypertension with SLE, fetal growth restriction, diabetes, or pregnancy-induced hypertension	26 weeks	Twice-weekly NST with AFI
Mild pregnancy-induced hypertension	At diagnosis	Twice-weekly MBPP
Severe pregnancy-induced hypertension	At diagnosis	Daily NST with BPP if nonreactive and AFI twice-weekly
Suspected fetal growth restriction	At diagnosis	Weekly NST plus AFI
Suspected fetal growth restriction	At diagnosis	UAD 1–2 times weekly
Confirmed fetal growth restriction	At diagnosis	Twice-weekly MBPP

Continued

TABLE 9.1   Recommendations for Initiation of Antepartum Testing—cont'd

Maternal and Fetal Indications	Reported Gestational Age at Initiation	Reported Options for Testing Mode and Schedule
Confirmed fetal growth restriction	At diagnosis	UAD 1–2 times weekly
Concordant twins	32 weeks	Weekly NST plus AFI
Discordant twins	At diagnosis	Twice-weekly MBPP
Triplets	28 weeks	Twice-weekly BPP
Oligohydramnios	At diagnosis	Twice-weekly NST plus AFI
Preterm premature rupture of membranes	At diagnosis	Daily NST or daily BPP
Gestational age 41 weeks	41 weeks	Twice-weekly BPP or weekly MBPP
Gestational age ≥42 weeks	42 weeks	Twice-weekly MBPP
Previous stillbirth	32 weeks	Twice-weekly MBPP or weekly BPP or weekly CST
Previous stillbirth	34 weeks or 1 week before previous stillbirth	Weekly MBPP
Decreased fetal movement	At diagnosis	MBPP
SLE	26 weeks	Weekly CST, BPP, or NST
Renal disease	30–32 weeks	Twice-weekly BPP
Cholestasis of pregnancy	34 weeks	Weekly MBPP

Source: C. Signore, R.K. Freeman, C.Y. Spong, Antenatal testing—a reevaluation: executive summary of a Eunice Kennedy Shriver National Institute of Child Health and Human Development workshop, Obstet. Gynecol. 113 (3) (2009) 687–701. Available at: www.ncbi.nlm.nih.gov/pmc/articles/PMC2771454/.
BPP, biophysical profile; *CST,* contraction stress test; *MBPP,* modified biophysical profile; *NST,* nonstress test; *SLE,* systemic lupus erythematosus; *UAD,* umbilical artery Doppler.

and frequency of testing are summarized in ACOG Practice Bulletin Number 145 [2]. Examples of indications for antepartum testing identified by ACOG are listed as follows.

Maternal conditions:
- Pregestational diabetes
- Hypertension
- Systemic lupus erythematosus
- Chronic renal disease
- Antiphospholipid syndrome

- Hyperthyroidism (poorly controlled)
- Hemoglobinopathies (sickle cell, sickle cell–hemoglobin C, or sickle cell–thalassemia disease)
- Cyanotic heart disease
  Pregnancy-related conditions:
- Gestational hypertension
- Preeclampsia
- Decreased fetal movement
- Gestational diabetes mellitus (poorly controlled or medically treated)
- Oligohydramnios
- Fetal growth restriction
- Late term or postterm pregnancy
- Isoimmunization
- Previous fetal demise (unexplained or recurrent risk)
- Monochorionic multiple gestation (with significant growth discrepancy)

METHODS OF TESTING

CONTRACTION STRESS TEST AND OXYTOCIN CHALLENGE TEST

The first antepartum testing technique, the contraction stress test or oxytocin challenge test, arose from intrapartum observations linking late decelerations with poor perinatal outcome. The test sought to identify transient fetal hypoxemia by demonstrating late decelerations in fetuses exposed to the stress of spontaneous (contraction stress test) or induced (oxytocin challenge test) uterine contractions. Kubli and associates reported that late decelerations occurring during spontaneous uterine contractions were associated with increased rates of fetal death, growth restriction, and neonatal depression [3]. Similar observations were made by other investigators using oxytocin or nipple stimulation to provoke uterine contractions.

Interpretation and Management

The contraction stress test is considered *negative* if there are at least three uterine contractions in a 10-minute period with no late decelerations on the tracing. In this case the routine weekly testing schedule usually is resumed. Failure to produce three contractions within a 10-minute window, or inability to trace the FHR, results in an *unsatisfactory* test. Prolonged decelerations, variable decelerations, or late decelerations occurring with less than 50% of the contractions constitute a *suspicious* or *equivocal* test. Decelerations that occur in the presence of contractions more frequent than every 2 minutes or lasting longer than 90 seconds constitute an equivocal test. Unsatisfactory, suspicious, or equivocal tests usually are managed by further evaluation in the form of prolonged monitoring or repeat testing after a reasonable interval, often the following day.

The contraction stress test or oxytocin challenge test is considered *positive* when at least half of the contractions during a 10-minute window are associated with late decelerations. Usually, a positive contraction stress test or oxytocin challenge test warrants hospitalization for further evaluation and/or delivery. Freeman and colleagues tested more than 4600 women with the contraction stress test and reported a false-negative rate of 0.4/1000 [4]. When the last test before delivery was a negative contraction stress test, the perinatal mortality rate was 2.3/1000, compared with a mortality rate of 176.5/1000 when the last test was a positive contraction stress test. Reported false-positive rates for the contraction stress test range from 8% to 57%, with an average of approximately 30% [5].

Interpretation summary of the contraction stress test is as follows:

- Negative: No late or significant variable decelerations
- Positive: Late decelerations with 50% or more of contractions (even if there are fewer than three contractions in 10 minutes)
- Equivocal-suspicious: Intermittent late decelerations or significant variable decelerations
- Equivocal: Fetal heart rate decelerations that occur in the presence of contractions more frequently than every 2 minutes or lasting longer than 90 seconds
- Unsatisfactory: Fewer than three contractions in 10 minutes or an uninterpretable tracing

Advantages and Limitations

Principal advantages of the contraction stress test include excellent sensitivity and a weekly testing interval. Limitations include a high rate of equivocal results requiring repeat testing, increased expense and inconvenience (particularly if oxytocin is required), and increased time requirement compared with the nonstress test.

Procedures for Contraction Stress Testing

The contraction stress test can be performed by breast or nipple stimulation or by administering an intravenous infusion with oxytocin. Note that the contraction stress test is contraindicated in several clinical situations, including preterm labor, placenta previa, vasa previa, cervical incompetence, multiple gestation, and previous classical cesarean delivery. The procedure for performing the contraction stress test follows.

Procedure for Nipple-Stimulated Contraction Stress Test

1. Assist the woman to a semi-Fowler's position with a lateral tilt.
2. Position the tocodynamometer above the uterine fundus.
3. Place the ultrasound transducer on the maternal abdomen where the clearest fetal signal can be obtained.
4. Monitor baseline FHR and uterine activity until 10 minutes of interpretable data are obtained (defer nipple stimulation if three spontaneous contractions of more than 40 seconds' duration occur within a 10-minute period).
5. Instruct woman to brush the surface of the fingers over the nipple of one breast through her clothes; continue four cycles of 2 minutes on and 2 to 5 minutes off; stop when contraction begins and restimulate when contraction ends (if a 2-minute period has elapsed).
   a. If unsuccessful after four cycles, restimulate the breasts for 10 minutes, stopping when contraction begins and resuming when contraction ends.
   b. If unsuccessful, begin bilateral continuous stimulation for 10 minutes, stopping when contraction begins and resuming when contraction ends.
6. Discontinue nipple stimulation when three or more spontaneous contractions lasting longer than 40 seconds occur in a 10-minute period and are palpable to the examiner.
7. Interpret results and continue monitoring until uterine activity has returned to the prestimulation state.

If nipple stimulation does not produce the desired uterine activity, an oxytocin-stimulated contraction stress test may be necessary.

Procedure for Oxytocin Challenge Test

The oxytocin challenge test is performed in the inpatient setting because labor may be stimulated in some sensitive women.

1. Assist the woman into a semi-Fowler's position with a lateral tilt.
2. Place the tocodynamometer above the uterine fundus.

3. Place the ultrasound transducer on the maternal abdomen where the clearest fetal signal can be obtained.

4. Monitor baseline FHR and uterine activity until 10 minutes of interpretable data are obtained.

5. Check the woman's blood pressure and pulse.

6. If fewer than three spontaneous contractions occur within a 10-minute period and if late decelerations do not occur with spontaneous contractions, oxytocin can be initiated.

7. Piggyback oxytocin into the primary intravenous line in the port nearest the intravenous insertion site.

8. Administer oxytocin, beginning with 0.5 to 2.0 mU/min, with a constant infusion pump per facility protocol.

9. Increase the dosage of oxytocin infusion by 0.5 to 1.0 mU/min at 15-minute intervals until the contraction frequency is three in 10 minutes of 40 seconds' or more duration and contractions are palpable to the examiner.

10. Discontinue the oxytocin when three contractions have occurred within a 10-minute period of interpretable data.

11. Discontinue the oxytocin any time there is evidence of excessive uterine activity, prolonged deceleration, or recurrent late decelerations; be prepared to administer terbutaline for tocolysis.

12. Continue to monitor until uterine activity and FHR return to baseline status.

THE NONSTRESS TEST

FHR accelerations that occur in association with fetal movements form the basis of the nonstress test (NST). Although many criteria have been reported, a normal or "reactive" nonstress test usually is defined by two or more accelerations in a 20-minute period, each lasting at least 15 seconds and peaking at least 15 bpm above the baseline. Before 32 weeks, an acceleration is defined as a rise of at least 10 bpm with an onset to offset of at least 10 seconds.

The NST is considered "nonreactive" if, *after 40 minutes of continuous monitoring,* the FHR tracing does not demonstrate at least two qualifying accelerations within any 20-minute window [2,6]. In most institutions, the test is repeated once or twice weekly. Boehm reported that twice-weekly testing yielded a threefold reduction in the incidence of fetal death [7].

Alternately, fetal acoustic stimulation testing (FAST) can be used. As discussed in Chapter 6, an FHR acceleration in response to fetal vibroacoustic stimulation is highly predictive of the absence of fetal metabolic acidemia and ongoing hypoxic injury [8–16]. Using an artificial larynx placed on the maternal abdomen near the fetal head, vibroacoustic stimulation is applied for 1 to 2 seconds. The test is considered *reactive* if stimulation results in an FHR acceleration. (NOTE: The gestational age–related criteria for acceleration peak and duration are the same for FAST as for the NST). Clinicians should note that with FAST, only one application of vibroacoustic stimulation is performed; if the fetus does not respond with an acceleration, the FAST is considered *nonreactive.*

Among 1542 women tested weekly with the nonstress test, Freeman reported a corrected fetal loss rate of 3.2/1000 and a false-negative rate of 1.9/1000 [4]. Assessment of FHR characteristics other than accelerations (baseline rate, variability, decelerations) may improve the sensitivity of the test. Decelerations may be observed in 33% to 50% of patients undergoing weekly nonstress tests [17–19]. In one study, reactive tests accompanied by variable decelerations were associated with rates of meconium passage and cesarean delivery for fetal indications that were similar to those encountered with nonreactive tests [18]. Manning and colleagues concluded that FHR decelerations during the nonstress test, regardless of reactivity, warrant consideration of delivery. Reported false-positive rates of the nonstress test vary widely, with an average rate of approximately 50%.

Interpretation and Management

The nonstress test is interpreted as reactive or nonreactive (see Figures 9.1 and 9.2).

- A reactive NST is defined as two accelerations in a 20-minute period, each lasting at least 15 seconds and peaking at least 15 bpm above the baseline. (Before 32 weeks an acceleration is defined as a rise of at least 10 bpm lasting at least 10 seconds from onset to offset.)
- A nonreactive NST is a test that does not demonstrate at least two qualifying accelerations within a 20-minute window.

A reactive nonstress test with no significant decelerations is considered normal, and the routine testing schedule is resumed (usually once or twice weekly). A nonreactive nonstress test requires further evaluation. In most cases, a backup test is performed (a contraction stress test or a biophysical profile) [2]. Management is guided by the results of the backup test. When performed twice weekly and

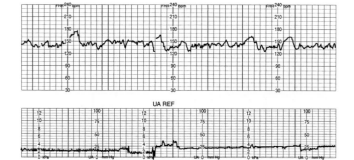

FIGURE 9.1 Reactive NST in term pregnancy. Note accelerations meet minimum criteria of 15 bpm or greater and last a minimum of 15 seconds or longer duration (onset to offset).

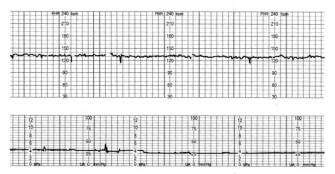

FIGURE 9.2 Segment of nonreactive NST in term pregnancy. The lack of accelerations meeting minimum criteria continued for 40 minutes.

interpreted in the context of associated FHR patterns, the nonstress test alone appears to be an acceptable, although not optimal, method of antepartum testing.

Advantages and Disadvantages

Advantages of the nonstress test include ease of use and interpretation, low cost, and minimal time requirement. The chief disadvantages include a twice-weekly testing interval, a high false-positive rate, and a higher false-negative rate than achieved with other methods. Management of the nonstress test is illustrated in Figure 9.3.

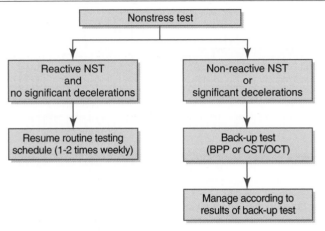

FIGURE 9.3 Management of the NST.

THE BIOPHYSICAL PROFILE

The biophysical profile, as described by Manning and colleagues [20], assesses five biophysical variables. Fetal heart rate reactivity, fetal movement, tone, and breathing reflect acute central nervous system function, while amniotic fluid volume serves as a marker of the longer term adequacy of placental function. Two points are assigned for each normal variable and zero points for each abnormal variable, for a maximum score of 10.

Interpretation and Management

Scoring the biophysical profile is outlined in Table 9.2. A biophysical profile score of 8 to 10, with normal amniotic fluid volume, is considered normal, and the routine testing schedule is resumed. A score of 6 is considered suspicious, and testing is usually repeated the next day. Scores less than 6 are associated with increased perinatal morbidity and mortality and usually warrant hospitalization for further evaluation or delivery.

The biophysical profile is a reliable predictor of fetal well-being. The false-negative rate is superior to that of the nonstress test alone and compares favorably with the false-negative rate of the contraction stress test. One study reported a false-negative rate of 0.6/1000

TABLE 9.2   Scoring the Biophysical Profile

Biophysical Variable	Score 2	Score 0
Fetal breathing movements	At least one episode of fetal breathing movements of at least 30-second duration in a 30-minute observation	Absent fetal breathing movements or less than 30 seconds of sustained fetal breathing movements in 30 minutes
Fetal movements	At least three trunk/limb movements in 30 minutes	Fewer than three episodes of trunk/limb movements in 30 minutes
Fetal tone	At least one episode of active extension with return to flexion of fetal limb or trunk; opening and closing of hand considered normal tone	Absence of movement or slow extension/flexion
Amniotic fluid	Deepest vertical pocket >2 cm	Deepest vertical pocket ≥2 cm
NST	Reactive	Nonreactive

among 12,620 women tested weekly with the biophysical profile [21]. Another study reported significantly lower rates of cesarean delivery for fetal distress (3% vs. 22%), low 5-minute Apgar scores (1.6% and 3.2% vs. 12.5%), and meconium aspiration syndrome when the last biophysical profile before delivery was normal versus when it was abnormal [22]. Among 19,221 referred high-risk pregnancies, Manning and colleagues [23] reported a false-negative rate of 0.7/1000. The false-positive rate of the biophysical profile varies with the score of the last test before delivery, ranging from 0% if the last biophysical profile score before delivery was 0, to more than 40% if the last biophysical profile score was 6.

Advantages and Limitations

Advantages of the biophysical profile include excellent sensitivity, a weekly testing interval, a low false-negative rate, and improved detection of structural fetal anomalies. The primary limitation is the requirement for personnel trained in sonographic visualization of the fetus. Additionally, although the duration of ultrasound observation is less than 10 minutes in the majority of cases, the complete bio-physical profile is more time-consuming than other noninvasive tests. However, when all ultrasound variables are normal, addition of the nonstress test does not appear to alter the discriminative accuracy of the test.

THE MODIFIED BIOPHYSICAL PROFILE

The modified biophysical profile (MBPP) combines the strengths of the nonstress test (ease of use, low cost) and the complete biophysical profile (improved sensitivity, low false-negative rate), while mini-mizing the requirement for additional training in sonographic visu-alization of the fetus. The test is performed once to twice weekly and uses the nonstress test as a short-term marker of fetal status and the amniotic fluid volume as a marker of longer term placental function. In 2014, ACOG changed the requirement for evaluation of amniotic fluid volume in an MBPP from the traditional 4-quadrant amniotic fluid index to a single deepest vertical pocket of greater than 2 cm [2].

Interpretation and Management

Interpretation of the nonstress test incorporates assessment of re-activity, baseline rate, variability, and FHR decelerations. Late, prolonged, or significant variable decelerations, particularly in the setting of low-normal amniotic fluid volume (single deepest vertical pocket 2 cm or less), are considered abnormal. The MBPP is con-sidered normal if the NST is reactive and the amniotic fluid volume measurement is a single deepest vertical pocket of greater than 2 cm [2]. Regardless of reactivity of the NST, oligohydramnios constitutes an abnormal test.

If the modified biophysical profile is normal, the routine testing schedule is resumed. If the modified biophysical profile is abnormal, a backup test is warranted. The biophysical profile and the contrac-tion stress test are the most common backup tests and perform sim-ilarly with respect to perinatal morbidity and mortality [2]. Further management is guided by the results of the backup test. Management of the modified biophysical profile is summarized in Figure 9.1.

Nageotte and coworkers [24] evaluated 2774 high-risk pregnan-cies with twice-weekly modified biophysical profiles and reported one unexplained fetal death within 1 week of a normal test result, for a false-negative rate of 0.36/1000. Another study, by Miller and col-leagues [25], reported 54,617 modified biophysical profiles in 15,482 high-risk pregnancies. Antepartum testing in high-risk pregnancies yielded a fetal death rate that was nearly sevenfold lower than that in the untested, "low-risk" population. When using the MBPP, amniotic fluid evaluation may be done weekly or twice-weekly, depending on gestational age and initial and ongoing evaluation of amniotic fluid volume [26,27]. The overall false-negative rate of the modified biophysical profile was 0.8/1000, and the false-positive rate was 60%. Abnormal test results prompted intervention in 15.5% of the tested population; however, iatrogenic prematurity occurred in only 1.5% of women tested before 37 weeks. Large studies reveal the false-negative rate of the modified biophysical profile to be similar to that of the contraction stress test and the complete biophysical profile.

Advantages and Limitations

Advantages of the modified biophysical profile are that it is easier to perform and less time-consuming than the contraction stress test or the complete biophysical profile. The sensitivity of the modified biophysical profile is superior to that of the nonstress test alone. Limitations include the need for backup testing in 10% to 50% of patients, a high false-positive rate, and a twice-weekly testing interval. Figure 9.4 depicts a schematic for management of the modified biophysical profile.

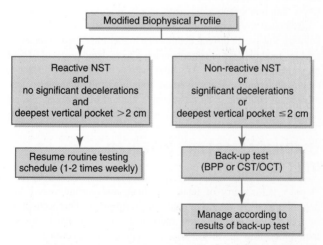

FIGURE 9.4 Management of the modified biophysical profile.

FETAL MOVEMENT COUNTS

Maternal perception of normal fetal movement has long been recognized as a reliable indicator of fetal well-being. Conversely, prolonged absence of fetal movement may signal fetal death. Cessation of fetal movement in response to hypoxia has been demonstrated in animal studies; however, controlled data in human fetuses are lacking. Nevertheless, any acute decrement in the number or strength of fetal movements should prompt further evaluation. Many clinicians recommend routine fetal movement counting, particularly in women who are considered high risk [28–30].

Interpretation and Management

A common approach is to recommend the pregnant woman count fetal movements for 1 hour each day.
- Ten fetal movements in a 1-hour period are considered reassuring.
- If fewer than 10 movements are perceived, counting is continued for another hour.
- Fewer than 10 movements in a 2-hour period should alert the patient to contact her physician for further evaluation.

Another approach calls for the pregnant woman to count movements for 1 hour three times per week. A third protocol calls for movement counting two to three times daily for 30 minutes. With this latter approach, further evaluation is recommended if there are fewer than four strong movements in a 30-minute period.

Evidence from one study using nonconcurrent controls demonstrated a lower rate of fetal death and a higher incidence of intervention for fetal distress in patients using a formalized protocol of fetal movement counting [29]. Although there is insufficient evidence to recommend routine fetal movement counting in all pregnancies, fetal movement counting is an inexpensive method of involving the patient in her own care and carries few if any risks [1].

UMBILICAL ARTERY DOPPLER VELOCIMETRY

Doppler velocimetry of fetal, umbilical, and uterine vessels has been the focus of intensive study in recent years. This technology utilizes systolic/diastolic flow ratios and resistance indices to estimate blood flow in various arteries. In pregnancies complicated by fetal growth restriction, addition of Doppler velocimetry has been shown to improve perinatal outcome [1,31,32]. Although severe restriction of umbilical artery blood flow—as evidenced by absent or reversed flow during diastole—has been correlated with fetal growth restriction, acidosis, and adverse perinatal outcome, the predictive values of less extreme deviations from normal remain undefined. In conditions other than fetal growth restriction, Doppler velocimetry does not appear to be a useful screening test for the detection of fetal compromise, and it is not recommended for use as a screening test in the general obstetric population.

Doppler velocimetry of the middle cerebral artery demonstrates increased diastolic flow in the setting of reduced fetal oxygenation, reflecting the brain-sparing effect of hypoxemia [33]. The peak systolic velocity in the middle cerebral artery has been shown to increase significantly in the setting of fetal anemia and can predict moderate to severe anemia with sensitivity and negative predictive values that equal or exceed those of the traditional method of amniocentesis for Delta OD 450 determination [22,34–39].

A number of studies have evaluated the utility of uterine artery Doppler waveform analysis in the prediction of fetal growth restriction [40]. In the setting of an abnormal uterine artery Doppler waveform, the pooled likelihood ratio was 3.67 for the development of fetal growth restriction. When Doppler velocimetry measurements are used in antepartum fetal surveillance, they should be interpreted in the context of the clinical setting and the results of other tests of fetal status. In the setting of fetal growth restriction, Doppler velocimetry used in conjunction with standard fetal surveillance, such as NST or BPP, is associated with improved outcomes [2].

BIOCHEMICAL ASSESSMENT

Amniocentesis for Fetal Lung Maturity

Amniocentesis is an invasive procedure in which a needle is introduced into the amniotic cavity to remove amniotic fluid for analysis. It is performed under ultrasound guidance using a 20- to 22-gauge spinal-type needle placed transabdominally to withdraw 5 to 20 mL of amniotic fluid (Figure 9.5). In the second trimester, amniocentesis is used frequently to detect a number of abnormalities, including aneuploidy. In the third trimester, it is used primarily to assess fetal lung maturity. Risks in the third trimester are relatively few and include bleeding, infection, membrane rupture, preterm labor, preterm

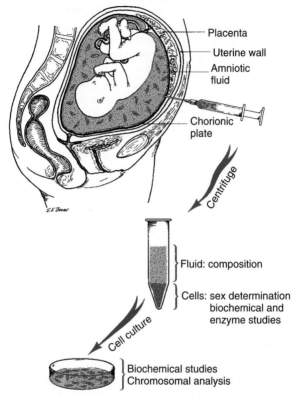

FIGURE 9.5 Amniocentesis. Amniotic fluid is aspirated with a sterile syringe. The sample is centrifuged to separate cells and fluid.

delivery, and alloimmunization in the setting of blood type incompatibility. Amniotic fluid can be used to assess fetal lung maturity by a number of methods.

Lecithin-to-Sphingomyelin Ratio

Pulmonary surfactant contains primarily phospholipids. Surfactant acts as a surface detergent at the air–liquid interface of the alveoli, preventing collapse at the end of expiration. The lecithin-to-sphingomyelin (L/S) ratio compares the concentrations of two phospholipids, lecithin and sphingomyelin, that are major components of surfactant. In the third trimester, an increase in lecithin causes a rise in the lecithin-to-sphingomyelin ratio. A ratio of 2.0 or greater is associated with a low risk of neonatal surfactant-deficient respiratory distress syndrome (RDS).

The following interpretation is generally accepted:

L/S Ratio	Fetal Lung	Risk for RDS
>2.0	Mature	Minimal
1.5–2.0	Transitional	Moderate
<1.5	Immature	High

Note that the presence of blood or meconium can interfere with the results of the lecithin-to-sphingomyelin ratio.

Foam Stability Test

This test is based on the ability of surfactant to generate stable foam when ethanol is added to the amniotic fluid specimen. Ethanol, isotonic saline, and amniotic fluid at varying dilutions are shaken together for 15 seconds. At the proper dilution, a ring of bubbles at the air–liquid interface after 15 minutes indicates probable fetal lung maturity (Figure 9.6).

Phosphatidylglycerol

The presence of phosphatidylglycerol can be ascertained quickly and is not affected by blood or meconium. The presence of phosphatidylglycerol indicates a low risk for respiratory distress syndrome.

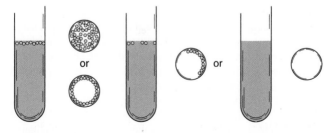

Positive foam test   Negative foam test

FIGURE 9.6 Foam stability test (shake test). For the test to be positive, bubbles must be seen around the entire circumference of the tube.

Whenever possible, fetal lung maturity assessment should be based on phosphatidylglycerol in combination with the lecithin-to-sphingomyelin ratio.

Fluorescence Polarization (FLM-II Assay)

The fetal lung maturity (FLM-II) assay uses fluorescence polarization to determine lipid membrane fluidity in amniotic fluid.

Interpretation of the FLM-II assay is summarized as follows:

Mature >55 mg/g
Transitional 40 to 54 mg/g
Immature <39 mg/g

Lamellar Body Count

Lamellar body counting measures the number of surfactant-containing particles in amniotic fluid directly by using the platelet channel of a standard hematology cell counter. The size and number of lamellar bodies in the amniotic fluid are predictive of fetal lung maturity [41]. Interpretation is summarized as follows:

Mature ≥50,000/μL
Transitional >15,000 to <50,000/μL
Immature ≤15,000/μL

SUMMARY

Our ability to assess the condition of the fetus has improved dramatically over the past 40 years. Although diagnostic precision is enhanced by electronic FHR monitoring and ultrasound technology, room for improvement remains. Electronic FHR monitoring is a very sensitive tool for the detection of interrupted fetal oxygenation; truly compromised fetuses rarely fail to exhibit abnormal FHR patterns. The converse, however, is not true. Fetal heart rate patterns such as decelerations, tachycardia, and intermittent reduction in variability and/or accelerations are frequently observed in the absence of fetal compromise. The limited positive predictive value is the principal shortcoming of FHR monitoring. Accuracy may be improved by combining FHR analysis with assessment of biophysical variables, such as amniotic fluid volume, fetal movement, breathing, tone, and blood flow characteristics. To date, the most effective combination of variables has not been defined, and no one approach to fetal surveillance has demonstrated clear superiority over the others. Despite the limitations, antepartum testing in high-risk pregnancies has been reported to yield a fetal death rate lower than that observed in untested, low-risk pregnancies [25]. If this observation is substantiated, future investigation will be needed to address the role of antepartum fetal surveillance in uncomplicated, low-risk pregnancies.

References

[1] C. Signore, R.K. Freeman, C.Y. Spong, Antenatal testing-a reevaluation: executive summary of a Eunice Kennedy Shriver National Institute of Child Health and Human Development workshop, Obstet. Gynecol. 113 (3) (2009) 687–701.

[2] American College of Obstetricians and Gynecologists, Antepartum fetal surveillance. ACOG Practice Bulletin No. 145, Obstet. Gynecol. 124 (2014) 182–192.

[3] F.W. Kubli, E.H. Hon, A.F. Khazin, et al., Observations on heart rate and pH in the human fetus during labor, Am. J. Obstet. Gynecol. 104 (8) (1969) 1190–1206.

[4] R.K. Freeman, G. Anderson, W. Dorchester, A prospective multi-institutional study of antepartum fetal heart rate monitoring. II. Contraction stress test versus nonstress test for primary surveillance, Am. J. Obstet. Gynecol. 143 (7) (1982) 778–781.

[5] D.C. Lagrew Jr., The contraction stress test, Clin. Obstet. Gynecol. 38 (1) (1995) 1–25.

[6] National Institute of Child Health and Human Development Research Planning Workshop, Electronic fetal heart rate monitoring: research guidelines for interpretation, Am. J. Obstet. Gynecol. 177 (6) (1997) 1385–1390.

[7] F.H. Boehm, S. Salyer, D.M. Shah, et al., Improved outcome of twice weekly nonstress testing, Obstet. Gynecol. 67 (4) (1986) 566–568.

[8] S.L. Clark, M.L. Gimovsky, F.C. Miller, Fetal heart rate response to scalp blood sampling, Am. J. Obstet. Gynecol. 144 (6) (1982) 706–708.

[9] S.L. Clark, M.L. Gimovsky, F.C. Miller, The scalp stimulation test: a clinical alternative to fetal scalp blood sampling, Am. J. Obstet. Gynecol. 148 (3) (1984) 274–277.

[10] T.G. Edersheim, J.M. Hutson, M.L. Druzin, et al., Fetal heart rate response to vibratory acoustic stimulation predicts fetal pH in labor, Am. J. Obstet. Gynecol. 157 (6) (1987) 1557–1560.

[11] A. Elimian, R. Figueroa, N. Tejani, Intrapartum assessment of fetal well-being: a comparison of scalp stimulation with scalp blood pH sampling, Obstet. Gynecol. 89 (3) (1987) 373–376.

[12] I. Ingemarsson, S. Arulkumaran, Reactive fetal heart rate response to VAS in fetuses with low scalp blood pH, Br. J. Obstet. Gynaecol. 96 (5) (1989) 562–565.

[13] G.B. Polzin, K.J. Blakemore, R.H. Petrie, et al., Fetal vibro-acoustic stimulation: magnitude and duration of fetal heart rate accelerations as a marker of fetal health, Obstet. Gynecol. 72 (4) (1988) 621–626.

[14] D.W. Skupski, C.R. Rosenberg, G.S. Eglington, Intrapartum fetal stimulation tests: a meta-analysis, Obstet. Gynecol. 99 (1) (2002) 129–134.

[15] C.V. Smith, H.N. Nguyen, J.P. Phelan, et al., Intrapartum assessment of fetal well-being: a comparison of fetal acoustic stimulation with acid-base determinations, Am. J. Obstet. Gynecol. 155 (4) (1986) 726–728.

[16] J.A. Spencer, Predictive value of a fetal heart rate acceleration at the time of fetal blood sampling in labour, J. Perinat. Med. 19 (3) (1991) 207–215.

[17] P.J. Meis, J.R. Ureda, M. Swain, et al., Variable decelerations during nonstress tests are not a sign of fetal compromise, Am. J. Obstet. Gynecol. 154 (3) (1986) 586–590.

[18] J.P. Phelan, P.E. Lewis Jr., Fetal heart rate decelerations during a non-stress test, Obstet. Gynecol. 57 (2) (1981) 228–232.

[19] J.P. Phelan, L.D. Platt, S.Y. Yseh, et al., Continuing role of the non-stress test in the management of post-dates pregnancy, Obstet. Gynecol. 64 (5) (1984) 624–628.

[20] F.A. Manning, L.D. Platt, L. Sipos, Antepartum fetal evaluation: development of a fetal biophysical profile, Am. J. Obstet. Gynecol. 136 (6) (1980) 787–795.

[21] F.A. Manning, I. Morrison, I.R. Lange, et al., Fetal assessment based upon fetal BPP scoring: experience in 12,620 referred high risk pregnancies. I. Perinatal mortality by frequency and etiology, Am. J. Obstet. Gynecol. 151 (3) (1985) 343–350.

[22] J.M. Johnson, C.R. Harman, I.R. Lange, et al., Biophysical profile scoring in the management of postterm pregnancy: an analysis of 307 patients, Am. J. Obstet. Gynecol. 154 (2) (1986) 269–273.

[23] F.A. Manning, I. Morrison, C.R. Harman, et al., Fetal assessment based on fetal biophysical profile scoring: experience in 19,221 referred high-risk pregnancies. II. An analysis of false-negative fetal deaths, Am. J. Obstet. Gynecol. 157 (4 Pt 1) (1987) 880–884.

[24] J.P. Nageotte, C.V. Towers, T. Asrat, et al., Perinatal outcome with the MBPP, Am. J. Obstet. Gynecol. 170 (6) (1994) 1672–1676.

[25] D.A. Miller, Y.A. Rabello, R.H. Paul, The modified biophysical profile: antepartum testing in the 1990s, Am. J. Obstet. Gynecol. 174 (3) (1996) 812–817.

[26] D.C. Lagrew, R.A. Pircon, M. Nageotte, et al., How frequently should the amniotic fluid index be repeated? Am. J. Obstet. Gynecol. 167 (4 Pt 1) (1992) 1129–1133.

[27] D.A. Wing, A. Fishman, C. Gonzalez, et al., How frequently should the amniotic fluid index be performed during the course of antepartum testing? Am. J. Obstet. Gynecol. 174 (1 Pt 1) (1996) 33–36.

[28] A. Grant, D. Elbourne, L. Valentin, et al., Routine formal fetal movement counting and risk of antepartum late death in normally formed singletons, Lancet 2 (8659) (1989) 345–349.

[29] T.R. Moore, K. Piacquadio, A prospective evaluation of fetal movement screening to reduce the incidence of antepartum fetal death, Am. J. Obstet. Gynecol. 60 (5 Pt 1) (1989) 1075–1080.

[30] S. Neldam, Fetal movements as an indicator of fetal well-being, Dan. Med. Bull. 30 (4) (1983) 274–278.

[31] Z. Alfirevic, J.P. Neilson, Doppler ultrasonography in high-risk pregnancies: systematic review with meta-analysis, Am. J. Obstet. Gynecol. 172 (5) (1995) 1379–1387.

[32] G. Mari, R.L. Deter, R.L. Carpenter, et al., Noninvasive diagnosis by Doppler ultrasonography of fetal anemia due to maternal red cell alloimmunization. Collaborative Group for Doppler Assessment of the Blood Velocity in Anemic Fetuses, N. Engl. J. Med. 342 (1) (2000) 9–14.

[33] R.O. Bahado-Singh, E. Kovanci, A. Jeffres, U. Oz, et al., The Doppler cerebroplacental ratio and perinatal outcome in intrauterine growth restriction, Am. J. Obstet. Gynecol. 180 (3 Pt 1) (1999) 750–756.

[34] D. Dukler, D. Oepkes, G. Seaward, et al., Noninvasive tests to predict fetal anemia: a study comparing Doppler and ultrasound parameters, Am. J. Obstet. Gynecol. 188 (5) (2003) 1310–1314.

[35] G. Mari, A. Adrignolo, A.Z. Abuhamad, et al., Diagnosis of fetal anemia with Doppler ultrasound in the pregnancy complicated by maternal blood group immunization, Ultrasound Obstet. Gynecol. 5 (6) (1995) 400–405.

[36] G. Mari, L. Detti, U. Oz, R. Zimmerman, et al., Accurate prediction of fetal hemoglobin by Doppler ultrasonography, Obstet. Gynecol. 99 (4) (2002) 589–593.

[37] G. Mari, F. Hanif, M. Kruger, et al., Middle cerebral artery peak systolic velocity: a new Doppler parameter in the assessment of growth-restricted fetuses, Ultrasound Obstet. Gynecol. 29 (3) (2007) 310–316.

[38] G. Mari, F. Rahman, P. Olofsson, et al., Increase of fetal hematocrit decreases the middle cerebral artery peak systolic velocity in pregnancies complicated by rhesus alloimmunization, J. Matern. Fetal Med. 6 (4) (1997) 206–208.

[39] D. Maulik, Doppler ultrasound in obstetrics, in: G. Cunningham, P. MacDonald, N. Gant, et al. (Eds.), Williams Obstetrics Supplement, Appleton & Lange, Stamford, CT, 1996.

[40] A.T. Papageorghiou, C.K. Yu, K.H. Nicolaides, The role of uterine artery Doppler in predicting adverse pregnancy outcome, Best Pract. Res. Clin. Obstet. Gynaecol. 18 (3) (2004) 383–396.

[41] M.G. Neerhof, J.C. Dohnal, E.R. Ashwood, et al., Lamellar body counts: a consensus on protocol, Obstet. Gynecol. 97 (2) (2001) 318–320.

Patient Safety, Risk Management, and Documentation

R isk reduction and risk mitigation are the two key components of risk management. Risk reduction seeks to avoid preventable adverse outcomes, thereby decreasing the risk of litigation, and risk mitigation relates to managing liability exposure after an adverse outcome (preventable or unpreventable) [1]. Safety initiatives in perinatal care have been successfully implemented both in the United States and internationally and have consistently demonstrated significant decreases in perinatal morbidity and mortality related to intrapartum asphyxia, low Apgar scores, hypoxic-ischemic encephalopathy, and suboptimal obstetric care [2–6]. Regardless of geographic location, patient safety initiatives share common themes, including a human factors approach to error, standardization of clinical practice, and emphasis on a team approach that places high value on communication. This chapter focuses on risk management specifically related to fetal monitoring, whether that is accomplished by electronic fetal monitoring (EFM) or intermittent auscultation (IA). Beginning with the background of human error and patient safety and continuing with a discussion of key legal issues related to fetal monitoring, including informed consent and refusal, documentation, and deposition testimony, this chapter highlights the relevant litigation issues faced by clinicians of all backgrounds.

HUMAN ERROR

Although progress has been made, errors in obstetrics continue to result in preventable morbidity and mortality, both maternal and neonatal [7]. Through the efforts of the Joint Commission for the Accreditation of Healthcare Organizations (The Joint Commission), the Agency for Healthcare Research and Quality, and other organizations engaged in quality improvement in healthcare, patient safety has been established as the first priority. The analysis of large numbers of injuries and reported errors confirms that adverse events most often result from error-prone systems and processes, not from error-prone individuals. Organizations must learn to avoid the "conspiracy of silence" and create systems in which errors can be identified and prevention strategies can be developed [8,9].

Healthcare providers are educated and socialized to "do the right thing"—that is, to provide safe and appropriate care that results in a positive outcome. However, healthcare providers are human, and humans make errors. Error is a normal part of the human experience and does not reflect laziness, bad intentions, or a personality defect [10]. Understanding the nature of human errors (human factor analysis) is essential to any effort to prevent them.

The *most common types of human errors are related to slips, trips, and lapses* [10], which occur throughout a wide range of human activity. The following lists these activities in decreasing order of probability of occurrence [11,12]:

- Stress (lack of time combined with high stakes—e.g., wrong sponge count in crash surgery)
- Change of shift (e.g., miscommunication)
- Inspection or monitoring (e.g., missing or not recognizing something)
- Arithmetic (e.g., miscalculating drug dosage)
- Omission (e.g., not doing or responding appropriately to something)
- Commission (doing something that is not consistent with an accepted standard of care)

Human errors *are more likely to occur in the presence of personal and environmental factors* known to increase the risk of error. Specific conditions have been identified that are known to increase the risk of error, and it is helpful to be aware of them. These conditions, listed in decreasing probability of risk of error, include the following [10–13]:

1. Lack of familiarity with a task
2. Shortage of time
3. Poor communication
4. Information overload
5. Misperception of risk
6. Lack of experience (not necessarily training)
7. Poor instructions or procedures
8. Inadequate checking
9. Educational mismatch of a person with the task
10. Disturbed sleep pattern

11. Hostile environment
12. Monotony and boredom

Being aware of the most common types of errors and error-producing conditions helps identify, reduce, and manage risks in the perinatal setting. It is also helpful to understand human performance as it relates to knowledge, application of rules, and skills. For example, nurses function from a specialized knowledge base. As they become more skilled and experienced, they process information rapidly in recurrent activities and perform many duties automatically [14].

Skill-based performance includes starting a routine intravenous line, applying the external fetal monitor, and performing Leopold's maneuvers. Errors can occur when nurses' routines change or their attention is diverted, or from physiologic (fatigue, illness), psychological (stress, family issues, frustration), or environmental (noise or unusual unit activity) factors.

Rule-based performance requires extra attention when an event differs from the routine. For example, when confronted with a commonly occurring problem, such as onset of fetal heart rate (FHR) variable decelerations, experienced nurses operate from known and practiced rules or a series of learned responses for doing X when Y happens. When an unfamiliar problem arises, a rule-based error may occur because the wrong rule is chosen, the situation is not accurately perceived, or the rule is misapplied [14].

Knowledge-based performance requires controlled and conscious thought when nurses encounter a completely new, unfamiliar, or infrequently occurring situation. Examples of this type of situation are acute uterine rupture, development of a rarely seen sinusoidal FHR pattern, unheralded prolonged FHR deceleration to 60 bpm or less, or maternal seizure in the absence of a known seizure-related condition. Errors can occur because of lack of information or data or from misdirected attempts to match this novel situation to previous and more familiar situations. As the expertise of the nurse increases, the focus of control moves from a knowledge-based and rule-based performance to skill-based functions. What was once novel has become routine, and the nurse does not usually have to resort to knowledge-based reasoning [14].

Not all errors are preventable. And although humans do err, errors do not always result in injury or adverse outcomes, and not all adverse outcomes are the result of error [14]. It is unreasonable to presume that any one individual is the only person responsible for an error that results in injury to a patient. *It is inappropriate to rely on prevention of error as the sole means of creating patient safety.*

Systems should be in place that will catch errors before they result in adverse outcomes; however, systems are subject to human and environmental variations. The role of risk management in the perinatal setting is twofold: (1) to reduce the probability that a given risk will result in a poor outcome and (2) to recognize, mitigate, or minimize the consequences of the event rather than relying on prevention of error as the sole means of creating patient safety [1,15].

Electronic fetal monitoring continues to be an area that has great potential for error, in part because of the wide variance in electronic fetal monitoring education both between and among the disciplines of nursing, midwifery, and medicine [16]. Electronic fetal monitoring interpretation issues have been linked to avoidable intrapartum fetal demise and "become the dominant litigation theme internationally" [16]. With a resurgence of the use of IA for low-risk pregnancies, there will likely be an uptick in allegations of error with IA, just as with EFM, when an unexpected outcome occurs. Clinicians are best served by advancing approaches *to both EFM and IA* that are based on patient safety principles, such as the development of high-reliability perinatal units.

ERROR PREVENTION AND RISK REDUCTION

High-Reliability Perinatal Units

Risk reduction and error prevention in perinatal care can be achieved when organizations direct their efforts to the avoidance of these common situations and foster high-reliability characteristics. *High reliability is defined as the technical ability to operate technologically complex systems essentially without error over long periods of time.* There are organizational characteristics and clinical practices that differentiate highly reliable perinatal units from those experiencing more error and injury. These organizations consider patient safety to be the first priority and have systems in place to prevent recognized sources of error and injury.

The primary characteristics of a high-reliability unit are as follows [17–20]:

- The organization creates and fosters a safety-oriented culture.
- Decision making to enhance safety occurs at every level of the organization.
- Alarms can be called by anyone; hierarchy is minimized, rank is not an issue; anyone can challenge the status quo.

- Jobs are designed for safety; there is minimal reliance on memory; protocols, checklists, and forcing functions are built into the system.
- Teams that are expected to work together (e.g., physicians, midwives, and nurses participating in the same advanced fetal monitoring workshops) are trained and educated together.
- Multidisciplinary teams carry out drills for high-risk situations such as emergency cesarean deliveries.
- Communication is continuous, valued, and highly rewarded.
- The organization promotes the development of competencies and evaluates ongoing competence using a variety of learning techniques such as simulations, computer tutorials, and case studies in fetal monitoring.

Knox and Simpson updated the concept of perinatal high reliability by discussing key concepts for patient safety initiatives. These include sensitivity to processes, avoidance of oversimplification when addressing failures, inclusion of near-miss analysis, and the importance of transparency in response to system failure [21]. There are many tools and resources for promoting high reliability in perinatal care, and hospitals should explore a variety of methods to reach these goals.

Guidelines to Promote Safety and Reduce Risks

Recommendations and guidelines to promote patient safety and to decrease risk exposure include the following [1,15,22–25]:

Policies, Procedures, and Protocols

- Develop policies, procedures, and protocols based on accepted standards of care [26–28].
- Create departmental policies (vs. nursing policies) for areas of practice that are interdisciplinary by nature (EFM, labor induction/augmentation) and attempt to standardize care whenever possible.
- Use guidelines promulgated by professional organizations (e.g., AWHONN, ACOG), journals, textbooks, and particularly evidence-based practice reports as sources for developing policies, procedures, and protocols [25].
- Institute a policy for obtaining cord blood gases [29].

Competency

- Verify nurses' qualifications at the time of hire to ensure that they meet the prerequisites of the institution.
- Develop tools to evaluate performance related to specific skills, knowledge base of physiology and pathophysiology, and the standard

of care to which nurses are held accountable, based on the facility's rules (i.e., policies, procedures, and protocols) [28].
- Promote and support certification of nurses in fetal monitoring [30].
- Require midwives and physicians to hold certification in EFM as part of their credentialing process [5,31,32].

Fetal Monitoring

- Standardize fetal assessment and monitoring language throughout the institution [31,33–37].
- Accurately monitor FHR and uterine activity; use instrumentation appropriately.
- Identify and interpret EFM and/or IA data accurately [38–40].
- Implement intrauterine resuscitation techniques appropriately; have reminders (printed or electronic) available for clinicians at bedside.
- Communicate findings and efforts to correct FHR changes to physician or midwife in a clear and unambiguous manner using SBAR (situation-background-assessment-recommendation) [41,42] or five-step assertiveness [43] (Boxes 10.1 and 10.2).
- Continue fetal assessment until birth, including monitoring until the abdominal preparation is begun on women who are having a cesarean delivery [33].

Neonatal Resuscitation

- Ensure availability of appropriately trained and certified staff; redeploy staff as necessary to provide optimal care.
- Prepare appropriate equipment and medications before delivery.

Organizational Resources and Systems to Support Timely Interventions

- Have sufficient staff or be able to redeploy staff as needed. During the intrapartum period, the nurse-to-patient ratio should be 1:2 or 1:1, depending on the stage of labor and the complexity of the situation [22,33,44]. Staffing should be sufficient to begin a cesarean delivery within 30 minutes of a physician's decision to operate. A more expeditious delivery (<30minutes) may be necessary in cases of abruptio placentae, prolapse of the umbilical cord, hemorrhage secondary to placenta previa, and uterine rupture [33].
- Utilize a perinatal patient safety nurse, a full-time position in nursing dedicated to implementation and evaluation of all perinatal safety activities for the institution [31].

BOX 10.1 Sample Communication Related to Electronic Fetal Monitoring Using SBAR

1. **Situation:** State what is happening at the present time; state the circumstances that prompted the communication. "Hi Dr. Johnson, it's Sue from L & D. Mrs. Smith, your patient in active labor who requested an epidural, is having an FHR pattern that is confusing to me. I can't tell if the changes are accelerations or decelerations."

2. **Background:** Put the situation into context; explain any pertinent background information. "She's a G2P1001, her last examination was 30 minutes ago, and she was 5 cm/100%/Vtx 1 with SROM clear since 0930. She has no noted risk factors."

3. **Assessment:** Explain what you think the problem is; include pertinent assessments. "I'm not sure the external monitor is picking up well. The prior baseline was 140 with moderate variability and no accels or decels. Now it's hard to tell, but I think the baseline has risen to 150, but it may have dropped to 130, there's minimal variability, and depending on where I read the baseline we have either accels or decels."

4. **Recommendation:** Express your thoughts on a solution. Be direct in asking for what you want to see happen. "If it's OK with you, I'd like to hold off on the epidural placement until I can get a clear reading on this tracing. I've paged the resident to come look at it with me, and if we can't figure it out, I may ask you to come to the bedside for an evaluation."

Adapted from M. Leonard, S. Graham, D. Bonacrum, The human factor: the critical importance of effective teamwork and communication in providing safe care, Qual. Saf. Health Care 13 (Suppl. 1) (2004) i85–i90; and K.M. Haig, S. Sutton, J. Whittington, SBAR: a shared mental model for improving communication between clinicians, Jt. Comm. J. Qual. Patient Saf. 32 (3) (2006) 167–175.

BOX 10.2 Sample Communication Related to Electronic Fetal Monitoring Using 5-Step Assertiveness

1. **Use a name or position to get the team member's attention.** "*Dr. Johnson.*"

2. **Express your discomfort.** "Dr. Johnson, I'm uncomfortable with proceeding with the epidural."

3. **Clearly and candidly state your concern.** "Dr. Johnson, I'm uncomfortable with proceeding with the epidural *because I can't determine whether these are accels or decels.*"

4. **Propose an alternative.** "Dr. Johnson, I'm uncomfortable with proceeding with the epidural because I can't determine whether these are accels or decels. *I'd like to adjust the monitor and have you come evaluate the tracing with me before we proceed with the epidural.*"

5. **Obtain acknowledgment.** "Dr. Johnson, I'm uncomfortable with proceeding with the epidural because I can't determine whether these are accels or decels. I'd like to adjust the monitor and have you come evaluate the tracing with me before we proceed with the epidural. *OK with you?*"

Adapted from L.A. Miller, Patient safety and teamwork in perinatal care, J. Perinat. Neonatal Nurs. 19 (1) (2005) 46–51.

BOX 10.3   Elements of Promoting Safety and Reducing Risk

1. Utilization of policies, procedures, and protocols to standardize care
2. Ensure competency of all clinicians via certification in EFM
3. Standardized definitions for fetal assessment and monitoring with clear and unambiguous communication among clinicians
4. Neonatal resuscitation-certified staff and appropriate equipment
5. Organizational resources, sufficient staff, and systems to support timely interventions by all clinicians
6. Perinatal teamwork with multidisciplinary collaboration and communication
7. Interdisciplinary focused case reviews, proactive approach to improving systems, and elimination of a blame-based environment
8. Chain of communication that supports quality and safe patient care to reduce risks and adverse outcomes
9. Conduct joint multidisciplinary education of the perinatal team

- Have systems in place that ensure a physician's timely response to the perinatal unit when needed and requested (e.g., in cases of an abnormal FHR tracing, excessive uterine activity or tachysystole, complications during vaginal birth after cesarean delivery). A policy that exists in high-reliability perinatal units is that "a physician will come to the unit when requested by a nurse" (Box 10.3) [17].
- Consider use of a hospitalist or laborist to ensure a physician is immediately available to labor and delivery [45].

Perinatal Teamwork: Collaboration and Communication

- Recognize multidisciplinary teams as the unifying principle that creates operational excellence and success. "In any situation requiring a real-time combination of multiple skills, experiences and judgment, *teams,* as opposed to individuals, create superior performance" [46].
- Engage in team building through a multidisciplinary clinical practice or performance improvement committee to come to consensus on both routine and problematic practices, to improve communication, to build trust and confidence in one another, and to achieve performance goals [46].
- Create a culture in which everyone feels free to ask for help [47,48] and questions are not viewed as challenges to authority [49].

- Implement strict policies on disruptive behavior for all disciplines, and provide education on effective and respectful interaction [50,51].
- Initiate formal team training, such as TeamSTEPPS, or Kaiser Permanente's Perinatal Patient Safety Project, which may prevent 40% or more malpractice-related events in labor and delivery [47,52].
- Utilize a variety of methodologies to measure and assess patient safety [53].

Interdisciplinary Case Reviews

- Eliminate a blame-based environment.
- Focus reviews on the *six most common allegations* of obstetric malpractice claims [48,54]. These are:
  1. Failure to recognize or respond to FHR changes, whether EFM or IA is employed
  2. Failure to do a timely delivery
  3. Failure to conduct proper resuscitation
  4. Negligently causing vacuum or forceps injuries
  5. Failure to prevent and manage shoulder dystocia
  6. Improper use of oxytocin
- Use a proactive approach, such as "failure to rescue" [55] to review processes related to EFM management. This approach does not require a sentinel event to trigger a review and allows hospitals to develop best-practice strategies as well as evaluate "near misses."
- Engage several reviewers from a variety of disciplines when reviewing and classifying adverse events [56].

Chain of Communication

- Develop a chain of communication (Figure 10.1) with key medical, nursing, administrative, and risk-management leaders.
- Implement the chain of communication when team members disagree (e.g., about tracing interpretation or management of the patient) or when the clinicians fail to respond [57].
- Report to the quality/performance improvement committee any incidence of provider behavior that does not support quality or safe patient care, that increases risk to the patient, or that could contribute to an adverse outcome. If retaliation or retribution occurs, it should be reported as well. "When people fail to engage in respectful interactions, things can get dangerous" [17].

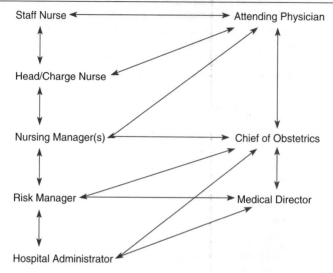

FIGURE 10.1 Sample chain of communication for resolution of conflicts in judgment between nurse and healthcare provider.

Joint Nurse/Provider Education

- Make EFM education a multidisciplinary event and teach all clinicians the standard management decision model presented in Chapter 6.
- Provide consistency of information and expectations, hold forums on skills (e.g., proper technique for IA, an emergency cesarean delivery drill), on conducting patient conferences, and on any other activities that involve multidisciplinary team members.
- Incorporate training on communication and teamwork into residency education [58].

ADVERSE OUTCOMES AND LITIGATION

The physician, midwife, hospital, and, often, individual perinatal nurses are named as defendants when litigation arises after an adverse maternal or neonatal outcome [59]. Healthcare providers by nature and education want to help and care for people, so they are particularly devastated when they are sued by a client. The word *malpractice* evokes a strongly negative response in all healthcare providers, particularly in obstetrics where the damages are likely catastrophic with economic damages in the millions. Care providers fear being involved in malpractice suits and judged by a jury as liable in a situation where the care was, in fact, reasonable. They are likely to become preoccupied because lawsuits can take 3 or more years to be resolved [60]. But medical errors and litigation are a reality of practice. Acknowledging the risk and developing systems to reduce the risk and/or consequence of error are the first steps in reducing medical-legal exposure. When risk issues or adverse outcomes are identified, the patient's medical record should be reviewed by the multidisciplinary healthcare team, using an approach that will objectively analyze the clinical course to identify errors and contributing factors that may have resulted in an adverse outcome. Additionally, disclosure of adverse or unanticipated events to the patient and family is the responsibility of the healthcare team and may result in a reduction in legal action [38].

Disclosure of Unanticipated Outcomes

When an injury occurs, The Joint Commission standards require that information about how the error occurred and remedies available be disclosed to the woman and her family [61]. During disclosure, the woman and her family should be informed that the factors involved in the injury will be investigated so that steps can be taken to reduce the likelihood of similar injury to other patients [62]. Disclosure should be made with the support of trained individuals; clinicians should refrain from discussing the details of the event with the patient and family without appropriate support through the organization's disclosure process. Institutions should provide education related to the components of disclosure, and several organizations have developed disclosure programs that can serve as models for disclosure in the perinatal setting [63].

Elements of Malpractice

Failure to do something that a reasonable and prudent clinician would do in the same circumstances is known as malpractice or professional negligence. Clinicians are held to national standards of care and practice within the "same or similar circumstances" and "reasonably expected" parameters. Inherent in this statement is the expectation that the clinician is knowledgeable about the standards of care and is fully competent to apply those standards when caring for patients [40].

Negligence is the failure to act in the required manner, causing harm to an individual. *Malpractice* is an unintentional act performed by a professional acting in a professional capacity that causes harm to an individual. Under the rule *respondeat superior,* "let the master answer," an employer is held liable for acts of malpractice committed by an employee while performing duties for which she or he was hired.

For an action to fit the *legal definition of malpractice,* the following four elements must be met:

- *Duty:* The patient is owed a specific duty or standard of care.
- *Breach of duty:* There was a failure to meet the required standard of care.
- *Proximate cause:* A direct causal relationship exists between the breach of duty and the harm or injury to the patient.
- *Harm or injury:* Actual harm or injury occurred to the woman, fetus, or neonate as a result of the breach of duty.

EFM, IA, and Informed Consent

Informed consent regarding mode of monitoring is the responsibility of the midwife or physician. To meet the legal requirements of informed consent, a discussion must include how a procedure is performed as well as risks, benefits, alternatives, and future implications [64]. Nurses may not be responsible for the elements of informed consent, but they have an independent duty to act as a patient advocate. Nurses are obligated to notify the provider if they believe a woman lacks an understanding regarding any procedure. This allows the provider to have further discussion and clarification before instituting the procedure. Although written informed consent is not a legal requirement for either IA or EFM, institutions may want to create written consent forms and/or fact sheets regarding EFM and IA, and interdisciplinary discussion regarding informed consent related to either IA or EFM is important. Box 10.4 provides a list of discussion points that a multidisciplinary team should address when developing fact sheets or consent forms. All clinicians should be comfortable discussing the evidence related to EFM and IA, including the significant limitations [65]. Including the views of various professional organizations when discussing IA can be helpful. ACOG has stated that in patients not experiencing complications, there is no clear benefit for EFM over IA [66]. AWHONN, in a position statement published in 2015, states that both a woman's preferences and her clinical presentation should be considered and that the least invasive method is generally preferred [67]. The

---

BOX 10.4   Discussion Points Regarding Informed Consent for EFM/IA

---

1. Indications for EFM or IA. This may be related to risk factors, and in the case of IA, it may actually be *a lack of indication* for EFM

2. Description of the procedure for EFM versus IA, which could include the technique (Doppler vs. fetoscope, abdominal fetal electrocardiogram or telemetry) as well as the frequencies of assessment for the different stages and phases of labor

3. Review of risks and benefits, which must include the serious quality limitations of the studies to date [65] and the grade levels of the recommendations being made

4. Alternatives to an absolute use of either IA or EFM; there are clinical situations that may warrant some combination of intermittent EFM with IA

5. Future implications for both EFM and IA; this may be currently developing evidence as new studies arise for both EFM and IA

American College of Nurse-Midwives goes a step further than either ACOG or AWHONN and states: "IA is the preferred method … for women at term who at the onset of labor are low risk for developing fetal acidemia" [68]. Regardless of which modality is used, both EFM and IA will likely be litigation issues in the event of an unexpected adverse outcome. Providing adequate informed consent on the topic is both ethically correct and sound risk management.

Notification and Clinical Review

When there is error, injury, or other adverse outcome, there should be written and well-understood procedures to guide staff. Notification of supervisory or management-level individuals should be timely, according to organizational policy. Appropriate quality assurance memos or incident reports should be completed for performance improvement purposes. The medical record should contain documentation of the facts surrounding the event and should be free from editorial commentary and potentially damaging, biased, or blaming comments.

When an adverse outcome occurs, the entire perinatal unit is usually aware of the event. There is great interest in finding out what happened, and the staff sincerely wants to support the team members involved by reviewing the event in detail. However, chart review and questions in the absence of a "need to know" basis must be avoided. Any discussions occurring outside an official quality improvement or risk management forum will be discoverable in the event of litigation and can be required to be repeated under oath. Perinatal care providers should be knowledgeable about the appropriate time and place to discuss events, and they should be compliant with the Health Insurance Portability and Accountability Act (HIPAA) regulations regarding protected patient information.

A critical incident debriefing by a skilled resource, such as an employee assistance program, a trained hospital-based team, a social worker, or a chaplain, provides an opportunity for staff to process feelings and concerns related to adverse outcomes and patient injuries in an environment free from discovery and blame. The critical incident debriefing is most effective when conducted as soon as possible after the occurrence of the event.

In the event of litigation, a plaintiff's attorney may attempt to make direct contact with nurses involved in the care of the allegedly injured patient. Hospital or unit orientation should include information about the correct response to such a request (refusal to discuss) and the requirement that the hospital's risk management department be notified and involved before any discussion with a plaintiff's attorney occurs.

Reporting of Sentinel Events

Adverse events that meet the definition of a sentinel event (i.e., an unexpected occurrence involving death or serious physical or psychological injury or the risk thereof) must be reported according to The Joint Commission and state department of health standards. A sentinel event signals the need for immediate investigation and response. The Joint Commission specifically lists "any intrapartum maternal death and any perinatal death unrelated to a congenital condition in an infant with birth weight >2500 grams" as voluntarily reportable events [61]. After the report of a sentinel event, the organization must conduct a root-cause analysis and report the findings of that process to The Joint Commission. The root-cause analysis identifies causal factors for the sentinel event and improvements in processes or systems that would decrease the likelihood of such events in the future. Root-cause analysis follows an event and focuses primarily on systems and processes, not individual performance.

DOCUMENTATION

The medical record and the terms used therein will be what attorneys, claim representatives, and reviewing expert physicians prejudge. The accuracy of terms and the consistency of terminology among providers will weigh in judging not only the competency but also the credibility of providers. In cases involving electronic fetal monitoring, clinician's use of the correct terminology in documentation as well as in communications under oath, such as deposition or trial testimony, can play a significant role in the outcome of litigation [69].

To reduce risk, appropriate documentation must be kept, including the frequency of, content reviewed, and nomenclature used for FHR evaluation. Providers must know, understand, and utilize institutional policies, guidelines, and resources in the delivery of appropriate care and documentation. These documents will form either the shield of the provider's defense or serve as a sword for the plaintiff's case.

Documentation in the patient's record is used to describe care and interventions provided in a sequential manner. This information may be stored or archived on an optical disk or other device (Figure 10.2). Increasing evidence indicates that documentation should be done only once, on the paper labor flow sheet or in the electronic record, to avoid duplication [70]. *Duplicative charting presents a significant risk of inconsistencies* that can be questioned or challenged by plaintiff attorneys in the event of future litigation. Furthermore, duplicative documentation in the medical record and on the fetal monitor strip is unnecessarily labor intensive for nurses who are frequently fully occupied in care of the woman and fetus.

To fully understand documentation issues in electronic fetal monitoring, the clinician must understand the difference between *assessment, communication,* and *documentation* (Figure 10.3). These are three distinct components of patient care, yet many nursing protocols fail to recognize the difference among these components, resulting in difficulty in compliance with documentation policies and excessive amounts of nursing time spent "nursing the chart" rather than providing patient care. A brief review is warranted here.

Components of Care: Assessment, Communication, Documentation

Assessment, the evaluation of patient status, is constant, ongoing, and very detailed. Clinicians notice many things about patients, not all of which are sufficiently clinically relevant to warrant communication or documentation. Indeed, much of what a nurse assesses

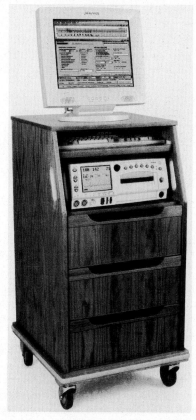

FIGURE 10.2 Corometrics 250cx Maternal/Fetal Monitor. The fetal strip and vital signs automatically flow to an electronic medical record, providing a backup or an alternative to the storage of paper FHR tracings. (Courtesy GE Medical Systems Information Technologies, Milwaukee, WI.)

and many activities a nurse performs are never communicated to other providers, nor do they appear in the medical record. Examples include the act of introducing oneself to the patient and family, changing a soiled gown or sheet, or simply offering support or encouragement to the patient and her family. *Thus the oft-quoted adage "if it wasn't charted, it wasn't done" has never been and will never be true.* Yet many clinicians readily agree with this statement when being deposed in relation to a malpractice suit. The reality is, there

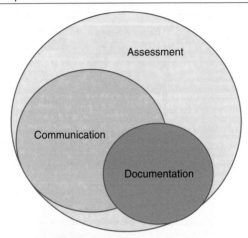

FIGURE 10.3 Illustration of the relationship between assessment, communication, and documentation in daily clinical practice. (Courtesy Lisa A. Miller, CNM, JD.)

is absolutely no rationale, and it would not be physically possible, to either communicate or document all the assessments and activities of any clinician, whether nurse, midwife, or physician. Assessment is simply too broad a category.

Communication is slightly less broad but still encompasses more than any clinician can, or needs, to document. Much communication in labor and delivery is routine, consisting of sharing information or giving instructions to patients and family members. It may include notification of the charge nurse or team leader regarding status changes or patient updates, not all of which needs to be placed in the medical record. Notification of the midwife or physician regarding labor progress and fetal status may be quite detailed but could be documented simply as "Provider updated as to patient status." There is no requirement, and it would not be effective use of a clinician's time, to document verbatim each and every conversation that occurs over the course of labor and birth.

Documentation, therefore, is the least broad of the three categories, and yet it is often the most important in relation to litigation. Evidence is presented in the courtroom in the form of exhibits or testimony. The primary exhibit in a malpractice case is the medical record. Accordingly, an accurate, contemporaneous record is the foundation of either the plaintiff or defense case.

The best evidentiary friend of a plaintiff attorney is either inaccurate or inconsistent documentation of the care provided. Inaccurate documentation can stem from a competency issue, for example, if an FHR tracing is not appropriately interpreted, or from inaccurate nomenclature, such as what is present on the tracing. In either situation, the healthcare provider is left with a narrative note or deposition testimony that is inconsistent with the objective evidence on the tracing. Inconsistencies within a courtroom do not favor the inconsistent party.

Conflicting or contradictory documentation and use of nomenclature create difficulties for clinicians in both the screening and testimonial phases of malpractice litigation. When a file is being *initially* reviewed by plaintiff's counsel to determine whether medical malpractice may have occurred, the medical record is the only documentation available. The narrative note supplied will be read against subsequent healthcare providers' notes and an FHR tracing. Accurate recognition and description of FHR assessments in the patient's chart demonstrate attentive and competent care. Inaccurate or incorrect terminology in a medical record when read and compared with the objective fetal heart tracing increases the likelihood of litigation.

Compounding the matter further, *inconsistent and inaccurate terminology* also creates difficult obstacles later, during the testimonial phase of litigation. When a witness uses modified or nonstandardized terminology, other healthcare providers and expert witnesses will not understand the full extent of what is meant. This creates unclear communication, which can result in medical errors or the appearance of errors within a medical record. This problem is exemplified by the following deposition excerpt.

Deposition Excerpt

A physician (MD) was questioned in deposition by the plaintiff's attorney (PA) regarding a nursing narrative note.

> PA: Dr. Doe, do you expect an intrapartum nurse to relay to you if there is any late component to a deceleration?
>
> MD: Any late decelerations should be relayed to me, particularly if there is more than one.
>
> PA: By late deceleration, do you mean if any portion of the deceleration is thought to be late?
>
> MD: I do not understand what that means. However, if a nurse sees something late, I want to know about it immediately, especially if it recurs.

The narrative notes within the case included the nurse documenting variable decelerations with "late components." Using the outdated terminology "late components" created a scenario in which the significance is undefined and suggests a call should have been made. Further testimony demonstrated that no information regarding this deceleration was relayed. The nurse (RN) testified as follows:

PA: Did you relay to Dr. Doe this deceleration had late components?

RN: No.

PA: Why not?

RN: Because I felt it was a variable deceleration with late components and was not nonreassuring.

PA: So you felt it was a variable and not a late?

RN: Yes.

PA: So when you chart the word *late,* you want the jury to believe it doesn't mean late?

RN: I guess.

The inappropriate utilization of nomenclature has created a scenario in which the physician has inadvertently criticized the nurse. Furthermore, the nurse must separate herself from her own charting of the word *late.* This makes the case more difficult to defend. With appropriate use of nomenclature, the nurse would have simply charted that this was a variable deceleration and could have answered that as it was not recurrent; it was her clinical judgment that it did not warrant immediate notification of the physician.

The use of standardized terminology not only supports the defense of a medical malpractice action; more importantly, it allows the physician and nurse to communicate clearly and make certain they are accurately discussing the findings and placing the same significance on each term.

Documentation Issues Specific to Electronic Fetal Monitoring

In 2008, the Eunice Kennedy Shriver National Institute of Child Health and Human Development (NICHD) reviewed and updated the standardized definitions for use in the interpretation of fetal heart tracings and created a three-tier categorization system [71]. Currently, all professional organizations in the United States support the use of standardized terminology [34,39,67]. Unfortunately, despite the attempts at standardization of terminology, many healthcare providers have been slow to adapt. This creates the risk of inaccurate communication among healthcare providers who misuse terms, and it creates the potential for a medical record replete with inconsistencies [72].

There are several documentation issues that relate specifically to electronic fetal monitoring. These include what should be included in electronic fetal monitoring documentation; definition and use of summary terms, such as FHR categories and use of normal/ tachysystole for uterine activity; further quantification of decelerations; and the frequency of documentation versus the frequency of assessment in FHR tracing review. Each institution must address these issues and provide guidance for staff members. There are few absolutes for any of these issues, and institutional approaches will naturally vary, but some general principles will provide a starting point for team discussion.

Components of Electronic Fetal Monitoring Evaluation

There are six components that should be included in evaluation of the FHR tracing [40,72]:
- Baseline rate
- Baseline variability
- Presence of accelerations
- Periodic or episodic decelerations
- Changes or trends over time
- Uterine activity

These six components form the basis of electronic fetal monitoring management and should be included in documentation related to the FHR tracing. If using a graphic flow sheet, the fifth component (changes or trends over time) is apparent by simple review of the flow sheet. However, when clinicians use narrative charting, as is the case for most doctors and midwives, changes or trends over time may need to be specifically identified. Documentation related to uterine activity should include mode of assessment (external or internal) and strength to palpation when using a tocodynamometer.

Use of FHR Categories

The 2008 NICHD workshop report introduced a three-tiered category system to replace the use of poorly defined summary terms, such as *reassuring* and *nonreassuring,* when classifying and discussing FHR tracings. For purposes of documentation, it is preferable that clinicians document the components of the FHR tracing rather than the category. Should an FHR tracing be lost or an electronic archival system fail, the clinician who documented the FHR components can always determine what the corresponding category was at the time in question, but the reverse is not true. The clinician who simply documents a category will not be able to later articulate the FHR components if the tracing is unavailable. Some institutions are requiring nurses to chart both the FHR components and the FHR tracing category, which is not only unnecessary but also counterproductive, considering the already burdensome paperwork responsibilities of the bedside nurse [69]. Clearly stated, *FHR categories are summary terms that clinicians should know and be able to apply and articulate if queried; they are not required documentation components.*

Documentation of Uterine Activity

Similar to the categories issue, clinicians should understand that the terms *normal* and *tachysystole* are summary terms used to describe uterine activity based on frequency of contractions over a 30-minute period. Clinicians are best served by documentation that provides a clear picture of uterine activity assessment as a whole, including frequency, duration, strength, and resting tone, the components of uterine activity (see Chapter 4). Although summary terms can be helpful in drafting policies and procedures, they are limited in usefulness during deposition or trial, where clinicians are expected to be able to provide specific answers regarding patient assessment. *There is no logical rationale for adding summary terms to documentation where documentation already includes the individual components assessed.*

Quantification of Decelerations

FHR decelerations may be further quantified by duration (onset to offset) and depth of nadir, but this is not mandatory [66,69]. Clinicians should think logically about the benefits (or lack thereof) further quantification provides within the clinical context of FHR monitoring. Given that early decelerations are not associated with hypoxemia and considered clinically insignificant, further quantification of early decelerations does not seem clinically indicated or logical. Late decelerations reflect transient hypoxemia and warrant a clinical response regardless of depth, making further quantification moot. However, management of variable and prolonged decelerations may differ on the basis of duration and depth of nadir, making it reasonable to further quantify these decelerations at least in communication with the team members, especially if the recipient of the communication does not have visual access to the FHR tracing. Communication is distinct from documentation and is often more detailed than what is documented in the medical record, as discussed earlier. Institutions will need to decide whether further quantification of decelerations is warranted in documentation practices and, if so, whether it is necessary for all deceleration types.

Frequency of Electronic Fetal Monitoring Assessment Versus Frequency of Electronic Fetal Monitoring Documentation

As discussed earlier in this chapter, assessment encompasses a clinical spectrum that is much larger than just documentation. Frequency of FHR tracing assessment may vary both by stage of labor as well as clinical context (antepartum vs. intrapartum, risk factors, previous FHR tracing, interventions). When using electronic fetal monitoring, a continuous permanent record is created and is often archived electronically in addition to (or as an alternative to) an actual paper strip. Institutional protocols should be in place to delineate both the frequency of assessment of FHR tracings as well as the frequency of documentation regarding FHR findings. It is reasonable that FHR assessments may be more frequent than FHR documentation, in keeping with the reality of clinical practice [69]. Although a detailed discussion of perinatal documentation policies is beyond the scope of this book, all documentation policies related to electronic fetal monitoring should address the following:

- Recognition of the difference between assessment, communication, and documentation
- The five components of FHR evaluation (baseline rate, baseline variability, presence of accelerations, periodic/episodic decelerations, changes/trends over time)
- Evaluation of uterine contractions (UC), including frequency, duration, strength, and resting tone
- Frequency of FHR and UC evaluation/assessment
- Minimum frequency of documentation of FHR and UC findings

It is imperative that institutions create reasonable and rational policies regarding all three areas: *assessment, communication,* and *documentation.* Although there is no one "right" way to accomplish this, the principles discussed in this chapter should serve as a starting point for clinicians, regardless of specialty. Documentation practices and policies will vary reasonably, based on type of system (computerized records vs. paper), style of charting (flow sheet vs. narrative), clinical context (labor evaluation vs. nonlabor complaint), and numerous other factors. Regardless of the method or clinical context, clinicians can remember the important aspects of documentation by use of the simple acronym CLEAR [69]:

- **Contemporaneous**—charted near the time of the occurrence, use of appropriate late entries
- **Logical**—easily understood and clear; consider SOAP (subjective, objective, assessment, plan) for progress notes
- **Explicit**—avoid vague or ambiguous terms; use standardized terminology
- **Accurate**—notes should reflect correct times and sequence of events; record must be truthful
- **Readable**—notes and entries must be legible; consider electronic documentation systems

Incorporating these concepts and addressing the key issues previously described will result in the development of sound, clinically realistic documentation policies that reflect interdisciplinary collaboration and patient care.

Electronic Medical Records and Information Systems

Computerized perinatal information systems are becoming more and more common as healthcare institutions strive to improve information flow and documentation practices. The options range from simple archiving of FHR tracings to completely integrated systems linking prenatal outpatient care to inpatient intrapartum and neonatal recordkeeping. Many systems offer remote viewing via computer intranet access, as well as real-time FHR tracing review via mobile phone. Another system uses several onscreen tools that provide graphic overlays to help clinicians correctly apply the NICHD definitions and reach consensus regarding FHR tracing components (Figure 10.4). Compared with traditional paper records, *computerized systems offer several benefits* [73,74], including the following:

- Single data entry for use on multiple forms/records
- Forced functions that promote user compliance with standardized terms and/or evaluations
- Ability to view information in several formats, such as timeline and graphic
- Automatic creation of notes and minimization of narrative/typing using preset scripts and drop-down menus
- Improved readability of records (avoidance of illegibility)
- Bedside access to protocols, policies, calculators, and other tools to improve or facilitate patient care

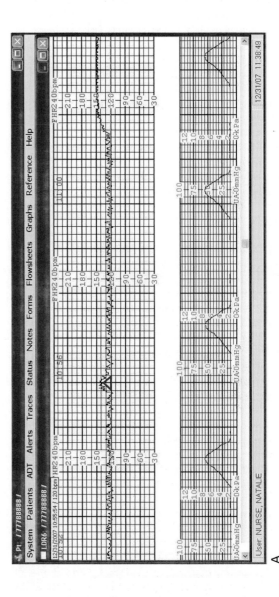

FIGURE 10.4 (A) "E-tools" allow clinicians to confirm FHR finding based on the NICHD terminology by overlaying them directly on the FHR tracing display on the computer. Pictured here is the Accel tool that identifies accelerations of the FHR. (Courtesy OBIX Perinatal System, Clinical Computer Systems, Inc., Elgin, IL.)

Continued

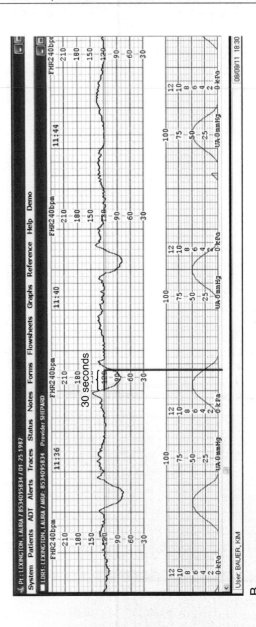

FIGURE 10.4, CONT'D (B) "E-tools" allow clinicians to confirm FHR finding based upon the NICHD terminology by overlaying them directly on the FHR tracing display on the computer. Pictured here is the Decel tool that helps evaluate the onset to nadir of decelerations as abrupt or gradual. (Courtesy OBIX Perinatal System, Clinical Computer Systems, Inc., Elgin, IL.)

- Access to multiple patient screens or multiple FHR tracings at a single computer display
- Facilitated data management and retrieval for reporting, statistics, and quality assurance activities

Although the popularity and acceptance of computerized perinatal information systems continue to grow, it is essential that institutions recognize the importance of appropriate training and an organized transition plan when moving from paper charting to electronic medical records. Setting a "go-live" date and providing adequate time for clinicians to become proficient with the system before that date are keys to a smooth transition. *Having clinicians "double-chart" over a transition period is a poor strategy* [70], replete with error potential and frustration for clinicians who are already burdened with documentation and administrative duties in addition to patient care.

Finally, it is important to note that computerized medical record systems vary with regard to transparency regarding documentation timing. Most systems provide the option to have medical record printouts that include keystroke data (i.e., the time the note was actually typed or entered) adjacent to the timing of the note. This information is sometimes referred to as the *history* or *audit trail*. When this information is included in the medical record printouts, the medical record is considered to be "transparent," meaning that a reviewer is able to clearly see the actual time the notation was entered. Problems can arise when the medical record printout does not include this information and clinicians have entered data that would normally be considered a late entry but do not identify it as such. If the computer printout of the medical record gives the appearance of contemporaneous charting but the audit trail or history reveals the actual time of the entry was hours or days after the notation time, it could be construed as a clinician's attempt to "buff" the chart. This can result in allegations of spoliation in medical malpractice cases. *Spoliation* refers to the withholding or hiding of evidence in legal proceedings and could include additions to the medical record with the purpose of falsification to avoid liability. These allegations can be devastating to the defense of a medical malpractice suit. They are easily avoided by providing medical records that are transparent as to data entry and by setting reasonable standards for late entries and addendums to medical records.

Record Storage and Retrieval

The fetal monitor tracing is a part of the patient's medical record; therefore, storage, security, and record retrieval are the responsibilities of the hospital's medical records department. If the paper strip is archived, each segment of the strip must be clearly identified per unit policy. The strips should be numbered sequentially and securely banded together for archiving. Confidentiality of the fetal monitor tracings must be maintained by storing them in a secure place until the woman's entire medical record is sent to the medical records department. A process must be in place to request and reliably retrieve all fetal monitoring tracings, whether on paper, microfilm, or electronic archive. In the event of litigation, any missing monitoring information makes a case difficult (if not impossible) to defend despite excellent care and complete compliance with established standards.

SUMMARY

A patient safety approach to risk management has been shown to improve outcomes and reduce liability, as well as improve safety climate and culture [5,31,37,75]. System analysis of risk and error must replace outdated punitive approaches that use blame and focus on individual behavior/error. There are specific perinatal risk reduction strategies related to fetal monitoring. An environment rich in competent care providers who practice as a team, use the same terminology, avoid variances in practice, and have systems in place for timely clinical intervention supports the likelihood of that organization being one of high reliability. Informed consent regarding EFM, IA, or combinations of monitoring modalities is ethical duty and a sound risk management strategy.

Guidelines for patient care and documentation must acknowledge the difference between assessment, communication, and documentation. All these areas have potential for error, but an approach that respects the realities of clinical practice and makes patient safety the top priority serves both patients and clinicians. Documentation issues specific to electronic fetal monitoring must be addressed, and any terminology used must be clearly defined, understood, and used consistently by all team members. Information technology and computerized perinatal information systems can assist clinicians in meeting this challenge.

Finally, clinicians have a duty to disclose unanticipated outcomes. Disclosure should be accomplished by trained individuals and should include a discussion of any errors in an honest and forthright manner. Through the combination of a core philosophy of patient safety, collaborative care and teamwork, and direct and open disclosure practices, patients and families can be assured that healthcare systems are working successfully toward improved outcomes. And nurses, midwives, and doctors can effectively abide by the ancient wisdom of *primum non nocere*—"first do no harm."

References

[1] K.R. Simpson, G.E. Knox, Risk management and EFM: decreasing risk of adverse outcomes and liability exposure, J. Perinat. Neonatal Nurs. 14 (3) (2000) 40–52.

[2] J. Becher, B. Stenson, A. Lyon, Is intrapartum asphyxia preventable? BJOG 114 (11) (2007) 1442–1444.

[3] T. Draycott, T. Sibanda, L. Owen, et al., Does training in obstetric emergencies improve neonatal outcome? BJOG 113 (2) (2006) 177–182.

[4] F. Mazza, J. Kitchens, S. Kerr, et al., Eliminating birth trauma at Ascension Health, Jt. Comm. J. Qual. Patient Saf. 33 (1) (2007) 15–24.

[5] S.D. Straub, Implementing best practice safety initiatives to diminish patient harm in a hospital-based family birth center, Newborn Infant Nurs. Rev. 10 (3) (2010) 151–156.

[6] P. Young, R. Hamilton, S. Hodgett, et al., Reducing risk by improving standards of intrapartum fetal care, J. R. Soc. Med. 94 (5) (2001) 226–231.

[7] P.J. Provonost, C.G. Holzmueller, C.S. Ennen, et al., Overview of progress in patient safety, Am. J. Obstet. Gynecol. 204 (1) (2011) 5–10.

[8] J.B. Conway, S.N. Weingart, Organizational change in the face of highly public errors. I: The Dana-Farber Cancer Institute Experience, AHRQ Perspectives on Safety (2005). [Serial online]. Available from: www.webmm.ahrq.gov/perspective.aspx?perspectiveID=3 (accessed 20.10.07).

[9] S. Downe, K. Finlayson, A. Fleming, Creating a collaborative culture in maternity care, J. Midwifery Womens Health 55 (3) (2010) 250–254.

[10] J.T. Reason, Understanding adverse events: the human factor, in: C. Vincent (Ed.), Clinical Risk Management, BMJ Books, London, 2001.

[11] K. Park, Human error, in: Handbook of Human Factors and Ergonomics, Wiley, New York, 1997.

[12] K.R. Simpson, G.E. Knox, Adverse perinatal outcomes: recognizing, understanding, and preventing common accidents, AWHONN Lifelines 7 (3) (2003) 224–235.

[13] A.A. White, J.W. Pichert, S.H. Bledsoe, et al., Cause and effect analysis of closed claims in obstetrics and gynecology, Obstet. Gynecol. 105 (5 Pt 1) (2005) 1031–1038.

[14] D. Raines, Making mistakes: prevention is key to error-free health care, AWHONN Lifelines 4 (1) (2000) 35–39.

[15] C. Rommal, Risk management issues in the perinatal setting, J. Perinat. Neonatal Nurs. 10 (3) (1996) 1–31.

[16] L.A. Miller, System errors in intrapartum electronic fetal monitoring: a case review, J. Midwifery Womens Health 50 (6) (2005) 507–517.

[17] G. Knox, K. Simpson, T. Garite, High reliability perinatal units: an approach to the prevention of patient injury and medical malpractice claims, J. Health Risk Manag. 19 (2) (1999) 24–32.

[18] L.A. Miller, Safety promotion and error reduction in perinatal care: lessons from industry, J. Perinat. Neonatal Nurs. 17 (2) (2003) 128–138.

[19] K.H. Roberts, Managing hazardous organizations, Calif. Manag. Rev. 32 (Summer) (1990) 101–113.

[20] K.H. Roberts, Some characteristics of high reliability organizations, Org. Sci 1 (2) (1990) 160–177.

[21] G. Knox, K.R. Simpson, Perinatal high reliability, Am. J. Obstet. Gynecol. 204 (5) (2011) 373–377.

[22] Association of Women's Health, Obstetric and Neonatal Nurses, Fetal Heart Monitoring: Principles and Practices, fifth ed., Kendall Hunt, Dubuque, IA, 2015.

[23] P. Baker, Medico-legal problems in obstetrics, Obstet. Gynaecol. Reprod. Med. 19 (9) (2009) 253–256.

[24] B.M. Dickens, R.J. Cook, The legal effects of fetal monitoring guidelines, Int. J. Gynecol. Obstet. 108 (2010) 170–173.

[25] Joint Commission on Accreditation of Healthcare Organizations, Preventing Infant Death during Delivery, Sentinel Event Alert No. 30, JCHAO, Oak Brook, IL, 2003.

[26] S. Gennaro, L.J. Mayberry, U. Kafulafula, The evidence supporting nursing management of labor, J. Obstet. Gynecol. Neonatal Nurs. 36 (6) (2007) 598–604.

[27] D. Koniak-Griffin, Strategies for reducing the risk of malpractice litigation in perinatal nursing, J. Obstet. Gynecol. Neonatal Nurs. 28 (3) (1999) 291–299.

[28] M. McRae, Fetal surveillance and monitoring: legal issues revisited, J. Obstet. Gynecol. Neonatal Nurs. 28 (3) (1999) 310–319.

[29] American College of Obstetricians and Gynecologists, Umbilical cord blood gas and acid–base analysis. ACOG committee opinion, Obstet. Gynecol. 108 (5) (2006) 1319–1322.

[30] M. Reeves, Building expertise: making the case for fetal heart monitoring certification, AWHONN Lifelines 5 (2) (2011) 71–72.

[31] C.M. Pettker, S.F. Thung, E.R. Norwitz, et al., Impact of a comprehensive patient safety strategy on obstetric adverse events, Am. J. Obstet. Gynecol. 200 (2009) 492.e1–492.e8.

[32] C.M. Pettker, S.F. Thung, C.A. Raab, et al., A comprehensive obstetrics patient safety program improves safety climate and culture, Am. J. Obstet. Gynecol. 204 (3) (2011) 216.e1–216.e6.

[33] American Academy of Pediatrics, American College of Obstetricians and Gynecologists: Guidelines for Perinatal Care, sixth ed., AAP, ACOG, Washington, DC, 2007.

[34] American College of Nurse-Midwives, Standard Nomenclature for Electronic Fetal Monitoring, Position Statement 2010, ACNM, Silver Spring, MD, 2010.

[35] R.L. Berkowitz, Of parachutes and patient care: a call to action, Am. J. Obstet. Gynecol. 205 (1) (2011) 7–9.

[36] D. Collins, Multidisciplinary teamwork approach in labor and delivery and electronic fetal monitoring, J. Perinat. Neonatal Nurs. 22 (2008) 125–132.

[37] A. Grunebaum, F. Chervenak, D. Skupski, Effect of a comprehensive obstetric patient safety program on compensation payments and sentinel events, Am. J. Obstet. Gynecol. 204 (2) (2011) 97–105.

[38] American College of Obstetricians and Gynecologists, Disclosure and Discussion of Adverse Events, Committee Opinion No. 380, ACOG, Washington, DC, 2007.

[39] American College of Obstetricians and Gynecologists, Management of intrapartum fetal heart rate tracings, ACOG Practice Bulletin No. 116, Obstet. Gynecol. 116 (2010) 1232.c–1240.c.

[40] L. Mahlmeister, Legal implications of fetal heart assessment, J. Obstet. Gynecol. Neonatal Nurs. 29 (5) (2000) 517–526.

[41] K.M. Haig, S. Sutton, J. Whittington, SBAR: a shared mental model for improving communication between clinicians, Jt. Comm. J. Qual. Patient Saf. 32 (3) (2006) 167–175.

[42] M. Leonard, S. Graham, D. Bonacrum, The human factor: the critical importance of effective teamwork and communication in providing safe care, Qual. Saf. Health Care 13 (Suppl. 1) (2004) i85–i90.

[43] L.A. Miller, Patient safety and teamwork in perinatal care, J. Perinat. Neonatal Nurs. 19 (1) (2005) 46–51.

[44] Association of Women's Health, Obstetric and Neonatal Nurses: Guidelines for Professional Registered Nurse Staffing for Perinatal Units, AWHONN, Washington, DC, 2010.

[45] H. Minkoff, D. Fridman, The immediately available physician standard, Semin. Perinatol. 34 (2010) 325–330.

[46] K.R. Simpson, G.E. Knox, Perinatal teamwork, AWHONN Lifelines 5 (5) (2001) 56–59.

[47] K.T. Harris, C.M. Treanor, M.L. Salisbury, Improving patient safety with team coordination: challenges and strategies of implementation, J. Obstet. Gynecol. Neonatal Nurs. 35 (4) (2006) 557–566.

[48] L. Veltman, Poor systems create liability for good providers, in: M. Garza, J.S. Piver (Eds.), Obstet. Gynecol. Malpract. Prevent. 10 (2003) 49–56.

[49] A. Lyndon, M.G. Zlatnick, R.M. Wachter, Effective physician-nurse communication: a patient safety essential for labor & delivery, Am. J. Obstet. Gynecol. 205 (2) (2011) 91–96, http://dx.doi.org/10.1016/j.ajog.2011.04.021.

[50] Joint Commission on Accreditation of Healthcare Organizations (The Joint Commission), Behaviors That Undermine a Culture of Safety, Sentinel Event Alert No. 40, JCHAO, Oak Brook, IL, 2008.

[51] A.H. Rosenstein, Managing disruptive behaviors in the health care setting: focus on obstetrics services, Am. J. Obstet. Gynecol. 204 (3) (2011) 187–192.

[52] S. McFerran, J. Nunes, D. Pucci, et al., Perinatal patient safety project: a multicenter approach to improve performance reliability at Kaiser Permanente, J. Perinat. Neonatal Nurs. 19 (1) (2005) 37–45.

[53] K.R. Simpson, Measuring perinatal patient safety: review of current methods, J. Obstet. Gynecol. Neonatal Nurs. 35 (3) (2006) 432–442.

[54] M. Jonsson, S.L. Nordén, U. Hanson, Analysis of malpractice claims with a focus on oxytocin use in labour, Acta Obstet. Gynecol. Scand. 86 (3) (2007) 315–319.

[55] K.R. Simpson, Failure to rescue: implications for evaluating quality of care during labor and birth, J. Perinat. Neonat Nurs. 19 (1) (2005) 24–34.

[56] A.J. Forster, E.K. O'Rourk, K.G. Shojania, et al., Combining ratings from multiple physician reviewers helped to overcome the uncertainty associated with adverse event classification, J. Clin. Epidemiol. 60 (9) (2007) 892–901.

[57] L. Greenwald, M. Mondor, Malpractice and the perinatal nurse, J. Perinat. Neonatal Nurs. 17 (2) (2003) 101–109.

[58] H. Singh, E.J. Thomas, L.A. Petersen, et al., Medical errors involving trainees: a study of closed malpractice claims from 5 insurers, Arch. Intern. Med. 167 (19) (2007) 2030–2036.

[59] B.P. Sinclair, Nurses and malpractice, AWHONN Lifelines 4 (5) (2000) 7.

[60] J.T. Queenan, Professional liability: storm warning, Obstet. Gynecol. 98 (2) (2001) 194–197.

[61] Joint Commission on Accreditation of Healthcare Organizations, Comprehensive Manual for Accreditation of Hospitals, JCAHO, Oak Brook, IL, 2003.

[62] National Patient Safety Foundation, Talking to Patients about Health Care Injury: Statement of Principle, NPSF, Chicago, IL, 2000.

[63] T. Gallagher, D. Studdert, W. Levinson, Disclosing harmful medical errors to patients, N. Engl. J. Med. 356 (26) (2007) 2713–2719.

[64] J.R. Woods, F.A. Rozovsky, Consent as a process, in: What Do I Say? Communicating Intended or Unanticipated Outcomes in Obstetrics, Jossey-Bass, San Francisco, CA, 2003, pp. 17–52.

[65] Z. Alfirevic, D. Devane, G.M.L. Gyte, Continuous cardiotocography (CTG) as a form of electronic fetal monitoring (EFM) for fetal assessment during labour, Cochrane Database Syst. Rev. (5) (2013). CD006066.

[66] American College of Obstetricians and Gynecologists, Intrapartum fetal heart rate monitoring: nomenclature, interpretation, and general management principles, ACOG Practice Bulletin No. 106, Obstet. Gynecol. 114 (2009) 192–202.

[67] Association of Women's Health, Obstetric and Neonatal Nurses, AWHONN Position Statement. Fetal heart monitoring, J. Obstet. Gynecol. Neonatal Nurs. 44 (5) (2015) 683–686, http://dx.doi.org/10.1111/1552-6909.12743.

[68] American College of Nurse-Midwives, Intermittent auscultation for intrapartum fetal heart rate surveillance. ACNM Clinical Bulletin Number 13, J. Midwifery Womens Health 60 (2015) 626–632.

[69] L. Miller, Intrapartum fetal monitoring: liability and documentation, Clin. Obstet. Gynecol. 54 (2011) 50–55.

[70] C.S. Kelly, Perinatal computerized patient record and archiving systems: pitfalls and enhancements for implementing a successful computerized medical record, J. Perinat. Neonatal Nurs. 12 (4) (1999) 1–14.

[71] G.A. Macones, G.D. Hankins, C.Y. Spong, et al., The 2008 National Institute of Child Health and Human Development workshop report on electronic fetal monitoring: update on definitions, interpretation, and research guidelines, J. Obstet. Gynecol. Neonatal Nurs. 37 (2008) 510–515.

[72] American College of Obstetricians and Gynecologists, Inappropriate Use of the Terms Fetal Distress and Birth Asphyxia, Committee Opinion No. 197, ACOG, Washington, DC, 1998.

[73] P.R. McCartney, Using technology to promote perinatal patient safety, J. Obstet. Gynecol. Neonatal Nurs. 35 (3) (2006) 424–431.

[74] T. Slagle, Perinatal information systems for quality improvement: visions for today, Pediatrics 103 (1 Suppl. E) (1999) 266–277.

[75] S.L. Clark, J.A. Meyers, D.K. Frye, et al., Patient safety in obstetrics—the Hospital Corporation of America experience, Am. J. Obstet. Gynecol. 204 (4) (2011) 283–287.

Obstetric Models and Electronic Fetal Monitoring in Europe

S tateside obstetric healthcare providers may travel abroad for employment or to volunteer professional services. In these situations, notable differences may be encountered, including model of care variations, use of electronic fetal monitoring (EFM), EFM terminology, and adjuncts to aid in intrapartum fetal assessment. This chapter provides a brief overview of models of care and the use of EFM, known by the term *cardiotocography* (CTG), in selected countries outside the United States. The international literature frequently refers to EFM as CTG, and the terms are used interchangeably in this chapter.

MODELS OF CARE

Various combinations of physician-led, midwifery-led, and shared models of care exist throughout the world. In some countries, obstetricians assume total responsibility for obstetric care. Other regions may have midwives as the main care providers for women, with patients only being transferred or referred to a physician or hospital when a complication is suspected or diagnosed. Lastly, the responsibility may be collectively shared among midwives, nurse practitioners, and physicians throughout the pregnancy course [1,2]. In fact, a more integrated interprofessional approach to obstetric care is becoming increasingly necessary in response to the rise in comorbidities such as diabetes [2]. For instance, Belgium, the Netherlands, and France enacted legislation in which the midwife oversees low-risk pregnancies and births while the physician assumes responsibility and management of high-risk pregnancies [3]. Furthermore, this model of care has the potential to lower healthcare costs, allow for increased access to obstetric care, and provide a higher level of quality care [4,5].

Midwifery-led care is a core part of universal healthcare coverage in many countries and is offered in a variety of settings [6]. In the United

Kingdom, for instance, women can give birth in physician-led hospital units, midwifery-supervised hospital-based or community-based birth centers, or at home [7]. Midwifery-led care can be differentiated from other models of care on the basis of variations in philosophy about pregnancy and birth, the goals and objectives of care, type of patient seeking midwifery-led care, provider–client relationships, use of interventions during labor, and the care setting [4,8,9]. Midwifery-led care is also distinctive from other models of care because this type of care merges public health and clinical health, while combining access to all women and newborns across the continuum of care in both community and clinical facilities [10]. In some countries, midwives attend as many as 80% of all births, compared with the United States in which certified nurse midwives attended less than 10% of births in 2013 [11]. This number may increase as changes occur in the healthcare plan system [5]. A systematic review of midwifery-led care demonstrated that women experienced fewer interventions, a reduction in the use of analgesia and regional anesthesia, more spontaneous vaginal births, and fewer episiotomies and operative vaginal births. There were no statistical differences in overall fetal loss or neonatal death compared with other models of care [1,5].

The physician-led model of care is a separate service from other healthcare disciplines [4]. Physician-led models of care can have an effective and powerful influence on women's care decisions in many countries [7]. In this type of care, physicians may take a more medicalized approach by treating pregnancy as a pathologic condition utilizing a "high-tech" approach, which can subsequently escalate into unnecessary interventions and procedures that potentially cause increased risk to the maternal–fetal dyad [4,7].

Interprofessional models of care, or shared models, are those in which groups or individuals that represent the same or similar field of work, such as obstetrics, come together to provide specific patient care services [5]. This model of care is essential to providing optimal care as certain experiences and skills can only be found in a broad range of healthcare professionals [2]. For example, a patient with gestational diabetes may be co-managed by a nurse practitioner and a physician. Interprofessional models of care also have a similar goal: providing safe, effective, patient-centered care for women and their families guided by shared rules and structures that govern a mutually beneficial relationship [5]. In fact, shared models of care between midwives and physicians have demonstrated decreased cesarean birth rates while maintaining similar neonatal outcomes compared with physician-led management of labor [8].

In addition, mounting global evidence demonstrates that countries utilizing skilled midwifery care within an environment that facilitates cohesive healthcare services in an interprofessional care model have achieved significant improvements in the survival rates of women and newborns [6,10].

ELECTRONIC FETAL MONITORING (EFM)–CARDIOTOCOGRAPHY (CTG)

International data regarding the exact percentage of intrapartum patients monitored with intrapartum auscultation (IA) versus EFM is lacking. The introduction of EFM in the 20th century resulted in a decreased use of IA as a primary fetal surveillance option during the intrapartum period in countries such as the United States [12–14]. IA is discussed in greater detail in Chapter 3. Outside of the United States, IA and intrapartum fetal surveillance clinical guidelines and recommendations have been published [13–16]. For example, the National Institute for Health and Clinical Excellence (NICE) is responsible for producing evidence-based guidelines and quality standards for the United Kingdom. Countries such as Australia and New Zealand have comparable guidelines on CTG.

NICE intrapartum guidelines now recommend routine CTG not be performed on every patient and that IA be offered to low-risk patients in the first stage of labor regardless of the birth setting. The NICE intrapartum guidelines also have an inclusive list of risk factors that indicate the need for CTG. For example, continuous CTG is recommended if any of the following risk factors occurs: suspected chorioamnionitis, sepsis, or maternal temperature of 38 °C or higher; severe hypertension (160/110 mm Hg or greater); oxytocin use; "significant" meconium; or vaginal bleeding that occurs in labor. Continuous CTG is also advised if two or more of the following are present: prolonged rupture of membranes (≥24 hours); moderate hypertension (150/100–159/109 mm Hg); delay in first or second stage labor; or the presence of "nonsignificant" meconium [17].

Quality of EFM-CTG

The international literature sometimes refers to FHR tracings or monitor strips as *obstetric registrations, registers,* or simply *"traces"*. Similar to the United States, other countries experience difficulties in CTG usage, which are assumed to be related to interpretation. Misinterpretation of the FHR trace, differentiating between maternal and FHR in the first and second stages of labor, and intervening for indeterminate and abnormal CTG traces have medicolegal significance [3,18]. Another shortcoming with interpretation is interobserver and intraobserver variability [19]. Thus the "human factor" is frequently blamed, whereas the monitor and the ability to deliver correct information are seldom questioned. Despite technological advances, errors directly related to the quality of the data acquisition and mistakes related to recognition of signal ambiguity continue to afflict obstetric management [18,20]. Solutions for this problem include using appropriate methods that optimize the quality of CTG traces, such as internal EFM [3,16]. For example, a fetal spiral electrode (FSE) is often used in European countries in second-stage labor and high-risk labors [21,22]. This offers the advantage of reducing signal loss [23]. Refer to Chapter 3 for further details.

Guidelines for Terminology and Interpretation

Numerous FHR pattern classification systems have been proposed by a number of countries [24]. At this time, a single universal standardized system of CTG and EFM terminology, interpretation, and management remains elusive. In 1987 a consensus development group presented a fetal monitoring document to the International Federation of Gynecology and Obstetrics (FIGO), which was subsequently adopted. The guidelines promulgated by FIGO were an important landmark in EFM history, and despite being dated, they still represent the sole international consensus document on the topic [24–26]. Subsequently, after the FIGO guidelines were released, other organizations such as NICE, which is supported by the Royal College of Obstetricians and Gynaecologists (RCOG), produced fetal monitoring guidelines aimed at a national level [17]. The definitions in the FIGO and NICE/RCOG guidelines differ from each other as well as the standardized definitions published in the United States by the National Institute of Child Health and Development [27]. Of note, when interpreting traces in other countries, international paper speeds are often 1 or 2 cm/minute, versus the typical 3 cm/minute seen in the United States.

In addition to definitions for various FHR components, FIGO and NICE have a three-tier classification systems for CTG patterns, with FIGO including a separate classification system for antepartum versus intrapartum tracings [17,25,26]. In general, there is agreement between the FIGO/NICE guidelines on CTG patterns being considered "normal" when baseline FHR is in a normal range, variability is 5 bpm or greater, and there are no decelerations. Likewise, for the guideline's agreement on "abnormal" when absent variability is coupled with recurrent late, variable, or prolonged decelerations or a bradycardia. Wide disagreement, which may potentially lead to conflict, is found among the different guidelines regarding the classification and management of intermediate or suspicious fetal monitoring patterns, equivalent to the Category II classification used in the United States. Integration of healthcare informatics including computer analysis of the FHR tracing and clinical decision support system can assist during these disagreements by helping clinicians with pattern interpretation and management [19,28–30].

Examples of 1- and 2-cm CTG Tracings

Figures 11.1 through 11.5 are examples of FHR tracings at 1- and 2-cm paper speeds. Consistent with the state of current practice, the figure legends reflect the terminology in use at the center where the tracing was obtained and do not necessarily coincide with FIGO or NICE/RCOG guidelines. They are provided to familiarize the reader with the appearance of tracings at different paper speeds.

Methods of Determining Fetal Acid–Base Status

Currently, there are three direct methods of fetal acid–base assessment in which blood sampling takes place: umbilical cord blood gases, fetal blood sampling (FBS) from the fetal scalp for pH, and FBS for fetal lactate [31,32]. FBS is no longer performed in the United States during the intrapartum period. ST analysis of the fetal electrocardiogram (FECG) may also be encountered as an adjunct

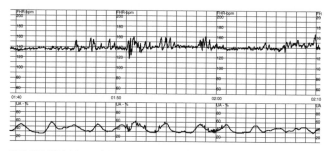

FIGURE 11.1 Normal CTG with accelerations, paper speed 1 cm/minute. (Courtesy Neoventa Medical, Mölndal, Sweden.)

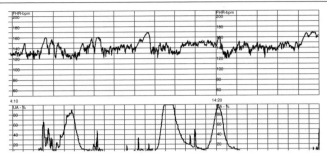

FIGURE 11.2 Normal CTG with accelerations, paper speed 2 cm/minute. (Courtesy Neoventa Medical, Mölndal, Sweden.)

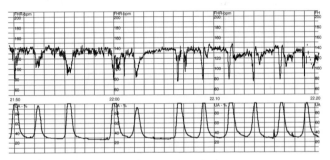

FIGURE 11.3 CTG with variable decelerations, paper speed 1 cm/minute. (Courtesy Neoventa Medical, Mölndal, Sweden.)

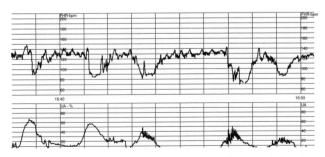

FIGURE 11.4 CTG with variable decelerations, paper speed 2 cm/minute. (Courtesy Neoventa Medical, Mölndal, Sweden.)

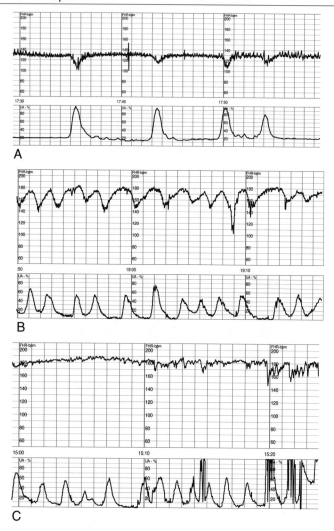

FIGURE 11.5 Examples of various CTG traces at 1 cm/min. (A) Early decelerations. (B) Late decelerations. (C) Tachycardia.

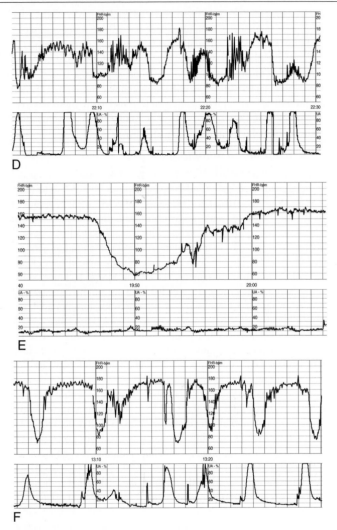

FIGURE 11.5, CONT'D (D) Prolonged decelerations. (E) Bradycardia. (F) "Complicated" or "atypical" variable decelerations. (Courtesy Neoventa Medical, Mölndal, Sweden.)

to CTG in terms of identifying cases of fetal hypoxia. Unlike the three prior methods, ST analysis does not require blood sampling. Umbilical cord blood gas evaluation is the most objective method of assessing the metabolic state of the newborn at the time of birth and is performed internationally. This method is discussed more thoroughly in Chapter 6. FBS is utilized in conjunction with CTG and can provide additional information on fetal metabolic status at a specific moment in time before critical decisions are made concerning the need for and timing of delivery [32–34].

Fetal Scalp Blood Sampling for pH

As mentioned previously, FBS for pH is a direct method of assessing fetal acid–base status and is considered an invasive procedure. A sample of fetal capillary blood is collected with heparinized glass tubes from the fetal scalp once the scalp surface has been punctured through an amnioscope with a small scalpel-like device. Approximately 30 to 50 microliters of blood is required to obtain a fetal blood pH value [35–37]. There are considerable clinical, facility, and equipment requirements, as well as precise technical skills for performing the procedure, which in turn potentially increases the inaccuracy rate of pH results [31,34,37]. For example, reported draw-to-result median time is 18 minutes with ranges of 12 to more than 30 minutes, which may result in a delay in delivering a compromised fetus [34]. The procedure must be repeated on a regular basis to guide FHR management. A pH value ≥7.25 is normal. Values between 7.21 and 7.24 are regarded as borderline and require corrective measures to improve fetal oxygenation; sampling is repeated within 20 to 30 minutes. Values of pH <7.20 (or <7.15 in the second stage of labor) are abnormal and require intervention [17,33,35]. Results should be interpreted in the entire clinical context that includes previous FBS results, stage of labor, progress in labor, and clinical characteristics of the FHR [34,37].

Clinicians need to correctly interpret the FHR using a standardized approach to identify the indication for FBS. Inappropriate FHR interpretation may result in FBS being performed unnecessarily or failing to be performed when indications warrant further action [17,24,33]. A systematic review of available evidence has questioned the continued use of fetal pH measurement as no reduction in cesarean delivery rates or neonatal seizures has been observed [15]. Nevertheless, professional organizations outside the United States continue to reference the use of FBS for fetal assessment as well as for the basis of clinical experience and indirect research.

Fetal Scalp Blood Sampling for Lactate

Fetal lactate measurement has been proposed as an alternative to fetal pH. Lactate is a marker or by-product of fetal dependence on anaerobic metabolism related to periods of hypoxia and appears to be more specific than pH in predicting fetal metabolic acidemia. Therefore, it is reasonable to assume that fetal lactate levels represent the metabolic stage of the acid–base balance, which is thought to be more closely related to the condition of the fetus rather than pH [32,36,38].

The procedure for lactate sampling is similar to pH sampling but requires a smaller volume of blood approximately 5 microliters [36,38]. Heparinized glass tubes, lactate test strips, and a lactate analyzer are utilized versus blood gas analysis equipment [34,38,39]. The test strips and lactate analyzer are similar to glucometers. Available data indicate that lactate levels >4.8 mmol/L are abnormal and require delivery, levels of 4.2 to 4.8 mmol/L are considered pre-acidemic and require repeat lactate testing 20 to 30 minutes later, and <4.2 mmol/L are normal [32,40]. The procedure for obtaining fetal blood for lactate level estimation is similar to FBS for pH evaluation but has been shown to provide more precise information on fetal acid–base status than does pH and base deficit, have quicker turnaround for sample results, be quicker and easier to perform, and yield results more often [32,39].

ST Analysis of the Fetal ECG

ST segment analysis of the fetal ECG is used in Europe as an adjunct to fetal monitoring for high-risk intrapartum patients. ST analysis requires a specialized FSE and software (STAN; Neoventa Medical, Göteborg, Sweden) that automatically analyzes the ratio of the T and QRS amplitudes, known as the T/QRS ratio as well as the ST interval, in situations in which fetal hypoxia may be occurring [21,41]. Using a combination of strict FHR interpretation and management guidelines as well as ST waveform analysis, this monitor provides clinicians with information on the fetal myocardial response to hypoxia based on fetal ECG changes [23,42–44]. The STAN system consists of a freestanding electronic fetal monitor with a special ST analysis feature. The monitor can be used with or without ST analysis, functioning as a standard fetal monitor with all gestational ages; however, use of the adjunctive ST analysis option requires several patient characteristics be met, as follows:

- Planned vaginal delivery
- >36 completed weeks' gestation

- Singleton fetus
- Vertex presentation
- Ruptured amniotic membranes

After appropriate patient selection and FSE application, fetal ECG data is analyzed to evaluate the T/QRS ratio and the ST interval so that clinicians can determine the fetal response to hypoxia and subsequent labor management [42,43]. These data are evaluated and appear on the monitor screen below the EFM tracing.

SUMMARY

Although IA is an accepted practice for low-risk laboring patients in some countries [14], the institutional culture may result in reliance on EFM over IA [45]. Like the United States, EFM utilization in other countries is fraught with challenges related to patient selection, standardization of terminology, interpretation, and management and appropriate application of adjunct tools. Simply making a single model of care and one specific fetal surveillance tool available for the intrapartum patient will never result in improved outcomes and quality care. Whether in the United States or abroad, clinicians will need to work together to identify approaches to obstetric care that make the best use of information provided by technology, keeping in mind the importance of the relationship among women, their families, and their caregivers. In the case of IA and EFM-CTG, standardization of guidelines and the simplification of management algorithms should be a priority regardless of geographic location.

References

[1] J. Sandall, H. Soltani, S. Gates, A. Shennan, D. Devane, Midwife-led continuity models versus other models of care for childbearing women, Cochrane Database Syst. Rev. (2013). CD004667.

[2] J. Shamian, Interprofessional Collaboration, The only way to save every woman and every child, Lancet 384 (9948) (2014) e41–e42.

[3] M. Eggermont, Intrapartum care and substandard care: juridical recommendations to reduce the risk of liability, Arch. Gynecol. Obstet. 292 (1) (2015) 1–9.

[4] A.B. Caughey, Midwife and obstetrician collaborative care: the whole is better than the parts, J. Midwifery Womens Health 60 (2) (2015) 120–121.

[5] D.C. SmithMidwife–Physician Collaboration, A conceptual framework for interprofessional collaborative practice, J. Midwifery Womens Health 60 (2) (2015) 128–139.

[6] R. Horton, O. Astudillo, The power of midwifery, Lancet 384 (9948) (2014) 1075–1076.

[7] E. Hadjigeorgiou, C. Kouta, E. Papastavrou, I. Papadopoulos, L.B. Mårtensson, Women's perceptions of their right to choose the place of childbirth: an integrative review, Midwifery 28 (3) (2012) 380–390.

[8] N.S. Carlson, N.K. Lowe, A concept analysis of watchful waiting among providers caring for women in labour, J. Adv. Nurs. 70 (3) (2014) 511–522.

[9] J.P. Rooks, The midwifery model of care, J. Nurse Midwifery 44 (4) (1999) 370–374.

[10] F. McConville, New global midwifery initiatives and why 2014 should be a good year for women and newborns, Midwifery 30 (5) (2014) 489–490.

[11] J.A. Martin, B.E. Hamilton, M.J.K. Osterman, et al., Births: final data for 2013, Natl. Vital Stat. Rep. 64 (1) (2015). National Center for Health Statistics, Hyattsville, MD.

[12] C.V. Ananth, S.P. Chauhan, H.Y. Chen, M.E. D'Alton, A.M. Vintzileos, Electronic fetal monitoring in the United States: temporal trends and adverse perinatal outcomes, Obstet. Gynecol. 121 (5) (2013) 927–933.

[13] N.F. Feinstein, A. Sprague, M.J. Trepanier, Fetal Heart Rate Auscultation, second ed., AWHONN, Washington, DC, 2008.

[14] S.L. Sholapurkar, Intermittent auscultation of fetal heart rate during labour—a widely accepted technique for low risk pregnancies: but are the current national guidelines robust and practical? J. Obstet. Gynaecol. 30 (6) (2010) 537–540.

[15] Z. Alfirevic, D. Devane, G.M. Gyte, Continuous cardiotocography (CTG) as a form of electronic fetal monitoring (EFM) for fetal assessment during labour, Cochrane Database Syst. Rev. 3 (2006). CD006066.

[16] J. Reinhard, B.R. Hayes-Gill, S. Schiermeier, et al., Intrapartum signal quality with external fetal heart rate monitoring: a two way trial of external Doppler CTG ultrasound and the abdominal fetal electrocardiogram, Arch. Gynecol. Obstet. 286 (5) (2012) 1103–1107.

[17] National Collaborating Centre for Women's and Children's Health, commissioned by the National Institute for Health and Clinical Excellence, Intrapartum Care, RCOG Press, London, 2014.

[18] T.R. Van Veen, M.A. Belfort, S. Kofford, Maternal heart rate patterns in the first and second stages of labor, Acta Obstet. Gynecol. Scand. 91 (5) (2012) 598–604.

[19] A. Costa, C. Santos, D. Ayres-de-Campos, et al., Access to computerised analysis of intrapartum cardiotocographs improves clinicians' prediction of newborn umbilical artery blood pH, BJOG 117 (10) (2010) 1288–1293.

[20] D.R. Neilson, R.K. Freeman, S. Mangan, Signal ambiguity in unexpected outcome with external fetal heart rate monitoring, Am. J. Obstet. Gynecol. 198 (6) (2008) 717–724.

[21] P.J. Steer, L.E. Hvidman, Scientific and clinical evidence for the use of fetal ECG ST segment analysis (STAN), Acta Obstet. Gynecol. Scand. 93 (6) (2014) 533–538.

[22] M.E. Westerhuis, G.H. Visser, K.G. Moons, et al., Cardiotocography plus ST analysis of fetal electrocardiogram compared with cardiotocography only for intrapartum monitoring: a randomized controlled trial, Obstet. Gynecol. 115 (6) (2010) 1173–1180.

[23] K.G. Rosén, I. Amer-Wåhlin, R. Luzietti, et al., Fetal ECG waveform analysis, Best Pract. Res. Clin. Obstet. Gynaecol. 18 (3) (2004) 485–514.

[24] X. Carbonell, E.F. Gonzalez, Recommendations and Guidelines for Perinatal Medicine (J.M. Carrera, Ed.), Matres Mundi, Barcelona, Spain, 2007.

[25] D. Ayres-de-Campos, J. Bernardes, FIGO Subcommittee, Twenty-five years after the FIGO guidelines for the use of fetal monitoring: time for a simplified approach? Int. J. Gynaecol. Obstet. 110 (1) (2010) 1–6.

[26] FIGO Subcommittee on Standards in Perinatal Medicine, Guidelines for the use of fetal monitoring 25 (3) (1987) 159–167.

[27] G.A. Macones, G.D. Hankins, C.Y. Spong, et al., The 2008 National Institute of Child Health and Human Development workshop report on electronic fetal monitoring: update on definitions, interpretation, and research guidelines, Obstet. Gynecol. 112 (2008) 661–666.

[28] S.K. Hasley, Decision support and patient safety: the time has come, Am. J. Obstet. Gynecol. 204 (6) (2011) 461–465.

[29] S. Smith, K. Bunting, E. Hamilton, Using intelligent electronic fetal monitoring software to reduce iatrogenic complications of childbirth: a case study, J. Healthc. Inf. Manag. 28 (4) (2014) 28–33.

[30] S. Weiner, Independent validation of a fetal heart rate pattern recognition software, Am. J. Obstet. Gynecol. 208 (1) (2013) S316–S317.

[31] R. Cypher, Assessment of fetal oxygenation and acid–base status, in: A. Lyndon, L. Usher Ali (Eds.), Fetal Heart Monitoring Principles and Practices, fifth ed., AWHONN, Washington, DC, 2015.

[32] Royal College of Obstetricians and Gynaecologists, Is It Time for UK Obstetricians to Accept Fetal Scalp Lactate as an Alternative to Scalp pH, Scientific Impact Paper, No. 47, RCOG Press, London, 2015.

[33] J.S. Jørgensen, T. Weber, Fetal scalp blood sampling in labor—a review, Acta Obstet. Gynecol. Scand. 93 (6) (2014) 548–555.

[34] D. Tuffnell, W. Haw, K. Wilkinson, How long does a fetal scalp blood sample take? BJOG 113 (3) (2006) 332–334.

[35] Z. Henderson, J.L. Ecker, Fetal scalp blood sampling—limited role in contemporary obstetric practice: part II, Lab. Med. 34 (8) (2003) 594–600.

[36] M. Westgren, K. Kruger, S. Ek, et al., Lactate compared with pH analysis at fetal scalp blood sampling: a prospective randomised study, BJOG 105 (1) (1998) 29–33.

[37] M.K. Whitworth, L. Bricker, How to perform intrapartum fetal blood sampling, Br. J. Hosp. Med. 67 (9) (2006) 162–164.

[38] L. Nordström, S. Achanna, K. Naka, S. Arulkumaran, Fetal and maternal lactate increase during active second stage, BJOG 108 (3) (2001) 263–268.

[39] A.M. Heinis, M.E. Spaanderman, J.M.K. Gunnewiek, F.K. Lotgering, Scalp blood lactate for intrapartum assessment of fetal metabolic acidosis, Acta Obstet. Gynecol. Scand. 90 (10) (2011) 1107–1114.

[40] K. Kruger, B. Hallberg, M. Blennow, M. Kublickas, M. Westgren, Predictive value of fetal scalp blood lactate concentration and pH as markers of neurologic disability, Am. J. Obstet. Gynecol. 181 (5) (1999) 1072–1078.

[41] K.G. Rosen, K. Lindencrantz, STAN—the Gothenburg model for fetal surveillance during labour by ST analysis of the fetal electrocardiogram, Clin. Phys. Physiol. Meas. 10 (Suppl. B) (1989) 51–56.

[42] I. Amer-Wåhlin, L.A. Miller, ST analysis as an adjunct to electronic fetal monitoring: an overview, J. Perinat. Neonatal Nurs. 24 (3) (2010) 231–237.

[43] M.A. Belfort, G.R. Saade, ST segment analysis as an adjunct to electronic fetal monitoring, part I: background, physiology, interpretation, Clin. Perinatol. 38 (2011) 143–157.

[44] M.A. Belfort, G.R. Saade, ST segment analysis (STAN) as an adjunct to electronic fetal monitoring, part II: clinical studies and future directions, Clin. Perinatol. 38 (2011) 143–157.

[45] M.E. Foley, M. Alarab, L. Daly, et al., The continuing effectiveness of active management of first labor, despite a doubling in overall nulliparous cesarean delivery, Am. J. Obstet. Gynecol. 191 (3) (2004) 891–895.

Amnioinfusion

Amnioinfusion is the administration of room temperature isotonic solution such as normal saline or Ringer's lactate via a double-lumen intrauterine pressure catheter (IUPC) by either a gravity flow or an infusion pump to restore amniotic fluid volume. The procedure is intended to relieve intermittent umbilical cord compression, which results in variable fetal heart rate decelerations and transient fetal hypoxemia. This procedure has no known effect on late decelerations and is no longer recommended for dilution of meconium.

An amnioinfusion generally begins by administering a bolus of fluid (250–500 mL) over 20 to 30 minutes. The maintenance dose is infused at a rate of 2 to 3 mL/min (maximum of 180 mL/hr), during which time it is imperative that the amount of fluid returning is approximated and documented to avoid overdistention of the uterus. Assessment of the output can be accomplished by weighing the absorbent pads underneath the woman (1 mL = 1 g) and counting the number of pads changed.

Assessment of uterine resting tone is also an important aspect of surveillance during the procedure, and it should not exceed 40 mm Hg. It is unlikely that more than 1000 mL of fluid need to be administered, and if variable decelerations persist even after this amount of fluid has been instilled into the uterus, other therapies should be used as treatment. Iatrogenic polyhydramnios may cause a placental abruption or pressure on the maternal diaphragm, causing shortness of breath, tachycardia, and a change in maternal blood pressure. A rapid release, or "gush," of fluid predisposes the woman to a prolapsed umbilical cord. The preterm fetus may benefit from a warmed solution, thus avoiding bradycardia. A blood warmer is the safest method for administering warmed fluid. *The fluid should not be heated in a microwave or blanket warmer.* Warmed fluid is also suggested if the rate of the amnioinfusion exceeds 15 mL/min.

There are a variety of ways to perform an amnioinfusion. It is important that the institution have a policy and procedure in place and these are followed.

INDICATIONS FOR AMNIOINFUSION

1. Laboring preterm women with premature rupture of the membranes (prophylactic)
2. Variable decelerations uncorrectable with conventional interventions
3. Significant oligohydramnios (amniotic fluid index ≤5) at term when labor is being induced

EQUIPMENT AND SUPPLIES

- Normal saline or Ringer's lactate solution, 1000 mL at room temperature
- Intrauterine catheter equipment, preferably with a double lumen and amnioport (if using single-lumen water-filled IUPC, intravenous [IV] extension tubing with twin sites or arterial line [12 inches] and a three-way stopcock are needed)
- Volumetric infusion pump and tubing or IV pole for gravity flow
- Blood warmer or blood/fluid warming set (optional)

PROCEDURE

Amnioinfusion should be initiated after insertion of the intrauterine catheter. Before the procedure, the intrauterine resting tone should be noted with the woman in the right and left lateral and supine positions for later comparison. Various procedures have been discussed in the literature, and each institution determines its own obstetric policies and procedures. A sample procedure follows:

1. Connect the 1000-mL bottle of amnioinfusion solution to the IV tubing.
2. Flush the tubing with the solution.
3. Connect the tubing to the woman's IUPC via the amnioport or double-lumen IUPC or via a three-way stopcock, depending on the type of IUPC used.
4. Initiate the flow of amnioinfusion and instill the initial bolus, usually 250 to 500 mL over a 20- to 30-minute period (10–15 mL/min) using either an infusion pump or gravity flow. If gravity flow is used, the solution must be hung about 3 to 4 feet above the level of the tip of the IUPC. If fluid will not run by gravity, check the position/placement of the IUPC.
5. When variable decelerations resolve, continue the infusion at a slower rate, usually about 2 to 3 mL/min (120–180 mL/hr), as

ordered by the care provider. If variable decelerations are not relieved after infusing 800 to 1000 mL of solution, discontinue the procedure and perform an alternative intervention.

6. Observe and evaluate for amount and character of vaginal drainage. Vaginal output is assessed and documented to demonstrate that the volume infused is also coming back out and not causing overdistention of the uterus. Be vigilant for sudden "gushes" of fluid and assess for cord prolapse.

NOTE: Intrauterine resting tone will appear higher than normal, from 25 to 40 mm Hg, because of resistance to outflow through the tiny holes in the tip of the catheter. The true resting tone can be checked by temporarily discontinuing the flow of infusion.

PATIENT CARE

Care of the woman undergoing amnioinfusion includes the following:

1. Stop the infusion periodically, approximately every 30 to 60 minutes, to note the baseline uterine pressure. If the resting tone of the uterus exceeds 40 mm Hg, discontinue the infusion and notify the physician.
2. Change the underpads frequently to ensure the woman's comfort.
3. Note the color and amount of fluid on the underpads. The underpads may be weighed. Amounts of fluid returned should be determined (1 mL = 1 g).
4. Monitor for signs and symptoms of infection.
5. Monitor for signs and symptoms of cardiac or respiratory compromise secondary to an overdistended uterus (maternal shortness of breath, hypotension, or tachycardia).
6. Monitor fetal heart rate patterns on the electronic fetal monitoring strip.

Instructions for Reviewing Appendix B FHR Tracings

Appendix B consists of 30 fetal heart rate (FHR) tracings clinicians can review for the purpose of improving competency in the application of both the National Institute for Child Health and Human Development terminology and the two central principles of FHR interpretation presented in Chapter 5. Clinicians should assume that all tracings are from term pregnancies unless otherwise noted. For purposes of identifying tachysystole as well as the issue of recurrence with decelerations, clinicians should assume the tracings have been present for 30 minutes.

Clinicians should review the tracings provided and determine the following:

1. The components of FHR (baseline rate, baseline variability, accelerations, decelerations)
2. The Category (1, 2, or 3) of each tracing
3. Whether uterine contraction frequency would be summarized as normal or tachysystole, as well as identify any possible excessive uterine activity, such as inadequate relaxation time (see Chapter 4)
4. Whether there is evidence of interruption of the oxygen pathway
5. Whether the possibility of evolving fetal metabolic acidemia/ongoing hypoxic injury can be ruled out

A key with the answers for each tracing is provided immediately after each tracing. Please note that because FHR tracing evaluation is a visual exercise, there may be valid differences of opinion among clinicians reviewing these tracings. Whenever possible, the authors have anticipated such differences and included them in the answer key for purposes of discussion.

Finally, specific management approaches are not included in the key that follows the tracings, primarily because application of the standardized management model presented in Chapter 6 would vary widely based on the patient's clinical context.

KEY FOR APPENDIX B FHR TRACINGS

Monitoring modes are identified as follows:
    US—external Doppler
    TOCO—external tocotransducer
    IFE—internal fetal electrode
    IUPC—intrauterine pressure catheter

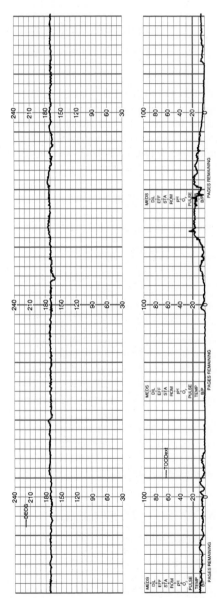

FIGURE B-1

1. **Monitoring Mode:** IFE/TOCO
   Baseline FHR: 170bpm. **Baseline variability:** Minimal. **Accelerations:** Absent. **Decelerations:** Absent. **Uterine activity:** None. **Accelerations:** Minimal. **Accelerations:** Absent. **Decelerations:** Absent. **Uterine activity:** Normal (vs. tachysystole), but it appears toco may need to be adjusted, and it is possible that palpation would reveal contraction duration that is excessive. **Category:** This is a Category 2 tracing.
   Interpretation
   Although there are no decelerations reflecting interruption of the oxygen pathway at one or more points; the lack of either acceleration(s) or moderate variability means clinicians are unable to rule out the possibility of evolving fetal metabolic acidemia/ongoing hypoxic injury. Clinicians should consider all causes of tachycardia when evaluating this tracing.

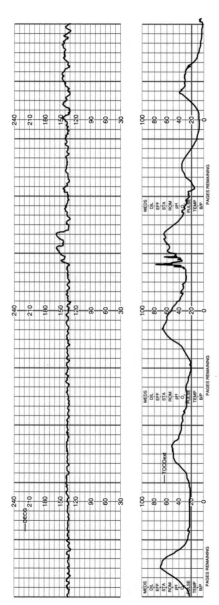

FIGURE B-2

2. **Monitoring Mode:** US/TOCO

    Baseline FHR: 135 bpm. **Baseline variability:** Moderate, although some clinicians may consider it minimal in the first minutes of the tracing. **Accelerations:** Present. **Decelerations:** Absent. **Uterine activity:** With six contractions in 10 minutes, this would be tachysystole. **Category:** This is a Category 1 tracing, unless the clinician believes the variability is minimal for the majority of the tracing, which would result in a Category II designation.

    Interpretation

    There is no evidence of interrupted oxygenation because there are no clinically significant decelerations. The possibility of evolving metabolic acidemia/ongoing hypoxic injury can be ruled out by the accelerations as well as the moderate variability. Remember, *either moderate variability or acceleration* of the FHR precludes the possibility of ongoing hypoxic injury.

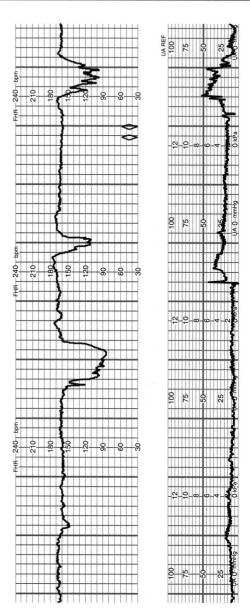

FIGURE B-3

3. **Monitoring Mode:** IFE/TOCO

Baseline FHR: 160 bpm. Although portions of the tracing appear to have a baseline of 165, the majority of the baseline is at 160 bpm. **Baseline variability:** Minimal. **Accelerations:** Absent. **Decelerations:** Recurrent variable decelerations; note that the deceleration at approximately minute 4 has a gradual onset but cannot be identified as late or early because of a lack of contraction data. **Uterine activity:** Normal, but it appears toco may need to be adjusted. **Category:** This is a Category 2 tracing.

Interpretation

Variable decelerations reflect interruption of the oxygen pathway at one or more points; unable to rule out the possibility of evolving fetal metabolic acidemia because of the lack of either acceleration(s) or moderate variability.

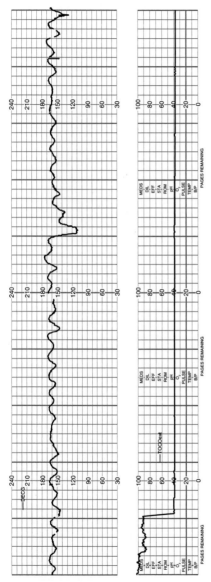

FIGURE B-4

4. **Monitoring Mode:** IFE/TOCO

Baseline FHR: 155 or 160 bpm, sinusoidal. **Baseline variability:** Not applicable because of sinusoidal tracing. **Accelerations:** Absent. **Decelerations:** Variable deceleration noted. **Uterine activity:** N/A, toco was removed as patient was being prepped for cesarean delivery. **Category:** This is a Category 3 tracing.

Interpretation

The sinusoidal pattern is rare, and this fetus was born with severe anemia due to a maternal–fetal hemorrhage, but the neonatal course went well after transfusion. Although the variable deceleration reflects interruption of the oxygen pathway at one or more points, the key finding here is the sinusoidal pattern.

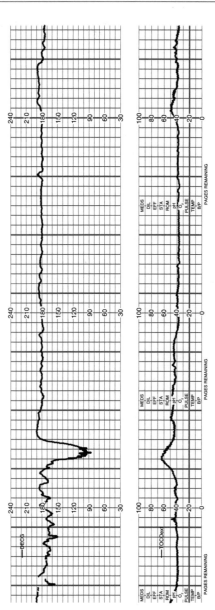

FIGURE B-5

5. **Monitoring Mode:** IFE/TOCO

Baseline FHR: 180bpm for the majority of the tracing. **Baseline variability:** Minimal for the majority of the tracing. **Accelerations:** Absent. **Decelerations:** Obvious variable deceleration at beginning of the tracing; however, immediately before the variable, it is unclear whether there is a deceleration, and clinicians would need to evaluate previous tracing portion to be certain. **Uterine activity:** Difficult to assess; the toco may need adjustment, and palpation should be used to assess for hypertonus and to evaluate the onset and offset of contractions because excessive contraction duration may be an issue at the beginning of the tracing. **Category:** This is a Category 2 tracing.

Interpretation

The variable deceleration reflects interruption of the oxygen pathway at one or more points; unable to rule out the possibility of evolving fetal metabolic acidemia because of the lack of either acceleration(s) or moderate variability. Additionally, tachycardia is noted.

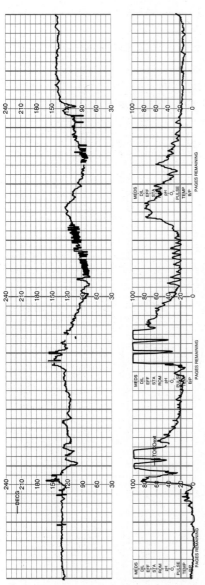

FIGURE B-6

6. **Monitoring Mode:** IFE/TOCO

Baseline FHR: 130 or 135bpm. **Baseline variability:** Minimal. **Accelerations:** Absent. **Decelerations:** Variable and prolonged decelerations. **Uterine activity:** Normal as to frequency; however, the contraction duration time may be excessive, resulting in inadequate relaxation time. **Category:** This is a Category 2 tracing.

Interpretation

The variable and prolonged decelerations reflect interruption of the oxygen pathway at one or more points; unable to rule out the possibility of evolving fetal metabolic acidemia/ongoing hypoxic injury because of the lack of either acceleration(s) or moderate variability. *Note the artifact during the prolonged deceleration. If this was persistent, it could represent an arrhythmia such as PACs.*

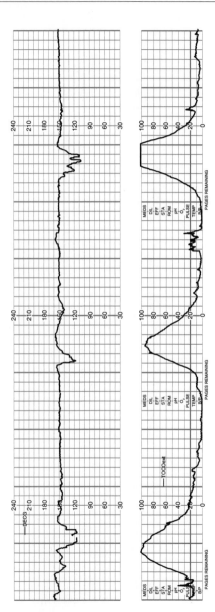

FIGURE B-7

7. **Monitoring Mode:** IFE/IUPC
Baseline FHR: 150 bpm. **Baseline variability:** Minimal. **Accelerations:** Absent. **Decelerations:** Variable decelerations. **Uterine activity:** Normal frequency, duration borders on excessive. **Category:** This is a Category 2 tracing.
Interpretation
The variable decelerations reflect interruption of the oxygen pathway at one or more points; unable to rule out the possibility of evolving fetal metabolic acidemia/ongoing hypoxic injury because of the lack of either acceleration(s) or moderate variability.

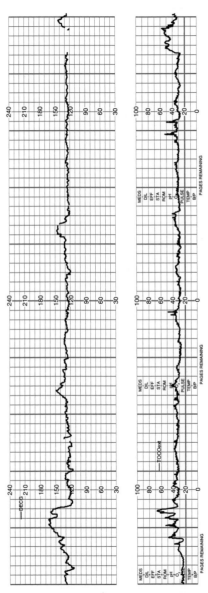

FIGURE B-8

8. **Monitoring Mode:** US/TOCO

Baseline FHR: 125 bpm. **Baseline variability:** Minimal for the majority of the tracing, although some clinicians may tend to call it moderate at first glance because of the accelerations. **Accelerations:** Present. **Decelerations:** Absent. **Uterine activity:** Difficult to determine; toco needs to be adjusted and palpation used to evaluate uterine activity thoroughly. **Category:** This is a Category 2 tracing (because of the lack of moderate variability).

Interpretation

There is no interruption of the oxygen pathway; the accelerations rule out the possibility of evolving fetal metabolic acidemia/ongoing hypoxic injury.

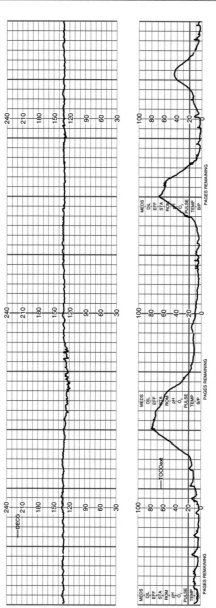

FIGURE B-9

9. **Monitoring Mode:** US/TOCO

Baseline FHR: 130 bpm. **Baseline variability:** Minimal. **Accelerations:** Absent. **Uterine activity:** Normal frequency; duration of contraction associated with late deceleration is excessive. **Decelerations:** Late deceleration. **Category:** This is a Category 2 tracing.

Interpretation

The late deceleration reflects interruption of the oxygen pathway at one or more points; unable to rule out the possibility of evolving fetal metabolic acidemia/ongoing hypoxic injury because of the lack of either acceleration(s) or moderate variability.

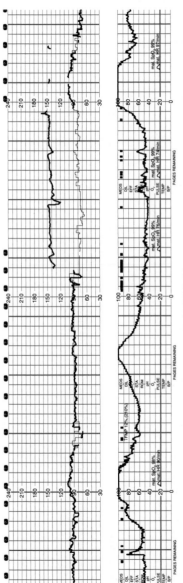

FIGURE B-10

10. **Monitoring Mode:** US/TOCO

Baseline FHR: 145bpm; note the limited segment (approximately 2½ minutes only) of FHR baseline due to the pickup of maternal heart rate (initial 5 minutes of tracing). Question marks at the top of the tracing alert the clinician to the possibility of signal coincidence, and maternal heart rate of 90bpm at the beginning of the tracing (see notation on lower portion of uterine activity panel) is consistent with the tracing showing a heart rate recorded in the 90s for the first 5 minutes of the tracing. **Baseline variability:** Moderate, but limited amount of FHR baseline to assess. **Accelerations:** Absent, but limited amount of tracing to assess. **Decelerations:** Absent, but limited amount of tracing to assess. **Uterine activity:** Probably normal, but toco needs to be adjusted and palpation used to assess contraction duration and uterine resting tone. **Category:** Of the limited portion of FHR available, it would fit into Category 1, but the majority of clinicians would wait for a clearer picture of FHR (adjust the Doppler and reassess) before committing to a Category designation.

Interpretation

Most clinicians would not provide an interpretation of such a limited amount of tracing; the correct action here is to adjust the Doppler and reassess the tracing when signal coincidence has been resolved.

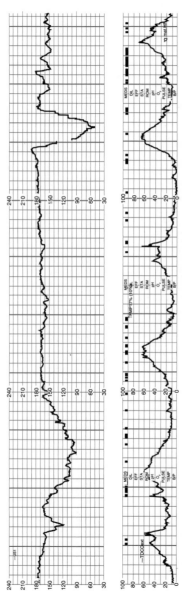

FIGURE B-11

11. **Monitoring Mode:** US/TOCO

Baseline FHR: The beginning and middle portions of this tracing reveal a FHR baseline of 170bpm; there may be a change in baseline near the end of the tracing, but this would require evaluation of the ongoing tracing to conclusively determine. **Baseline variability:** Minimal, for the portion of the tracing with a clearly identifiable baseline rate of 170 bpm. **Accelerations:** Absent. **Decelerations:** Present; a prolonged deceleration is seen at the beginning of the tracing, followed by a late deceleration in the middle of the tracing, and a variable deceleration is seen at the end of the tracing. This tracing clearly demonstrates that a variety of decelerations can be seen within a short period of time during labor. **Uterine activity:** Tachysystole, assuming this represents the average frequency over a 30-minute period. If this contraction pattern is new (<30 minutes), it would still qualify as excessive uterine activity because the relaxation time is not sufficient. During the first stage, relaxation time should be at least 60 seconds between contractions to avoid deterioration of fetal acid-base status. **Category:** This is a Category 2 tracing.

Interpretation

Three types of clinically significant decelerations (prolonged, late, and variable) reflect interruption of the oxygen pathway at one or more points; the possibility of evolving fetal metabolic acidemia cannot be ruled out because the tracing lacks either acceleration(s) or moderate variability.

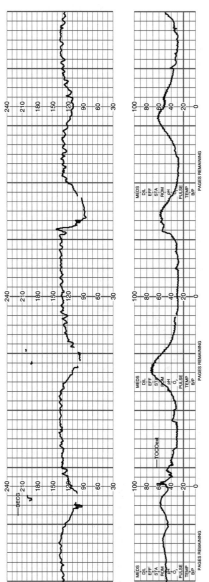

FIGURE B-12

12. **Monitoring Mode:** US/TOCO

Baseline FHR: 130bpm. **Baseline variability:** Minimal. **Accelerations:** Absent. **Decelerations:** Late and variable (third decel) decelerations. **Uterine activity:** Normal frequency, but there may be an issue with resting tone, and toco should be readjusted. **Category:** This is a Category 2 tracing.

Interpretation

The late and variable decelerations reflect interruption of the oxygen pathway at one or more points; unable to rule out the possibility of evolving fetal metabolic acidemia/ongoing hypoxic injury because of the lack of either acceleration(s) or moderate variability. *Note: maternal blood pressures were low (94–106/40–49mm Hg) during this tracing and should have been corrected.*

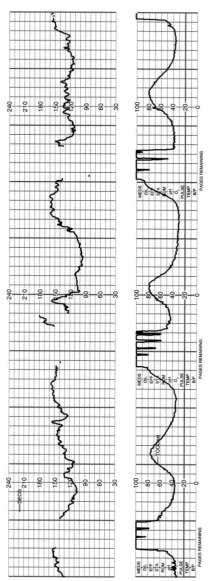

FIGURE B-13

13. **Monitoring Mode:** US/TOCO

Baseline FHR: Indeterminate. **Baseline variability, Accelerations, and Decelerations:** Unable to assess because of the indeterminate baseline. **Uterine activity:** Tachysystole.

Category: This is a Category 2 tracing.

Interpretation

The indeterminate baseline results in an inability to assess the FHR components, and therefore no interpretation can be provided. Clinicians will need to look to other portions of this tracing to assist in assessment and interpretation, and correcting the tachysystole is crucial because there is a strong likelihood of significant decelerations of the FHR (given the overall characteristics of the tracing).

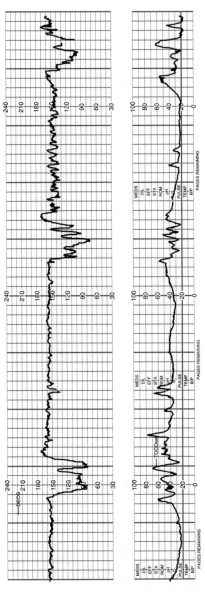

FIGURE B-14

14. **Monitoring Mode:** IFE/TOCO
Baseline FHR: 155 bpm. **Baseline variability:** Moderate. **Accelerations:** Absent. **Decelerations:** Variable decelerations. **Uterine activity:** Unable to accurately assess; toco should be readjusted. **Category:** This is a Category 2 tracing.
Interpretation
The variable decelerations reflect interruption of the oxygen pathway at one or more points; the moderate variability rules out the possibility of evolving fetal metabolic acidemia/ongoing hypoxic injury.

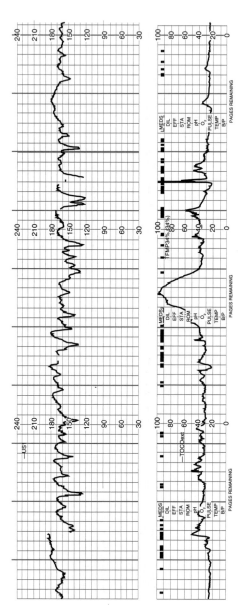

FIGURE B-15

15. **Monitoring Mode:** US/TOCO

Baseline FHR: Indeterminate, due to period of marked variability. **Baseline variability:** Marked. **Accelerations:** Unable to determine because of marked variability. **Decelerations:** None apparent but difficult to determine because of marked variability. **Uterine activity:** Appears normal, but toco may need to be adjusted and baseline resting tone should be evaluated by palpation. **Category:** This is a Category 2 tracing.

Interpretation

The significance (if any) of marked variability is unknown, and it is most frequently seen with fetal movement or fetal stimulation. Unlike moderate variability, it does not allow the clinician to rule out the possibility of evolving fetal metabolic acidemia/ongoing hypoxic injury.

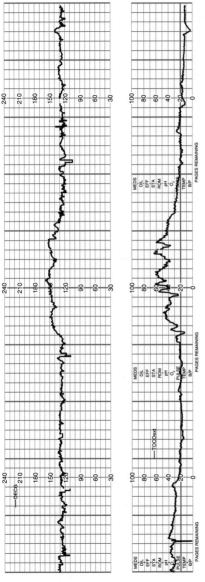

FIGURE B-16

16. **Monitoring Mode:** US/TOCO
Baseline FHR: 130 bpm. **Baseline variability:** Moderate. **Accelerations:** Prolonged acceleration present. **Decelerations:** Absent. **Uterine activity:** Normal frequency, but contraction duration appears excessive. **Category:** This is a Category 1 tracing.
Interpretation
There is no interruption of the oxygen pathway; the prolonged acceleration rules out the possibility of evolving fetal metabolic acidemia/ongoing hypoxic injury.

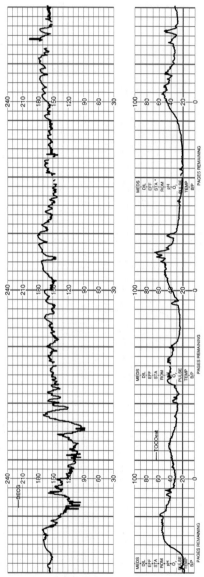

FIGURE B-17

17. **Monitoring Mode:** IFE/TOCO

Baseline FHR: 155 bpm. **Baseline variability:** Moderate. **Accelerations:** Present. **Decelerations:** Prolonged deceleration. **Uterine activity:** Normal frequency (five contractions in 10 minutes), but uterine activity should be considered excessive because of lack of relaxation time. **Category:** This is a Category 2 tracing.

Interpretation

The prolonged deceleration reflects an interruption of the oxygen pathway; the prolonged accelerations and moderate variability rule out the possibility of evolving fetal metabolic acidemia/ongoing hypoxic injury.

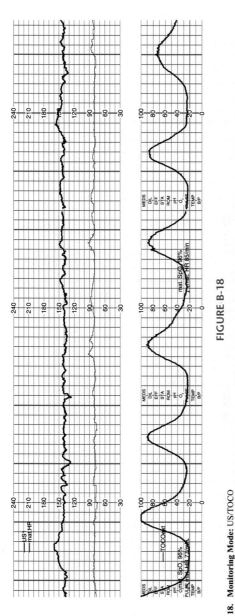

FIGURE B-18

18. **Monitoring Mode:** US/TOCO
Baseline FHR: 140bpm. **Baseline variability:** Moderate. **Accelerations:** Present. **Decelerations:** Absent. **Uterine activity:** Tachysystole. **Category:** This is a Category 1 tracing.
Interpretation
There is no evidence of interruption of the oxygen pathway; the possibility of evolving fetal metabolic acidemia can be ruled out by the presence of moderate variability and accelerations. Even though this is a Category 1 tracing, the tachysystole should be addressed to avoid deterioration of fetal acid–base status.

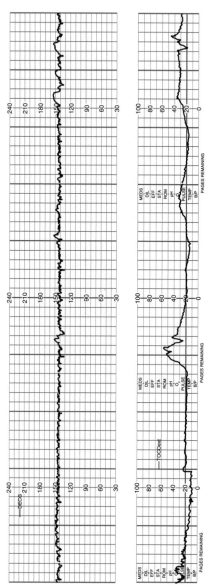

FIGURE B-19

19. **Monitoring Mode:** IFE/TOCO
Baseline FHR: 140bpm. **Baseline variability:** Minimal for majority of the tracing, changing to moderate near the end of the tracing. **Accelerations:** Absent. **Decelerations:** Absent.
Uterine activity: Unable to adequately assess; toco should be adjusted. **Category:** This is a Category 2 tracing.
Interpretation
Although there is no evidence of interruption of the oxygen pathway, the possibility of evolving fetal metabolic acidemia/ongoing hypoxic injury cannot be ruled out initially because of the lack of either accelerations or moderate variability. However, continued observation may reveal moderate variability as the tracing continues.

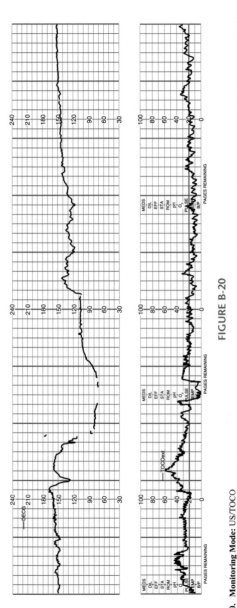

FIGURE B-20

20. **Monitoring Mode:** US/TOCO

Baseline FHR: 150 bpm. **Baseline variability:** Minimal. **Accelerations:** Absent. **Decelerations:** Prolonged deceleration. **Uterine activity:** Unable to adequately assess; toco should be adjusted. **Category:** This is a Category 2 tracing.

Interpretation

The prolonged deceleration is evidence of interruption of the oxygen pathway; the possibility of evolving fetal metabolic acidemia/ongoing hypoxic injury cannot be ruled out because of the lack of either accelerations or moderate variability.

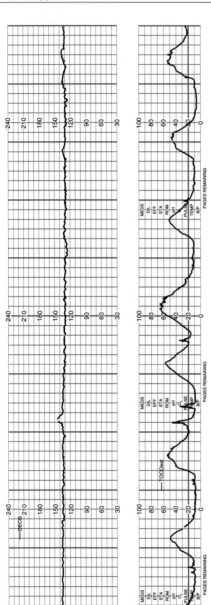

FIGURE B-21

21. **Monitoring Mode:** US/TOCO

Baseline FHR: 130 bpm. **Baseline variability:** Minimal. **Accelerations:** Absent. **Decelerations:** Absent. **Uterine activity:** Tachysystole. **Category:** This is a Category 2 tracing.

Interpretation

There is no evidence of interruption of the oxygen pathway; however, the possibility of evolving fetal metabolic acidemia/ongoing hypoxic injury cannot be ruled out because of the lack of either accelerations or moderate variability.

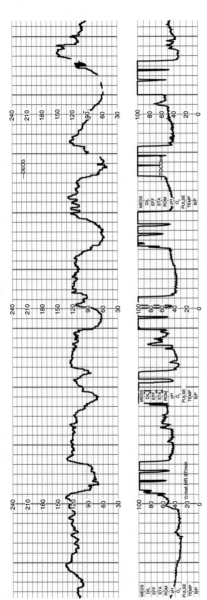

FIGURE B-22

22. **Monitoring Mode:** IFE/IUPC
Baseline FHR: 120 bpm (note baseline may be decreasing near the end of the tracing). **Baseline variability:** Moderate. **Accelerations:** Absent. **Decelerations:** Recurrent variable decelerations for the majority of the tracing. **Uterine activity:** Tachysystole. Also note the hypertonus and the apparent use of closed glottis pushing. **Category:** This is a Category 2 tracing.

Interpretation
The variable decelerations reflect interruption of the oxygen pathway at one or more points; the possibility of fetal metabolic acidemia/ongoing hypoxic injury can be ruled out because of the presence of moderate variability. Although this type of tracing is fairly common in second-stage labor, and the moderate variability allows one to rule out evolving fetal metabolic acidemia, which may not continue to be the case unless clinicians intervene to decrease uterine activity and alter pushing technique.

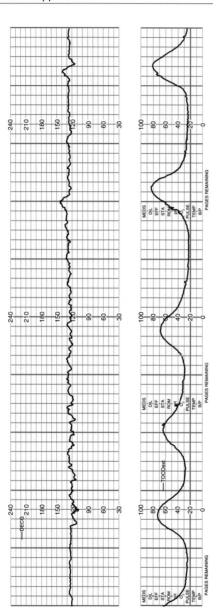

FIGURE B-23

23. **Monitoring Mode:** US/IUPC
Baseline FHR: 125bpm. **Baseline variability:** Moderate. **Accelerations:** Absent. **Decelerations:** Absent. **Uterine activity:** Tachysystole, with the possibility of hypertonus during initial portion of tracing. Note that total Montevideo units may be less than adequate, but without adequate relaxation time, steps to adjust uterine activity should be instituted. **Category:** This is a Category 1 tracing.

Interpretation
There is no evidence of interruption of the oxygen pathway; the possibility of fetal metabolic acidemia/ongoing hypoxic injury can be ruled out because of the presence of moderate variability.

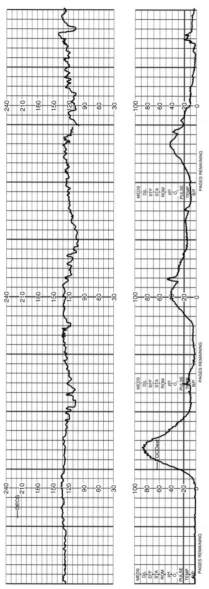

FIGURE B-24

24. **Monitoring Mode:** US/TOCO

Baseline FHR: 130bpm. **Baseline variability:** Moderate. **Accelerations:** Absent. **Decelerations:** Late decelerations. **Uterine activity:** Normal, although toco may need adjustment.

Category: This is a Category 2 tracing.

Interpretation

The late decelerations are evidence of interruption of the oxygen pathway; however, the possibility of fetal metabolic acidemia/ongoing hypoxic injury can be ruled out because of the presence of moderate variability.

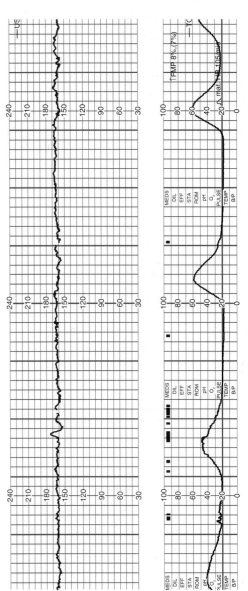

FIGURE B-25

25. **Monitoring Mode:** US/IUPC

Baseline FHR: 160bpm. **Baseline variability:** Minimal. **Accelerations:** Absent. **Decelerations:** Absent. **Uterine activity:** Normal. **Category:** This is a Category 2 tracing.

Interpretation

Although there is no evidence of interruption of the oxygen pathway, the possibility of evolving fetal metabolic acidemia/ongoing hypoxic injury cannot be ruled out because of the absence of moderate variability or accelerations. Although the baseline is not technically tachycardic for a term pregnancy, it should be evaluated as such because it is the high end of normal and not expected at term.

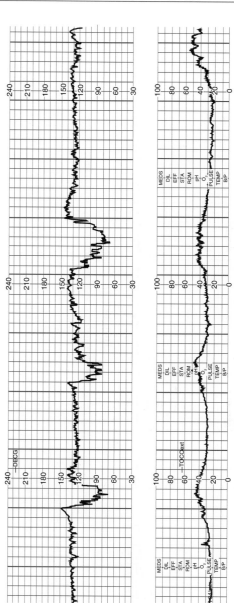

FIGURE B-26

26. **Monitoring Mode:** IFE/TOCO

Baseline FHR: 130bpm. **Baseline variability:** Moderate. **Accelerations:** Absent. **Decelerations:** Recurrent variable decelerations. **Uterine activity:** Normal frequency, but palpation should be used to rule out hypertonus. **Category:** This is a Category 2 tracing.

Interpretation

The variable decelerations reflect interruption of the oxygen pathway; the possibility of evolving fetal metabolic acidemia/ongoing hypoxic injury can be ruled out because of the presence of moderate variability.

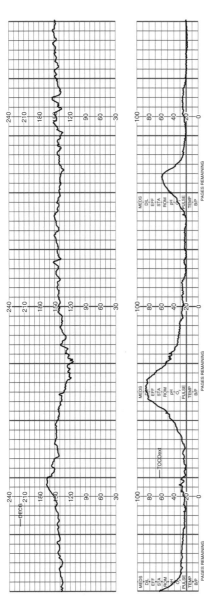

FIGURE B-27

27. **Monitoring Mode:** IFE/TOCO
Baseline FHR: 145 bpm. **Baseline variability:** Moderate. **Accelerations:** Absent (see note). **Decelerations:** Prolonged deceleration. **Uterine activity:** Normal. **Category:** This is a Category 2 tracing.
Interpretation
The prolonged deceleration reflects interruption of the oxygen pathway; the possibility of evolving fetal metabolic acidemia/ongoing hypoxic injury can be ruled out because of the presence of moderate variability. *Note:* Some clinicians may believe there is an acceleration immediately preceding the prolonged deceleration, but it appears that the deceleration begins before a return to baseline. Although an argument can be made for either view, it does not alter the interpretation of the tracing because there is moderate variability.

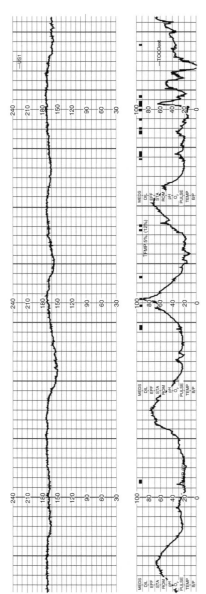

FIGURE B-28

28. **Monitoring Mode:** US/TOCO

Baseline FHR: 170bpm. **Baseline variability:** Absent (although some clinicians may believe this is minimal variability, most would consider this to be absent). **Accelerations:** Absent. **Decelerations:** Recurrent late decelerations. **Uterine activity:** Although the uterine activity here may be considered normal rather than tachysystole based on frequency, it should be viewed as excessive because of the inadequate relaxation time between several of the contractions. **Category:** This is a Category 3 tracing; it may be seen as a Category 2 tracing if the clinician believes the variability is minimal. Regardless of category, the interpretation (as follows) will be the same.

Interpretation

The late decelerations reflect interruption of the oxygen pathway; the possibility of evolving fetal metabolic acidemia/ongoing hypoxic injury cannot be ruled out because of the absence of either moderate variability or accelerations.

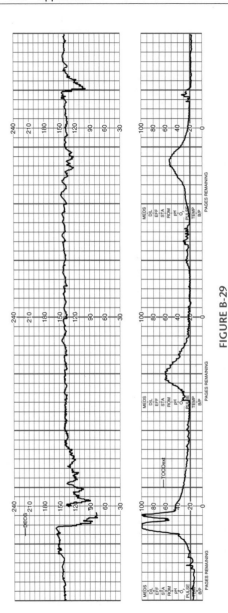

FIGURE B-29

29. **Monitoring Mode:** IFE/TOCO
Baseline FHR: 140 bpm. **Baseline variability:** Moderate. **Accelerations:** Absent. **Decelerations:** Variable decelerations. **Uterine activity:** Normal. **Category:** This is a Category 2 tracing.
Interpretation
The variable decelerations reflect interruption of the oxygen pathway; the possibility of evolving fetal metabolic acidemia/ongoing hypoxic injury can be excluded because of the presence of moderate variability.

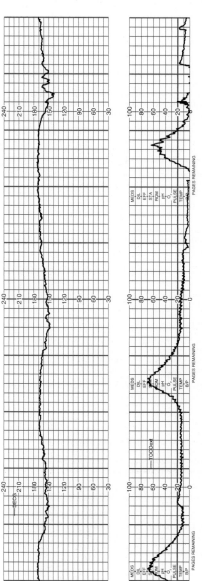

FIGURE B-30

30. **Monitoring Mode:** US/TOCO
Baseline FHR: 170 bpm. **Baseline variability:** Minimal. **Accelerations:** Absent. **Decelerations:** Recurrent prolonged decelerations. *Note: Some clinicians may identify these as late decelerations, depending on the visual points identified as onset and offset.* **Uterine activity:** Normal. **Category:** This is a Category 2 tracing.

Interpretation

The prolonged (or late) decelerations reflect interruption of the oxygen pathway; the possibility of evolving fetal metabolic acidemia/ongoing hypoxic injury cannot be excluded because of the absence of either moderate variability or accelerations.

APPENDIX C

Self-Assessment

1. Prior to 32 weeks' gestation, a fetal heart rate (FHR) acceleration is defined as an increase in FHR that must be at least
   a. 15 bpm above the baseline and the acceleration must last at least 10 seconds.
   b. 10 bpm above the baseline and the acceleration must last at least 10 seconds.
   c. 10 bpm above the baseline and the acceleration must last at least 15 seconds.

2. FHR variability can be interpreted with an external monitor
   a. only after 32 weeks' gestation.
   b. but not as clearly as with an internal monitor.
   c. using a Doppler technology called autocorrelation.

3. Use of the terms "beat-to-beat" variability and "long-term" variability is not recommended by the NICHD because in actual practice, they are
   a. visually determined as a unit.
   b. not really very different from each other.
   c. of no consequence to management or outcome.

4. Variable deceleration of the fetal heart rate is defined as a visually apparent *abrupt* decrease in FHR. *Abrupt* is defined as an onset of the deceleration to the nadir (lowest point) that is less than
   a. 15 seconds.
   b. 20 seconds.
   c. 30 seconds.

5. According to NICHD definitions of FHR variability, which of the following is accurate?
   a. Range visually detectable but ≤5 bpm = reduced variability
   b. Range 6 to 25 bpm = average variability
   c. Range visually detectable but ≤5 bpm = minimal variability

6. According to standardized NICHD terminology, the normal FHR baseline range is:
   a. 120 to 160 beats per minute regardless of gestational age.
   b. 110 to 160 beats per minute after 32 weeks of gestation.
   c. 110 to 160 beats per minute regardless of gestational age.

7. According to the 2008 NICHD consensus report, at the time it observed, moderate FHR variability is highly predictive of the absence of fetal
   a. metabolic acidemia.
   b. respiratory acidemia.
   c. hypoxemia.

8. Late deceleration of the FHR is associated most specifically with
   a. transient fetal tissue hypoxia during a uterine contraction.
   b. transient fetal tissue metabolic acidosis during a uterine contraction.
   c. transient fetal hypoxemia during a uterine contraction.

9. Clinically significant FHR decelerations (late, variable, prolonged) are associated with interruption of the normal delivery of oxygen from the environment to the fetus along a pathway including:
   a. lungs, heart, vasculature, kidneys, uterus, placenta, umbilical cord
   b. lungs, heart, vasculature, uterus, placenta, umbilical cord
   c. heart, vasculature, kidneys, uterus, umbilical cord

10. According to standardized NICHD nomenclature, decelerations that occur with at least 50% of uterine contractions in a 20-minute window are defined as:
    a. Repetitive
    b. Recurrent
    c. Persistent

11. Which setting is most appropriate for fetal vibroacoustic stimulation?
    a. 38 weeks, active labor, FHR baseline 140 bpm, minimal variability, no accelerations, no decelerations
    b. 40 weeks, active labor, FHR baseline 150 bpm, moderate variability, prolonged deceleration to 60 bpm for 8 minutes
    c. 39 weeks, active labor, FHR baseline 115 beats per minute, minimal variability, frequent accelerations, occasional late decelerations

12. An intrapartum FHR tracing demonstrates a baseline rate of 125 bpm, moderate variability, accelerations, and intermittent late and variable decelerations. Which of the following statements is most accurate?
    a. Moderate variability and accelerations are highly predictive of the absence of metabolic acidemia at the time they are observed.
    b. Late decelerations reflect transient fetal asphyxia during uterine contractions.
    c. Variable decelerations are caused by respiratory acidosis during cord compression.

13. According to the 2008 NICHD consensus report, a Category I FHR tracing requires which of the following?
    a. Baseline rate 120 to 160 bpm
    b. Moderate variability
    c. Accelerations
    d. All of the above
    e. a and b only

14. According to standardized the 2008 NICHD consensus report, which of the following would be classified as a Category III FHR tracing:
    a. Baseline 180 bpm, absent variability, no accelerations, no decelerations
    b. Baseline 180 bpm, minimal variability, no accelerations, recurrent late decelerations
    c. Baseline rate 140 bpm, absent variability, recurrent late decelerations
    d. b and c
    e. a and c

15. According to the 2008 NICHD consensus report, the normal frequency of uterine contractions is
    a. ≤5 contractions in 10 minutes averaged over 30 minutes
    b. <5 contractions in 10 minutes averaged over 30 minutes
    c. <6 contractions in 10 minutes averaged over 30 minutes

16. Which of the following most closely approximates normal umbilical artery pH at term?
    a. 6.9-7.0
    b. 7.0-7.1
    c. 7.1-7.2
    d. 7.2-7.3
    e. 7.3-7.4

17. According to the 2008 NICHD consensus report, the "overshoot" FHR pattern is highly predictive of
    a. fetal asphyxia.
    b. fetal hypoxia.
    c. fetal cerebral ischemia.
    d. preexisting fetal neurologic injury.
    e. None of the above.

18. Which of the following statements is accurate regarding the FHR tracing below?
    a. The absence of decelerations indicates the absence of interruption of fetal oxygenation.
    b. Accelerations and moderate variability reliably predict the absence of fetal metabolic acidemia.
    c. The absence of metabolic acidemia reliably excludes ongoing hypoxic injury.
    d. This is a Category I tracing.
    e. All of the above.

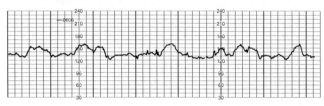
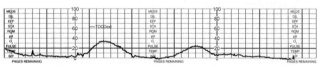

19. Which of the following statements is accurate regarding the FHR tracing below?
    a. Decelerations reflect interruption of oxygen transfer from the environment to the fetus.
    b. Moderate variability reliably predicts the absence of fetal hypoxemia.
    c. The absence of accelerations predicts fetal hypoxemia and metabolic acidemia.
    d. Normal baseline FHR excludes chorioamnionitis.

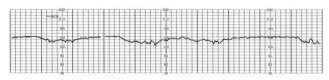
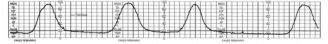

20. Which of the following is most accurate regarding the FHR tracing below?
    a. Variable decelerations can be caused by umbilical cord compression.
    b. Variable decelerations reflect interruption of oxygen transfer from the environment to the fetus at one or more points.
    c. Variability is moderate.
    d. Accelerations are present.
    e. All of the above.
    f. Only a, b, and c.

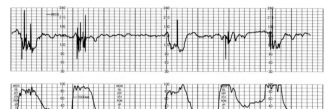

21. Appropriate management of the FHR pattern identified below includes all of the following *except*
    a. supplemental oxygenation.
    b. confirm maternal heart rate and blood pressure.
    c. maternal position changes.
    d. correct maternal hypotension if present.
    e. scalp stimulation.

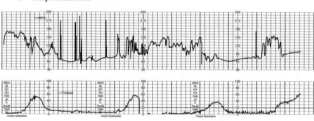

22. Which of the following statements most accurately interprets change to the tracing below?
    a. Baseline FHR 150 bpm
    b. Highly predictive of fetal metabolic acidemia
    c. Highly predictive of abnormal neurologic outcome
    d. Cannot exclude fetal metabolic acidemia at this time
    e. Subtle early decelerations present

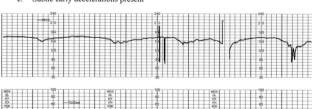

23. Umbilical vein pH is normally lower than umbilical artery pH
    a. True
    b. False
    c. Only when late decelerations are present and recurrent

24. Fetal scalp stimulation is used to
    a. elicit FHR accelerations.
    b. correct prolonged decelerations.
    c. stimulate FHR variability during a prolonged deceleration.
    d. All of the above.

25. A key point regarding the occurrence of tachysystole is that
    a. it can occur in spontaneous or stimulated labor.
    b. it requires FHR decelerations to be clinically significant.
    c. it should be documented only if oxytocin is being used.

26. According to the algorithm for delivery decision making authored by Clark and colleagues, the proper management of a patient with intermittent late decelerations and moderate variability in second stage labor with normal progress is
    a. expedited delivery by operative vaginal delivery or cesarean delivery.
    b. performance of fetal scalp stimulation to rule out acidemia.
    c. continued observation.

27. Which of the following is true about EFM documentation?
    a. If something is not documented, it is legally considered not to have occurred.
    b. Documentation frequency should be every 5 minutes in second stage if a patient has risk factors.
    c. Categories of the EFM tracing should be regularly documented.
    d. None of the above.
    e. All of the above.

28. The FHR dysryhthmia that can be associated with fetal hydrops is
    a. supraventricular tachycardia.
    b. atrioventricular heart block.
    c. persistent premature ventricular contractions.

29. Chemoreceptors are
    a. located in the aortic arch and carotid sinus.
    b. sensitive to changes in fetal blood pressure.
    c. sensitive to changes in fetal oxygenation.
    d. Both a and c.
    e. Both a and b.

30. When a FHR tracing is Category II, this means
    a. it requires further evaluation.
    b. it will progress to a Category III if no intervention.
    c. the fetus is at risk for acidemia.

ANSWER KEY FOR SELF ASSESSMENT

1. b		16. d	
2. c		17. e	
3. a		18. e	
4. c		19. a	
5. c		20. f	
6. c		21. e	
7. a		22. d	
8. c		23. b	
9. b		24. a	
10. b		25. a	
11. a		26. c	
12. a		27. d	
13. b		28. a	
14. c		29. d	
15. a		30. a	

INDEX

Note: Page numbers followed by *b* indicate boxes, *f* indicate figures, and *t* indicate tables.